# Working *together* for health

The World Health Report **2006** 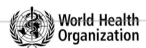 World Health Organization

WHO Library Cataloguing-in-Publication Data

World Health Organization.
    The world health report 2006: working together for health.

    1. World health – trends. 2. Health personnel – education. 3. Education, Medical. 4. Health manpower.
    5. National health programs – organization and administration. 6. World Health Organization.
    I. Title. II. Title: Working together for health.

    ISBN 92 4 156317 6        (NLM classification: WA 530.1)
    ISBN 978 92 4 156317 8
    ISSN 1020-3311

This report was produced under the overall direction of Tim Evans (Assistant Director-General, Evidence and Information for Policy). The principal authors were Lincoln Chen, David Evans, Tim Evans, Ritu Sadana, Barbara Stilwell, Phyllida Travis, Wim Van Lerberghe and Pascal Zurn, assisted by Christie Aschwanden and Joanne McManus. Organizational supervision of the report was provided by Manuel M. Dayrit and Carmen Dolea. The Managing Editor of the report was Thomson Prentice.

Valuable inputs in the form of contributions, peer-review, suggestions and criticisms were received from the Director-General's Office, and from Maia Ambegaokar, Dina Balabanova, James Buchan, Gilles Dussault, Martin McKee and Barbara McPake. Significant contributions to the analytical work were received from Mario Dal Poz, Sigrid Draeger, Norbert Dreesch, Patricia Hernandez, Yohannes Kinfu, Teena Kunjumen, Hugo Mercer, Amit Prasad, Angelica Souza and Niko Speybroek. Additional help and advice were kindly provided by Regional Directors and members of their staff.

Other contributors were Sabine Ablefoni, Taghreed Adam, Alayne Adams, Chris Afford, Alan Leather, Fariba Aldarazi, Ghanim Al'Sheick, Ala Alwan, Sarah Barber, Kisalaya Basu, Jacques Baudouy, Robert Beaglehole, Habib Benzian, Karin Bergstrom, Isa Bogaert, Paul Bossyns, Jean-Marc Braichet, Hilary Brown, Paul Bunnell, Francisco Campos, Eleonora Cavagnero, Xuanhao Chan, Amélina Chaouachi, Ottorino Cosivi, Nadia Danon-Hersch, Khassoum Diallo, Alimata Diarra, Marjolein Dieleman, Dela Dovlo, Nathalie Drew, Sambe Duale, Steeve Ebener, Dominique Egger, JoAnne Epping-Jordan, Marthe-Sylvie Essengue, Edwige Faydi, Paulo Ferrinho, Noela Fitzgerald, Martin Fletcher, Helga Fogstad, Gilles Forte, Kathy Fritsch, Michelle Funk, Charles Godue, Sandy Gove, Alexandre Griekspoor, Steffen Groth, Anil Gupta, Piya Hanvoravongchai, Hande Harmanci, Lisa Hinton, Sue Ineson, Anwar Islam, Anna Iversen, PT Jayawickramarajah, Patrick Kadama, Hans Karle, Julia Karnaukhova, Guy Kegels, Meleckidzedeck Khayesi, Mireille Kingma, Stephen Kinoti, Etienne Krug, Yunkap Kwankam, Chandrakant Laharyia, Gaert Laleman, Jean Pierre Lokonga, Ana Lopes Temporão, Alessandro Loretti, Pat McCarty, Judith Mandelbaum-Schmid, Annick Manuel, Bruno Marchal, Tim Martineau, Liz Mason, Zoe Matthews, Sandra McGinnis, Abdelhay Mechbal, Remo Meloni, Nata Menabde, Phillipa Mladovski, Dominic Montagu, Jean Moore, Krishnan Natarajan, Mwansa Nkwane, John Norcini, Ezekiel Nukoro, Isabelle Nuttal, Jennifer Nyoni, Cornelius Oepen, Judith Oulton, Francis Omaswa, Mary O'Neill, Ariel Pablos-Mendez, Fred Peccaud, Margie Peden, Galina Perfilieva, Bob Pond, Raymond Pong, Amit Prasad, Usha Raman, Tom Ricketts, Robert Ridley, Arjanne Rietsema, Felix Rigoli, Barbara Rijks, Salif Samake, Benedetto Saraceno, Shekhar Saxena, Robert Scherpbier, Lee-Martin Shook-Pui, Kit Sinclair, Alaka Singh, Ronald Skeldon, Susan Skillman, Ajay Tandon, Tessa Tan-Torres Edejer, Linda Tawfik, Michel Thieren, Anke Tijstma, Nicole Valentine, Wim Van Damme, Dirk Van der Roost, Mark van Ommeren, Paul Verboom, Marko Vujicic, Lis Wagner, Eva Wallstam, Diane Whitney, Marijke Wijnroks, Paul Wing, Christiane Wiskow, Tana Wuliji, Jean Yan, Sandy Yule, Manfred Zahorka, Diana Zandi, and Lingling Zhang.

Contributors to statistical tables not already mentioned were Endre Bakka, Dorjsuren Bayarsaikhan, Ties Boerma, Eduard Bos, Thomas Buettner, Veneta Cherilova, Trevor Croft, Driss Zine Eddine Elidrissi, Anton Fric, Charu Garg, Peter Ghys, Amparo Gordillo, Eleanor Gouws, Attila Hancioglu, Kenneth Hill, Chandika Indikadahena, Mie Inoue, Gareth Jones, Joses Kirigia, Jan Klavus, Joseph Kutzin, Eduardo Levcovitz, Edilberto Loaiza, Doris Ma Fat, François Pelletier, Ravi Rannan-Elyia, Hossein Salehi, Cheryl Sawyer, Kenji Shibuya, Karen Stanecki, Rubén Suárez, Emi Suzuki, Nathalie Van de Maele, Jakob Victorin, Neff Walker, Tessa Wardlaw, Charles Waza, Jens Wilkens, John Wilmoth, and many staff in WHO country offices, governmental departments and agencies, and international institutions.

The report was edited by Leo Vita-Finzi, assisted by Barbara Campanini. Editorial, administrative and production support was provided by Shelagh Probst and Gary Walker, who also coordinated the photographs. Figures and tables were provided by Gael Kernen who also was responsible for the web site version, and other electronic media. Proofreading was by Marie Fitzsimmons. The index was prepared by June Morrison.

Design: Reda Sadki
Layout: Steve Ewart and Reda Sadki
Figures: Christophe Grangier
Printing coordination: Raphaël Crettaz
Printed in France

# contents

## Tables – Overview

## Tables – Chapters

## Boxes – Chapters

# Message from the Director-General

In 2003, before I took up the position of Director-General, I asked many leaders and decision-makers in health what they saw as the most important issues in their countries. One common theme, whether in developed or developing countries, was the crisis in human resources.

There is a chronic shortage of well-trained health workers. The shortage is global, but most acutely felt in the countries that need them most. For a variety of reasons, such as the migration, illness or death of health workers, countries are unable to educate and sustain the health workforce that would improve people's chances of survival and their well-being.

People are a vital ingredient in the strengthening of health systems. But it takes a considerable investment of time and money to train health workers. That investment comes both from the individuals and from institutional subsidies or grants. Countries need their skilled workforce to stay so that their professional expertise can benefit the population. When health workers leave to work elsewhere, there is a loss of hope and a loss of years of investment.

The solution is not straightforward, and there is no consensus on how to proceed. Redressing the shortages in each individual country involves a chain of cooperation and shared intent between the public and private sector parties which fund and direct educational establishments; between those who plan and influence health service staffing; and between those able to make financial commitments to sustain or support the conditions of service of health workers.

This report aims to provide clarity through presentation of the evidence gathered, as a first step towards addressing and resolving this urgent crisis.

**Dr LEE Jong-wook**
Director-General
World Health Organization

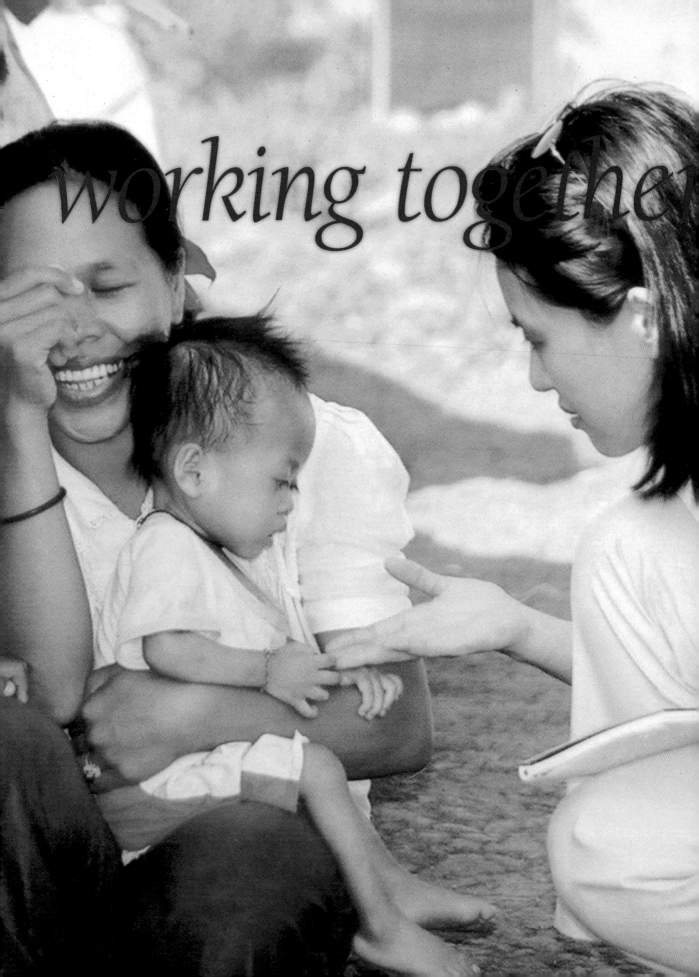

working together

# overview

# *for health*

> *"We have to work together to ensure access to a motivated, skilled, and supported health worker by every person in every village everywhere."*
>
> LEE Jong-wook
> High-Level Forum, Paris, November 2005

## WHY THE WORKFORCE IS IMPORTANT

In this first decade of the 21st century, immense advances in human well-being coexist with extreme deprivation. In global health we are witnessing the benefits of new medicines and technologies. But there are unprecedented reversals. Life expectancies have collapsed in some of the poorest countries to half the level of the richest – attributable to the ravages of HIV/AIDS in parts of sub-Saharan Africa and to more than a dozen "failed states". These setbacks have been accompanied by growing fears, in rich and poor countries alike, of new infectious threats such as SARS and avian influenza and "hidden" behavioural conditions such as mental disorders and domestic violence.

The world community has sufficient financial resources and technologies to tackle most of these health challenges; yet today many national health systems are weak, unresponsive, inequitable – even unsafe. What is needed now is political will to implement national plans, together with international cooperation to align resources, harness knowledge and build robust health systems for treating and preventing disease and promoting population health. Developing capable, motivated and supported health workers is essential for overcoming bottlenecks to achieve national and global health goals. Health care is a labour-intensive service industry. Health service providers are the personification of a system's core values – they heal and care for people, ease pain and suffering, prevent disease and mitigate risk – the human link that connects knowledge to health action.

At the heart of each and every health system, the workforce is central to advancing health. There is ample evidence that worker numbers and quality are positively associated with immunization coverage, outreach of primary care, and infant, child and maternal survival (see Figure 1). The quality of doctors and the density of their distribution have been shown to correlate with positive outcomes in cardiovascular diseases. Conversely, child malnutrition has worsened with staff cutbacks during health sector reform. Cutting-edge quality improvements of health care are best initiated by workers themselves because they are in the unique

Figure 1  Health workers save lives!

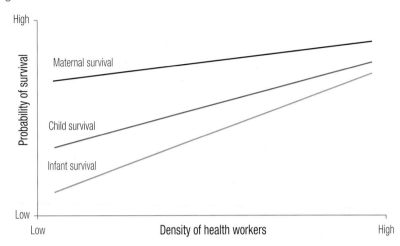

position of identifying opportunities for innovation. In health systems, workers function as gatekeepers and navigators for the effective, or wasteful, application of all other resources such as drugs, vaccines and supplies.

## Picture of the global workforce

All of us at some stage work for health – a mother caring for her child, a son escorting his parents to a hospital, or a healer drawing on ancient wisdom to offer care and solace. This report considers that *"Health workers are all people primarily engaged in actions with the primary intent of enhancing health"*. This is consistent with the WHO definition of health systems as comprising all activities with the primary goal of improving health – inclusive of family caregivers, patient–provider partners, part-time workers (especially women), health volunteers and community workers.

Based on new analyses of national censuses, labour surveys and statistical sources, WHO estimates there to be a total of 59.2 million full-time paid health workers worldwide (see Table 1). These workers are in health enterprises whose primary role is to improve health (such as health programmes operated by government or nongovernmental organizations) plus additional health workers in non-health organizations (such as nurses staffing a company or school clinic). *Health service providers* constitute about two thirds of the global health workforce, while the remaining third is composed of *health management and support workers*.

Workers are not just individuals but are integral parts of functioning health teams in which each member contributes different skills and performs different functions. Countries demonstrate enormous diversity in the skill mix of health teams. The ratio of nurses to doctors ranges from nearly 8:1 in the African Region to 1.5:1 in the Western Pacific Region. Among countries, there are approximately four nurses per doctor in Canada and the United States of America, while Chile, Peru, El Salvador and Mexico have fewer than one nurse per doctor. The spectrum of essential worker competencies is characterized by imbalances as seen, for example, in the dire shortage of public health specialists and health care managers in many countries. Typically, more than 70% of doctors are male while more than 70% of nurses are female – a marked gender imbalance. About two thirds of the workers are in the public sector and one third in the private sector.

## Table 1 Global health workforce, by density

| WHO region | Total health workforce Number | Total health workforce Density (per 1000 population) | Health service providers Number | Health service providers Percentage of total health workforce | Health management and support workers Number | Health management and support workers Percentage of total health workforce |
|---|---|---|---|---|---|---|
| Africa | 1 640 000 | 2.3 | 1 360 000 | 83 | 280 000 | 17 |
| Eastern Mediterranean | 2 100 000 | 4.0 | 1 580 000 | 75 | 520 000 | 25 |
| South-East Asia | 7 040 000 | 4.3 | 4 730 000 | 67 | 2 300 000 | 33 |
| Western Pacific | 10 070 000 | 5.8 | 7 810 000 | 78 | 2 260 000 | 23 |
| Europe | 16 630 000 | 18.9 | 11 540 000 | 69 | 5 090 000 | 31 |
| Americas | 21 740 000 | 24.8 | 12 460 000 | 57 | 9 280 000 | 43 |
| World | 59 220 000 | 9.3 | 39 470 000 | 67 | 19 750 000 | 33 |

Note: All data for latest available year. For countries where data on the number of health management and support workers were not available, estimates have been made based on regional averages for countries with complete data.

Data source: World Health Organization. *Global Atlas of the Health Workforce* (http://www.who.int/globalatlas/default.asp).

## Driving forces: past and future

Workers in health systems around the world are experiencing increasing stress and insecurity as they react to a complex array of forces – some old, some new (see Figure 2). Demographic and epidemiological transitions drive changes in population-based health threats to which the workforce must respond. Financing policies, technological advances and consumer expectations can dramatically shift demands on the workforce in health systems. Workers seek opportunities and job security in dynamic health labour markets that are part of the global political economy.

The spreading HIV/AIDS epidemic imposes huge work burdens, risks and threats. In many countries, health sector reform under structural adjustment capped public sector employment and limited investment in health worker education, thus drying up the supply of young graduates. Expanding labour markets have intensified profes-

## Figure 2 Forces driving the workforce

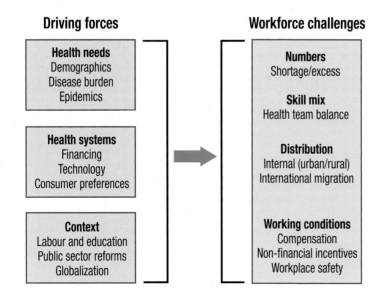

| Driving forces | Workforce challenges |
|---|---|
| **Health needs** Demographics Disease burden Epidemics | **Numbers** Shortage/excess |
| | **Skill mix** Health team balance |
| **Health systems** Financing Technology Consumer preferences | **Distribution** Internal (urban/rural) International migration |
| **Context** Labour and education Public sector reforms Globalization | **Working conditions** Compensation Non-financial incentives Workplace safety |

Figure 3 Countries with a critical shortage of health service providers
(doctors, nurses and midwives)

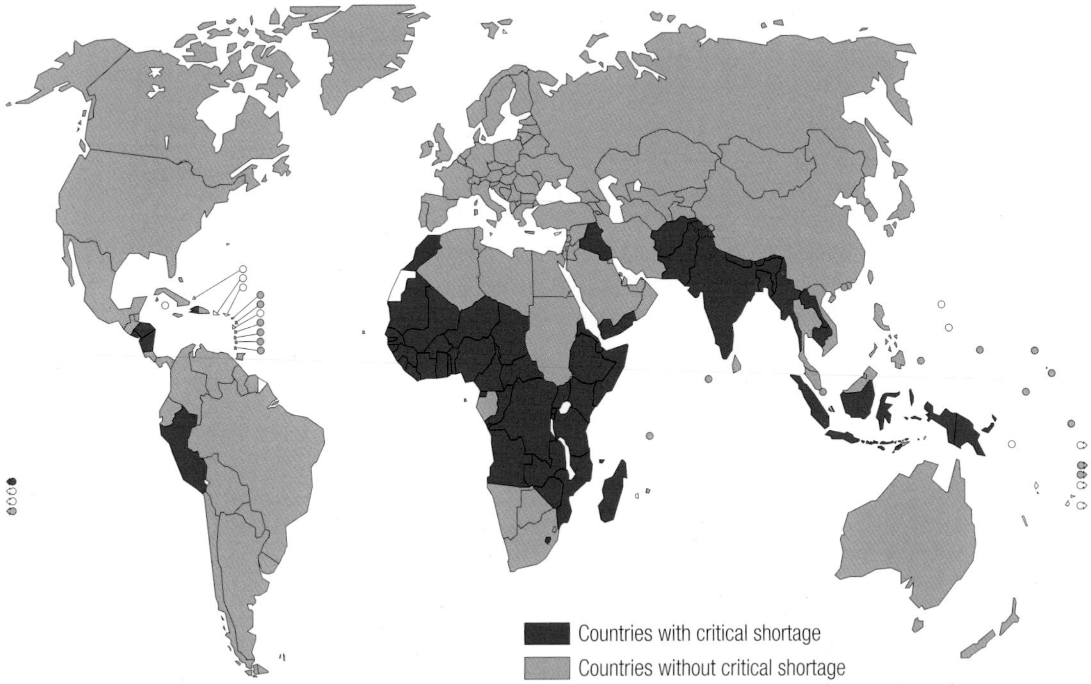

Data source: World Health Organization. *Global Atlas of the Health Workforce* (http://www.who.int/globalatlas/default.asp).

sional concentration in urban areas and accelerated international migration from the poorest to the wealthiest countries. The consequent workforce crisis in many of the poorest countries is characterized by severe shortages, inappropriate skill mixes, and gaps in service coverage.

WHO has identified a threshold in workforce density below which high coverage of essential interventions, including those necessary to meet the health-related Millennium Development Goals (MDGs), is very unlikely (see Figure 3). Based on these estimates, there are currently 57 countries with critical shortages equivalent to a global deficit of 2.4 million doctors, nurses and midwives. The proportional shortfalls are greatest in sub-Saharan Africa, although numerical deficits are very large in South-East Asia because of its population size. Paradoxically, these insufficiencies often coexist in a country with large numbers of unemployed health professionals. Poverty, imperfect private labour markets, lack of public funds, bureaucratic red tape and political interference produce this paradox of shortages in the midst of underutilized talent.

Skill mix and distributional imbalances compound today's problems. In many countries, the skills of limited yet expensive professionals are not well matched to the local profile of health needs. Critical skills in public health and health policy and management are often in deficit. Many workers face daunting working environments – poverty-level wages, unsupportive management, insufficient social recognition, and weak career development. Almost all countries suffer from maldistribution characterized by urban concentration and rural deficits, but these imbalances are perhaps most disturbing from a regional perspective. The WHO Region of the Americas, with 10% of the global burden of disease, has 37% of the world's health workers spending more than 50% of the world's health financing, whereas the African Region has 24% of the burden but only 3% of health workers commanding less than 1% of world health expenditure. The exodus of skilled professionals in the midst of so much unmet health need places Africa at the epicentre of the global health workforce crisis.

This crisis has the potential to deepen in the coming years. Demand for service providers will escalate markedly in all countries – rich and poor. Richer countries face a future of low fertility and large populations of elderly people, which will cause a shift towards chronic and degenerative diseases with high care demands. Technological advances and income growth will require a more specialized workforce even as needs for basic care increase because of families' declining capacity or willingness to care for their elderly members. Without massively increasing training of workers in this and other wealthy countries, these growing gaps will exert even greater pressure on the outflow of health workers from poorer regions.

In poorer countries, large cohorts of young people (1 billion adolescents) will join an increasingly ageing population, both groups rapidly urbanizing. Many of these countries are dealing with unfinished agendas of infectious disease and the rapid emergence of chronic illness complicated by the magnitude of the HIV/AIDS epidemic. The availability of effective vaccines and drugs to cope with these health threats imposes huge practical and moral imperatives to respond effectively. The chasm is widening between what can be done and what is happening on the ground. Success in bridging this gap will be determined in large measure by how well the workforce is developed for effective health systems.

These challenges, past and future, are well illustrated by considering how the workforce must be mobilized to address specific health challenges.

■ **The MDGs** target the major poverty-linked diseases devastating poor populations, focusing on maternal and child health care and the control of HIV/AIDS, tuberculosis and malaria. Countries that are experiencing the greatest difficulties in meeting the MDGs, many in sub-Saharan Africa, face absolute shortfalls in their health workforce. Major challenges exist in bringing priority disease programmes into line with primary care provision, deploying workers equitably for universal access to HIV/AIDS treatment, scaling up delegation to community workers, and creating public health strategies for disease prevention.

■ **Chronic diseases,** consisting of cardiovascular and metabolic diseases, cancers, injuries, and neurological and psychological disorders, are major burdens affecting rich and poor populations alike. New paradigms of care are driving a shift from acute tertiary hospital care to patient-centred, home-based and team-driven care requiring new skills, disciplinary collaboration and continuity of care – as demonstrated by innovative approaches in Europe and North America. Risk reduction, moreover, depends on measures to protect the environment and the modification of lifestyle factors such as diet, smoking and exercise through behaviour change.

■ **Health crises** of epidemics, natural disasters and conflict are sudden, often unexpected, but invariably recurring. Meeting the challenges requires coordinated planning based on sound information, rapid mobilization of workers, command-and-control responses, and intersectoral collaboration with nongovernmental organizations, the military, peacekeepers and the media. Specialized workforce capacities are needed for the surveillance of epidemics or for the reconstruction of societies torn apart by ethnic conflict. The quality of response, ultimately, depends upon workforce preparedness based on local capacity backed by timely international support.

These examples illustrate the enormous richness and diversity of the workforce needed to tackle specific health problems. The tasks and functions required are extraordinarily demanding, and each must be integrated into coherent national health systems. All of the problems necessitate efforts beyond the health sector. Effective strategies therefore require all relevant actors and organizations to work together.

## STRATEGIES: WORKING LIFESPAN OF ENTRY–WORKFORCE–EXIT

In tackling these world health problems, the workforce goal is simple – *to get the right workers with the right skills in the right place doing the right things!* – and in so doing, to retain the agility to respond to crises, to meet current gaps, and to anticipate the future.

A blueprint approach will not work, as effective workforce strategies must be matched to a country's unique history and situation. Most workforce problems are deeply embedded in changing contexts, and they cannot be easily resolved. These problems can be emotionally charged because of status issues and politically loaded because of divergent interests. That is why workforce solutions require stakeholders to be engaged in both problem diagnosis and problem solving.

This report lays out a "working lifespan" approach to the dynamics of the workforce. It does so by focusing on strategies related to the stage when people enter the workforce, the period of their lives when they are part of the workforce, and the point at which they make their exit from it. The road map (see Figure 4) of training, sustaining and retaining the workforce offers a worker perspective as well as a systems approach to strategy. Workers are typically concerned about such questions as: How do I get a job? What kind of education do I need? How am I treated and how well am I paid? What are my prospects for promotion or my options for leaving? From policy and management perspectives, the framework focuses on modulating the roles of both labour markets and state action at key decision-making junctures:

- Entry: preparing the workforce through strategic investments in education and effective and ethical recruitment practices.
- Workforce: enhancing worker performance through better management of workers in both the public and private sectors.
- Exit: managing migration and attrition to reduce wasteful loss of human resources.

### Entry: preparing the workforce

A central objective of workforce development is to produce sufficient numbers of skilled workers with technical competencies whose background, language and social attributes make them accessible and able to reach diverse clients and populations. To do so requires active planning and management of the health workforce production pipeline with a focus on building strong training institutions, strengthening professional regulation and revitalizing recruitment capabilities.

- **Building strong institutions** for education is essential to secure the numbers and qualities of health workers required by the health system. Although the variations are enormous among countries, the world's 1600 medical schools, 6000

## Figure 4  Working lifespan strategies

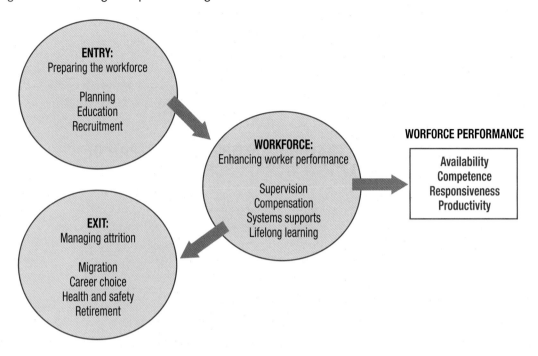

nursing schools and 375 schools of public health in aggregate are not producing sufficient numbers of graduates. Addressing shortfalls will require building new institutions and ensuring a more appropriate mix of training opportunities – for example, more schools of public health are needed. Commensurate with the shift in expectations of graduates from "know-all" to "know-how", improving education calls for attention to both curricular content and pedagogical learning methods. Teaching staff, too, require training as well as more credible support and career incentives so that a better balance with the competing demands of research and service can be achieved. Greater access to education at lower cost can be achieved by regional pooling of resources and expanding the use of information technologies such as telemedicine and distance education.

■ **Assuring educational quality** involves institutional accreditation and professional regulation (licensing, certification or registration). Rapid growth of the private sector in education calls for innovative stewardship to maximize the benefits of private investments while strengthening the state's role in regulating the quality of education. Too often lacking or ineffective in low income countries, structures for regulation are rarely developed sufficiently to ensure quality, responsiveness and ethical practice. State intervention is necessary in order to set standards, protect patient safety, and ensure quality through provision of information, financial incentives and regulatory enforcement.

■ **Revitalizing recruitment capabilities** is necessary in order to broker more effectively demands from the labour market that often overlook public health needs. Recruitment and placement services should aim not only to get workers with the right skills to the right place at the right time but also to achieve better social compatibility between workers and clients in terms of gender, language, ethnicity and geography. Institutional weaknesses related to recruitment information and effective deployment of health workers merit serious attention, especially where there are expectations in scaling up the health workforce.

## Workforce: enhancing performance

Strategies to improve the performance of the health workforce must initially focus on existing staff because of the time lag in training new health workers. Substantial improvements in the availability, competence, responsiveness and productivity of the workforce can be rapidly achieved through an array of low-cost and practical instruments.

- **Supervision makes a big difference.** Supportive yet firm – and fair – supervision is one of the most effective instruments available to improve the competence of individual health workers, especially when coupled with clear job descriptions and feedback on performance. Moreover, supervision can build a practical integration of new skills acquired through on-the-job training.
- **Fair and reliable compensation.** Decent pay that arrives on time is crucial. The way workers are paid, for example salaried or fee-for-service, has effects on productivity and quality of care that require careful monitoring. Financial and non-financial incentives such as study leave or child care are more effective when packaged than provided on their own.
- **Critical support systems**. No matter how motivated and skilled health workers are, they cannot do their jobs properly in facilities that lack clean water, adequate lighting, heating, vehicles, drugs, working equipment and other supplies. Decisions to introduce new technologies – for diagnosis, treatment or communication – should be informed in part by an assessment of their implications for the health workforce.
- **Lifelong learning** should be inculcated in the workplace. This may include short-term training, encouraging staff to innovate, and fostering teamwork. Frequently, staff devise simple but effective solutions to improve performance and should be encouraged to share and act on their ideas.

## Exit: managing migration and attrition

Unplanned or excessive exits may cause significant losses of workers and compromise the system's knowledge, memory and culture. In some regions, worker illness, deaths and migration together constitute a haemorrhaging that overwhelms training capacity and threatens workforce stability. Strategies to counteract workforce attrition include managing migration, making health a career of choice, and stemming premature sickness and retirement.

- **Managing migration of health workers** involves balancing the freedom of individuals to pursue work where they choose with the need to stem excessive losses from both internal migration (urban concentration and rural neglect) and international movements from poorer to richer countries. Some international migration is planned, for example the import of professionals into the Eastern Mediterranean Region, while other migrations are unplanned with deleterious health consequences. For unplanned migration, tailoring education and recruitment to rural realities, improving working conditions more generally and facilitating the return of migrants represent important retention strategies. Richer countries receiving migrants from poorer countries should adopt responsible recruitment policies, treat migrant health workers fairly, and consider entering into bilateral agreements.

- **Keeping health work as a career of choice for women.** The majority of health workers are women and "feminization" trends are well established in the male dominated field of medicine. To accommodate female health workers better, more attention must be paid to their safety, including protecting them from violence. Other measures must be put in place. These include more flexible work arrangements to accommodate family considerations, and career tracks that promote women towards senior faculty and leadership positions more effectively.

- **Ensuring safe work environments.** Outflows from the workforce caused by illness, disability and death are unnecessarily high and demand priority attention especially in areas of high HIV prevalence. Strategies to minimize occupational hazards include the recognition and appropriate management of physical risks and mental stress, as well as full compliance with prevention and protection guidelines. Provision of effective prevention services and access to treatment for all health workers who become HIV-positive are the only reasonable way forward in the pursuit of universal access to HIV prevention, treatment and care.

- **Retirement planning.** In an era of ageing workforces and trends towards earlier retirement, unwanted attrition can be stemmed by a range of policies. These policies can reduce incentives for early retirement, decrease the cost of employing older people, recruit retirees back to work and improve conditions for older workers. Succession planning is central to preserving key competencies and skills in the workforce.

## MOVING FORWARD TOGETHER

### An imperative for action

The unmistakable imperative is to strengthen the workforce so that health systems can tackle crippling diseases and achieve national and global health goals. A strong human infrastructure is fundamental to closing today's gap between health promise and health reality and anticipating the health challenges of the 21st century.

Momentum for action has grown steadily over recent years. Member States of WHO, spearheaded by health leaders from Africa, adopted two resolutions at recent World Health Assemblies calling for global action to build a workforce for national health systems, including stemming the flow of unplanned professional emigration. Europe and Latin America have promoted regional observatories in human resources for health, and the South-East Asia and Eastern Mediterranean Regional Offices have launched new public health training initiatives. One hundred global health leaders in the Joint Learning Initiative recommended urgent action to overcome the crisis of human resources for health. Calls for action have come from a series of High-Level Forums for the health-related MDGs in Geneva, Abuja and Paris, and two Oslo Consultations have nurtured a participatory stakeholder process to chart a way forward. A clear mandate has emerged for a global plan of action bringing forth national leadership backed by global solidarity.

### National leadership

Strong country strategies require both solid technical content and a credible political process. This involves embracing the breadth of issues inherent in the entry–workforce–exit framework while cultivating trust and brokering agreements through effective engagement of stakeholders in planning and implementation. In addition, national strategies are likely to be more successful if they adopt three priorities: acting now, anticipating the future, and acquiring critical capabilities.

- **Acting now for workforce productivity** by cutting waste (such as eliminating ghost workers and absenteeism) and improving performance through compensation adjustments, work incentives, safer working conditions, and worker mobilization efforts. Better intelligence gathering is crucial in order to understand national situations and monitor progress or setbacks.
- **Anticipating the future** by engaging stakeholders to craft national strategic plans through evidence-based information and scenarios on likely future trends. Significant growth of private education and services should be anticipated, necessitating the targeting of public funds for health equity, promotion and prevention. Public action in information, regulation and delegation are key functions for mixed public and private systems.
- **Acquiring critical capacities** by strengthening core institutions for sound workforce development. Leadership and management development in health and other related sectors such as education and finance is essential for strategic planning and implementation of workforce policies. Standard setting, accrediting and licensing must be effectively established to improve the work of worker unions, educational institutions, professional associations and civil society.

## Global solidarity

National strategies on their own, however well conceived, are insufficient to deal with the realities of health workforce challenges today and in the future. Strategies across countries are similarly constrained by patchy evidence, limited planning tools and a scarcity of technical expertise. Outbreaks of disease and labour market inflections transcend national boundaries, and the depth of the workforce crisis in a significant group of countries requires international assistance. National leadership must therefore be complemented by global solidarity on at least three fronts: knowledge and learning; cooperative agreements; and responsiveness to workforce crises.

- **Catalysing knowledge and learning.** Low-cost but significant investments in the development of better metrics for the workforce, agreement on common technical frameworks, and the identification of and support for priority research will accelerate progress in all countries. Effective pooling of the diverse technical expertise and breadth of experiences can assist countries in accessing the best talent and practices.
- **Striking cooperative agreements.** The growing international nature of the health workforce related to the flows of migrants, relief workers and volunteers calls for cooperative agreements to protect the rights and safety of workers and to enhance the adoption of ethical recruitment practices. The current global situation regarding avian influenza is indicative of a more fundamental need for effective international capacity to marshal the requisite human resources for acute health and humanitarian emergencies.
- **Responding to workforce crises.** The magnitude of the health workforce crisis in the world's poorest countries cannot be overstated and requires an urgent, sustained and coordinated response from the international community. Donors must facilitate the immediate and longer-term financing of human resources as a health systems investment. A 50:50 guideline is recommended, whereby 50% of all international assistance funds are devoted to health systems, with half of this funding devoted to national health workforce strengthening strategies. Development financing policies must find ways to ensure that hiring ceilings are not the primary constraint to workforce expansion. All partners should critically evaluate their modalities for supporting the workforce with a view to shedding inefficient practices and aligning more effectively with national leadership.

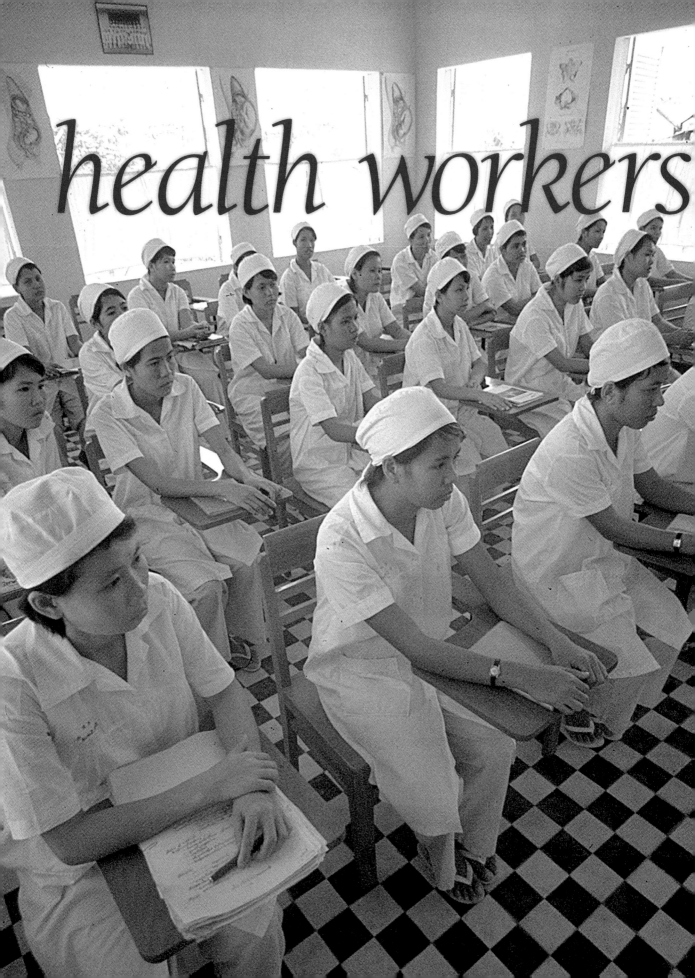

health workers

Figure 5  Global stakeholder alliance

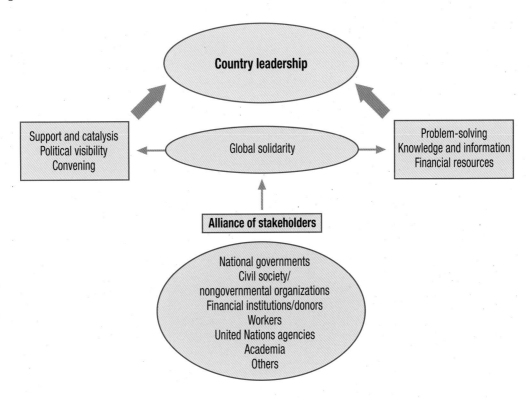

a full range of evidence-based guidelines should inform good practice for health workers. Effective cooperative agreements will minimize adverse consequences despite increased international flows of workers. Sustained international financing should be in place to support recipient countries for the next 10 years as they scale up their workforce.

## Moving forward together

Moving forward on the plan of action necessitates that stakeholders work together through inclusive alliances and networks – local, national and global – across health problems, professions, disciplines, ministries, sectors and countries. Cooperative structures can pool limited talent and fiscal resources and promote mutual learning. Figure 5 proposes how a global workforce alliance can be launched to bring relevant stakeholders to accelerate core country programmes.

A premier challenge is advocacy that promotes workforce issues to a high place on the political agenda and keeps them there. The moment is ripe for political support as problem awareness is expanding, effective solutions are emerging, and various countries are already pioneering interventions. Workforce development is a continuous process that is always open for improvement. However, immediate acceleration of performance can be attained in virtually all countries if well-documented solutions are applied. Some of the work should be implemented immediately; other aspects will take time. There are no short cuts and there is no time to lose. Now is the time for action, to invest in the future, and to advance health – rapidly and equitably.

National leadership and global solidarity can result in significant structural improvements of the workforce in all countries, especially those with the most severe crises. Such advances would be characterized by universal access to a motivated, competent and supported health workforce, greater worker, employer and public satisfaction, and more effective stewardship of the workforce by the state, civil society and professional associations.

## Plan of action

National leadership must urgently jump-start country-based actions and sustain them for at least a decade. Table 2 summarizes targets in the plan of action over the decade 2006–2015.

■ Immediate actions over the next few years should consist of lead countries pioneering national plans for scaling up effective strategies, increasing investments, cutting waste, and strengthening educational institutions. Global support should accelerate progress in countries, with immediate policy attention given to intelligence, technical cooperation, policy alignment of fiscal space and migration, and harmonization of priority initiatives and donor assistance.

■ At the decade's mid-point, over half of all countries should have sound national plans with expanded execution of good policies and management practices concerned with workforce incentives, regulation and institutions. Global advances will include shared norms and frameworks, strong technical support, and improved knowledge management. Responsible recruitment and alignment of priority programmes and development instruments to support the health workforce should be in place.

■ The decade goal in all countries is to build high-performing workforces for national health systems to respond to current and emerging challenges. This means that every country should have implemented national strategic plans and should be planning for the future, drawing on robust national capacity. Globally,

## Table 2 Ten-year plan of action

| | | 2006 Immediate | 2010 Mid-point | 2015 Decade |
|---|---|---|---|---|
| **Country leadership** | **Management** | Cut waste, improve incentives | Use effective managerial practices | Sustain high performing workforce |
| | **Education** | Revitalize education strategies | Strengthen accreditation and licensing | Prepare workforce for the future |
| | **Planning** | Design national workforce strategies | Overcome barriers to implementation | Evaluate and redesign strategies, based on robust national capacity |
| **Global solidarity** | **Knowledge and learning** | Develop common technical frameworks | Assess performance with comparable metrics | Share evidence-based good practices |
| | | Pool expertise | Fund priority research | |
| | **Enabling policies** | Advocate ethical recruitment and migrant workers' rights | Adhere to responsible recruitment guidelines | Manage increased migratory flows for equity and fairness |
| | | Pursue fiscal space exceptionality | Expand fiscal space for health | Support fiscal sustainability |
| | **Crisis response** | Finance national plans for 25% of crisis countries | Expand financing to half of crisis countries | Sustain financing of national plans for all countries in crisis |
| | | Agree on best donor practices for human resources for health | Adopt 50:50 investment guideline for priority programmes | |

# chapter one
# a global profile

**Health workers are people whose job it is to protect and improve the health of their communities. Together these health workers, in all their diversity, make up the global health workforce. This chapter gives an overview of what is known about them. It describes the size and distribution of the workforce, and some of its characteristics, including how much it costs. It shows that there is a substantial shortage of health workers to meet health needs, but that shortages are not universal, even across low income countries. The chapter then considers how much it would cost to scale up training to meet this shortfall and pay health workers subsequently.**

The data used in this chapter are drawn from many different sources, with varying degrees of completeness by country and by year. WHO supplemented this information with written requests to numerous agencies as well as with special country surveys requesting information about the numbers and types of health workers and training institutions. Substantial gaps remain, however, in the information, and the picture painted here is based on incomplete data which means that it needs to be interpreted carefully.

## WHO ARE THE HEALTH WORKERS?
This report defines health workers to be all people engaged in actions whose primary intent is to enhance health. This meaning extends from WHO's definition of the health system as comprising activities whose primary goal is to improve health. Strictly speaking, this means that mothers looking after their sick children and other unpaid carers are in the health workforce.

They make important contributions and are critical to the functioning of most health systems. However, the data available on health worker numbers are generally limited to people engaged in paid activities, so the numbers reported in this chapter are limited to such workers.

> *" This report defines health workers to be all people engaged in actions whose primary intent is to enhance health "*

Even then, the definition of a health action for classifying paid workers is not straightforward. Consider a painter employed by a hospital: the painter's own actions do not improve health, though the actions of the painter's employer, the hospital, do. Then take the case of a doctor employed by a mining company to care for its employees: the actions of the doctor improve health, though the actions of the employer do not. A classification system that considers the actions of the individual alone, or those of the employer alone, cannot place them both in the health workforce.

In principle, the report argues that the actions of the individual are most important, so that the painter is not a health worker while the mine's doctor is. However, in practice, it is not yet possible to fully apply this rule because much of the data on health worker numbers do not provide sufficient detail to allow people directly engaged in improving health to be separated from other employees *(1)*. For this reason, the report takes a pragmatic approach and includes all paid workers employed in organizations or institutions whose primary intent is to improve health as well as those whose personal actions are primarily intended to improve health but who work for other types of organizations. This means that the painter working for a hospital is included as is the doctor working for a mine. WHO is working to devise a more detailed, standard classification system for health workers that should permit the gold standard definition to be applied in the future (see Box 1.1).

The system of counting used in this chapter allows two types of health workers to be distinguished. The first group comprises the people who deliver services – whether personal or non-personal – who are called "health service providers"; the second covers people not engaged in the direct provision of services, under the term "health management and support workers" (details are given in Box 1.1; see also Box 1.2). The report sometimes presents information for different types of health service providers, although such detail is often available only for doctors and nurses. Further explanation of the sources of the data, classification issues, and the triangulation and harmonization applied to make the data comparable across countries is found in the Statistical Annex.

The available data do not allow reporting on the people working for a part of their time to improve health, such as social workers who work with mentally ill patients. In addition, the report has chosen not to include workers in other types of occupations who contribute in vital ways to improving population health, if their main function lies elsewhere. This category includes, for instance, police officers who enforce seat-belt laws. Finally, current methods of identifying health workers do not allow unpaid carers of sick people or volunteers who provide other critical services to be counted. This exclusion is simply because of a lack of data, and all these valuable contributions are acknowledged in subsequent chapters.

Furthermore, official counts of the health workforce often omit people who deliver services outside health organizations, for example doctors employed by mining companies or agricultural firms, because they classify these employees under the

# Box 1.1  Classifying health workers

The third version of the International Standard Classification of Occupations (ISCO), an international classification system agreed by members of the International Labour Organization, was adopted in 1987 and is known as ISCO-88 *(2)*. Many national occupational classifications, and most censuses and labour force surveys, use one of the three ISCO versions. Because the system is used to classify all types of workers, the breakdown provided for health workers is not very detailed, so many ministries of health have developed their own classification systems. WHO is now working on a process to devise a more detailed, standard classification system for health workers that is consistent with the ISCO. This work coincides with the update of ISCO-88, which is expected to be ready in 2008.

The table below shows the health-specific occupational classification used in the South African census of 2001, which is typical of many countries using a three-digit ISCO coding system (four-digit codes break down each of the categories listed into subcategories). Note that traditional healers are part of the official occupational classification and are included in counts in this report where data are available.

At the same time, another internationally agreed classification system – the International Standard Industrial Classification of all Economic Activities (ISIC) – is commonly used to define the different types of economic activity in a country. In ISIC, health is considered a separate industry. Vast numbers of workers with different training and occupational classifications are found in the health industry: many more than the health service providers themselves. These include professionals such as statisticians, computer programmers, accountants, managers and administrators and also various types of clerical staff as well as support staff such as drivers, cleaners, laundry workers and kitchen staff. Examples of the various types of occupations included for the health industry classification in the South African census are provided below.

Some health service providers work in industries other than health, such as mining or manufacturing. Accordingly, for this report, health workers include all occupations listed under the health industry, plus people in occupational groups 1–5 working in other industries.

The report groups health workers into two categories that map directly into the ISCO codes. People covered by occupational codes for groups 1–5 in the table are "health service providers"; other workers in the health industry are called "health management and support workers". This is shown in the figure, where health workers make up the first three of the four occupational boxes.

## Occupational classifications for the health industry, South African census, 2001

| ISCO groups of health service providers | Type | ISCO code no. |
|---|---|---|
| 1. Health professionals (except nursing) | Professionals | 222 |
| 2. Nursing and midwifery professionals | Professionals | 223 |
| 3. Modern health associate professionals (except nursing) | Associates | 322 |
| 4. Nursing and midwifery associate professionals | Associates | 323 |
| 5. Traditional medicine practitioners and faith healers | Associates | 324 |
| **Examples of other occupations involved in the health industry** | | |
| 6. Computing professionals | Professionals | 213 |
| 7. Social science and related professionals | Professionals | 244 |
| 8. Administrative associate professionals | Associates | 343 |
| 9. Secretaries and keyboard operating clerks | Clerks | 411 |
| 10. Painters, building structure cleaners and related trades workers | Craft and related trades workers | 714 |

Data source: *(2)*.

## Health workers in all sectors

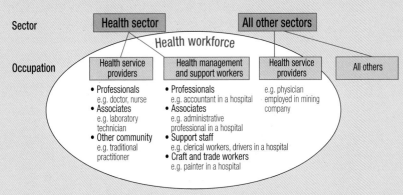

> ❝*The global health workforce is conservatively estimated to be just over 59 million workers*❞

industries that employ them. An accurate count of such workers is difficult to obtain, but they make up between 14% and 37% of all health service providers in countries with available census data. Excluding them from official counts results in a substantial underestimation of the size of the health workforce and its potential to improve health. Such undercounting also prevents consideration of the complex labour market links between different sectors that could inform planning, recruitment, retention and career paths.

## HOW MANY HEALTH WORKERS ARE THERE?

The work undertaken for this report allowed WHO to update the information contained in its *Global Atlas of the Health Workforce (3)* for some countries and to find previously unavailable data for others. Data are generally more complete for health service providers than for health management and support workers but, using the best available information from various sources, a conservative estimate of the size of the health workforce globally is just over 59 million workers (see Table 1.1). This figure is conservative in so far as it is likely to undercount health workers outside the health industry in countries where census information is not available.

Health service providers account for 67% of all health workers globally, though only 57% in the Region of the Americas. A breakdown by the level of national income in a country shows that health management and support workers slightly outnumber health service providers in high income countries, while the opposite is the case in low and middle income settings where health service providers typically constitute over 70% of the total health workforce.

Within the category of health service providers, attention is often focused on the ratio of nurses (and midwives) to doctors, though the exact numbers and mix necessary for a health system to run efficiently and effectively remains unclear *(4–8)*. The number of nurses per 1000 doctors for a typical country is highest in the WHO African Region, partly because of the very low number of doctors per 1000 population in that region. The ratio is lowest in the Western Pacific Region. There is also considerable heterogeneity among countries within regions. For example, there are approximately four nurses per doctor in Canada and the United States of America, while some other countries in the Region of the Americas, such as Chile, El Salvador, Mexico and Peru, have more doctors than nurses. Similarly, in the European Region, there is nearly one physician for every nurse in Bulgaria, Portugal and Turkey, but around five nurses for each physician in Norway and the United Kingdom.

## Box 1.2 The invisible backbone of the health system: management and support worker

People who help the health system to function but do not provide health services directly to the population are often forgotten in discussions about the health workforce. These individuals perform a variety of jobs, such as distributing medicines, maintaining essential buildings and equipment, and planning and setting directions for the system as a whole. Health management and support workers provide an invisible backbone for health systems; if they are not present in sufficient numbers and with appropriate skills, the system cannot function – for example, salaries are not paid and medicines are not delivered.

## Table 1.1 Global health workforce, by density

| WHO region | Total health workforce | | Health service providers | | Health management and support workers | |
|---|---|---|---|---|---|---|
| | Number | Density (per 1000 population) | Number | Percentage of total health workforce | Number | Percentage of total health workforce |
| Africa | 1 640 000 | 2.3 | 1 360 000 | 83 | 280 000 | 17 |
| Eastern Mediterranean | 2 100 000 | 4.0 | 1 580 000 | 75 | 520 000 | 25 |
| South-East Asia | 7 040 000 | 4.3 | 4 730 000 | 67 | 2 300 000 | 33 |
| Western Pacific | 10 070 000 | 5.8 | 7 810 000 | 78 | 2 260 000 | 23 |
| Europe | 16 630 000 | 18.9 | 11 540 000 | 69 | 5 090 000 | 31 |
| Americas | 21 740 000 | 24.8 | 12 460 000 | 57 | 9 280 000 | 43 |
| World | 59 220 000 | 9.3 | 39 470 000 | 67 | 19 750 000 | 33 |

Note: All data for latest available year. For countries where data on the number of health management and support workers were not available, estimates have been made based on regional averages for countries with complete data.

Data source: *(3)*.

Information has also been obtained on the relative availability of dentists and pharmacists, though fewer countries report this information. There is close to parity between the number of pharmacists and doctors in the South-East Asia Region, substantially more than in the other regions. The ratio of dentists to doctors is highest in the Region of the Americas. These data should be interpreted carefully, however, because of the difficulties involved in counting dentists and pharmacists, many of whom are likely to work in the private sector.

## Public and private sector workers

Most data on the distribution of health workers between the public and private sectors describe who is the primary employer of the worker rather than where the money to pay the salary or most of the worker's income comes from. This information suggests that the majority of health service providers in low and middle income countries report their primary site of employment as the public sector: over 70% of doctors and over 50% of other types of health service providers. Insufficient information is available from high income countries to allow similar analysis; it is likely, however, that the proportions officially employed by governments are lower, because many providers are officially in private practice despite much of their income coming directly from the public purse. This is also true for providers employed by faith-based and nongovernmental organizations in many settings.

These broad averages hide considerable variation across countries with the same level of income or in the same geographical region. For example, while 70% of doctors in sub-Saharan Africa are officially employed in the public sector, in six countries in the region more than 60% of them are formally employed in the private sector. Furthermore, even in countries where the public sector is the predominant employer, public sector employees often supplement their incomes with private work or receive a large part of their income directly from patients rather than from the government *(9–11)*. The data presented here on the relative importance of the public sector need, therefore, to be supplemented with information on health expenditures, as discussed below.

### Sex and age of health workers

Figure 1.1 illustrates the average distribution of women health service providers across countries. Insufficient information is available on the sex distribution of health management and support workers for them to be included. Men continue to dominate the medical profession, while other health service providers remain predominantly female. Notable exceptions exist, however. Mongolia, the Russian Federation, a number of other former Soviet republics and Sudan report more female than male doctors. Moreover, women are making substantial progress in some regions. The proportion of female doctors in Europe increased steadily during the 1990s, as did the proportion of female students in medical schools *(12)*. In the United Kingdom, for example, women now constitute up to 70% of medical school intakes *(13)*.

> ❝ *The proportion of female doctors in Europe increased steadily during the 1990s* ❞

From the limited information that exists on the ages of health workers in different settings, no general patterns can be observed, though some information is available for specific countries. For example, an increase in the average age of the nursing workforce over time has been noted in a number of OECD countries, including the United Kingdom and the United States *(14, 15)*. Policies relating to the official age of retirement are considered in Chapter 5.

It has not been possible to document trends over time in the mix of health professionals or their characteristics in enough countries to allow a global analysis. Systems for recording and updating health worker numbers often do not exist, which presents a major obstacle to developing evidence-based policies on human resource development.

Figure 1.1 Distribution of women in health service professions, by WHO region

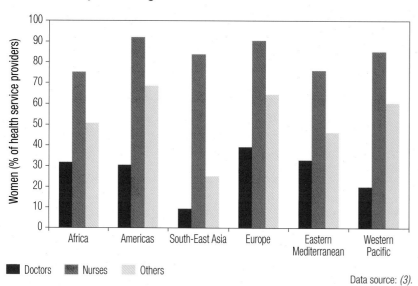

Data source: *(3)*.

Table 1.2 Proportion of government health expenditure paid to health workers

| WHO region | Wages, salaries and allowances of employees as percentage of general government health expenditure (GGHE) | Number of countries with available data |
|---|---|---|
| Africa | 29.5 | 14 |
| South-East Asia | 35.5 | 2 |
| Europe | 42.3 | 18 |
| Western Pacific | 45 | 7 |
| Americas | 49.8 | 17 |
| Eastern Mediterranean | 50.8 | 5 |
| World | 42.2 | 64 |

Note: Grouped proportions are simple averages of the country proportions, showing the ratio in a typical country in the region.

## HOW MUCH IS SPENT ON THE HEALTH WORKFORCE?

The large numbers of health workers in the world make up an important part of the total labour force. In general, the relative importance of the health workforce is higher in richer countries than in poorer ones and can account for up to 13% of the total workforce. Payments of salaries and other benefits to health workers are also a significant component of total government health expenditure (including capital costs) (Table 1.2). A typical country devotes just over 42% of total general government health expenditure to paying its health workforce, though there are regional and country variations around this average *(16)*. For example, governments in Africa and South-East Asia typically devote lower proportions than do those in other regions.

Information on the non-government (i.e. private) sector by itself is not available. Data have been obtained, however, from 43 countries on the share of total health expenditure (including capital costs) from all sources, government and non-government, paid in salaries and other allowances. On average, payments to the health workforce account for just under 50% of total health expenditure, suggesting that payments to health workers in the non-government sector make up a higher proportion of total expenditures than in the government sector. However, there is little overlap between the 43 countries described here and those included in Table 1.2 because of the way data are reported by different countries, so this information should be interpreted carefully. It should also be remembered that payments made by households directly to providers, and which are not captured in official records of salaries, are not included in this analysis.

Trends over time (1998–2003) in the ratio of wages, salaries and allowances to government health expenditure are available for only 12 countries. Trends in the share of total health expenditure paid to health workers as wages, salaries and allowances are available for another 24. Neither set of figures shows any consistent pattern. The share rose in some countries and fell in others, and the average across all countries is remarkably stable.

> *"A typical country devotes just over 42% of total general government health expenditure to paying its health workforce"*

# WHERE ARE THE HEALTH WORKERS?

## Uneven distribution across the globe

Health workers are distributed unevenly *(17)*. Countries with the lowest relative need have the highest numbers of health workers, while those with the greatest burden of disease must make do with a much smaller health workforce. This pattern is summarized in Figure 1.2, where the vertical axis shows burden of disease, the horizontal axis the number of health workers, and the size of the dots represents total health expenditure. The Region of the Americas, which includes Canada and the United States, contains only 10% of the global burden of disease, yet almost 37% of the world's health workers live in this region and spend more than 50% of the world's financial resources for health. In contrast, the African Region suffers more than 24% of the global burden of disease but has access to only 3% of health workers and less than 1% of the world's financial resources – even with loans and grants from abroad.

> " *Countries with the lowest relative need have the highest numbers of health workers* "

## Uneven spread within countries

Within regions and countries, access to health workers is also unequal. For example, Viet Nam averages just over one health service provider per 1000 people, but this figure hides considerable variation. In fact, 37 of Viet Nam's 61 provinces fall below this national average, while at the other extreme one province counts almost four health service providers per 1000 *(20)*. Similar variations exist in other countries *(21)*.

Many factors influence the geographical variation that is observed in health worker density. Areas with teaching hospitals and a population that can afford to pay for health services invariably attract more health workers than regions without such facilities or financial support. As a result, health worker density is generally highest in urban centres where teaching hospitals and high incomes are most common. Although the extent of urbanization increases across countries with increasing income, in countries of all income levels the proportion of health professionals living in urban areas exceeds the proportion of the general population found there. This is particularly the case for doctors, as shown in Figure 1.3, where the red dotted line shows that, while under 55% of all people live in urban areas, more than 75% of doctors, over 60% of nurses and 58% of other health workers also live in urban areas.

In many countries, female health service providers are particularly scarce in rural areas, a situation that may arise in part because it is unsafe for female workers to live alone in some isolated areas. The picture may well be different if traditional birth attendants and village volunteers could be included in the calculations, as these are the domains of women in many countries, but this information is rarely routinely available. Moreover, there are some notable exceptions. For example, Ethiopia and Pakistan are among the countries that have actively sought to recruit and train female health workers in rural areas: they are called health extension workers in Ethiopia and lady health workers and lady health visitors in Pakistan.

WHO is developing a tool to help countries to identify their health service resources, including where their health workers are to be found (see Box 1.3).

Figure 1.2  Distribution of health workers by level of health expenditure and burden of disease, by WHO region

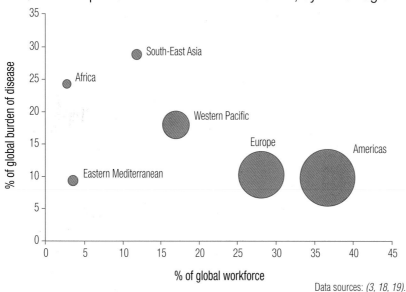

Data sources: *(3, 18, 19).*

## ARE THERE ENOUGH HEALTH WORKERS?

How important is the uneven geographical distribution of health workers within countries? Perfect equality is not feasible, and in some cases it is not even desirable. For instance, teaching hospitals must be strategically located, and a concentration of certain types of health workers around hospitals can be completely acceptable. But while some degree of geographical variation in health worker numbers is appropriate, the question remains: to what degree?

Although available data do not allow a simple response, coverage rates of key interventions are generally lower in areas with relatively low numbers of health workers, compared with those that have higher concentrations. This relationship can be observed across countries and within them. For example, researchers have recently found that countries with a higher density of health workers attain higher levels of measles vaccination and coverage with antenatal care *(23–25).*

Figure 1.3  Rural–urban distribution of health service providers

Data sources: *(3, 22).*

The correlation between the availability of health workers and coverage of health interventions suggests that the public's health suffers when health workers are scarce *(20, 21, 25–27)*. This raises the more fundamental issue of whether there are enough health workers. Methodologically, there are no gold standards for assessing sufficiency. The following section examines sufficiency from the perspective of essential health needs.

## Box 1.3  Where are the health workers?  Service Availability Mapping

To help national decision-makers obtain information rapidly, WHO is working with countries to develop a tool called Service Availability Mapping (SAM). Using WHO's Health Mapper (a Geographic Information System-based software package) and a questionnaire loaded on personal digital assistants, district health teams collect critical information on health resources, public health risks and programme implementation, in order to provide updated maps of health services. For more information, see http://www.who.int/healthinfo/systems/serviceavailabilitymapping/en/index.html.

A rapid version of a national SAM has been applied in a dozen countries, providing a rich picture of services across districts. Data on human resources include the density and distribution of health workers by major cadre and training exposure in the last two years, unfilled posts and absentee rates. The figure shows the density of doctors, clinical officers, registered and enrolled nurses and midwives, combined, per 1000 population in Zambia.

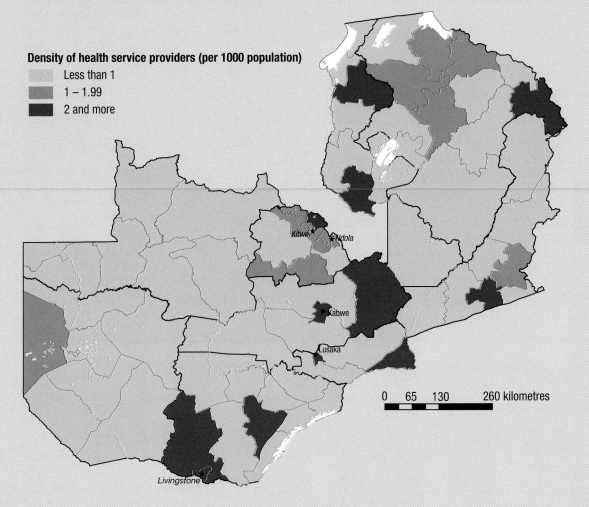

**Density of health service providers (per 1000 population)**
- Less than 1
- 1 – 1.99
- 2 and more

Source: Ministry of Health, Zambia, in collaboration with WHO.
Map production: Public Health Mapping and GIS/WHO.

Figure 1.4  Population density of health care professionals required to ensure skilled attendance at births

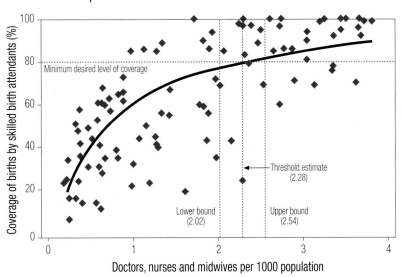

Data sources: *(3, 30, 31)*.

## Needs-based sufficiency

Various estimates of the availability of health workers required to achieve a package of essential health interventions and the Millennium Development Goals (including the scaling up of interventions for HIV/AIDS) have resulted in the identification of workforce shortfalls within and across mostly low income countries. In the HIV/AIDS literature, scaling up treatment with antiretrovirals was estimated to require between 20% and 50% of the available health workforce in four African countries, though less than 10% in the other 10 countries surveyed *(28)*. In more general terms, analysts estimated that in a best case scenario for 2015 the supply of health workers would reach only 60% of the estimated need in the United Republic of Tanzania and the need would be 300% greater than the available supply in Chad *(29)*. Furthermore, *The world health report 2005* estimated that 334 000 skilled birth attendants would have to be trained globally over the coming years merely to reach 72% coverage of births *(18)*.

To achieve a global assessment of shortfall, the Joint Learning Initiative (JLI), a network of global health leaders, launched by the Rockefeller Foundation, suggested that, on average, countries with fewer than 2.5 health care professionals (counting only doctors, nurses and midwives) per 1000 population failed to achieve an 80% coverage rate for deliveries by skilled birth attendants or for measles immunization *(24)*. This method of defining a shortage, whether global or by country, is driven partly by the decision to set the minimum desired level of coverage at 80% and partly by the empirical identification of health worker density associated with that level of coverage. Using a similar "threshold"

*"WHO estimates a shortage of more than 4 million doctors, nurses, midwives and others"*

Figure 1.5 Countries with a critical shortage of health service providers (doctors, nurses and midwives)

Countries with critical shortage

Countries without critical shortage

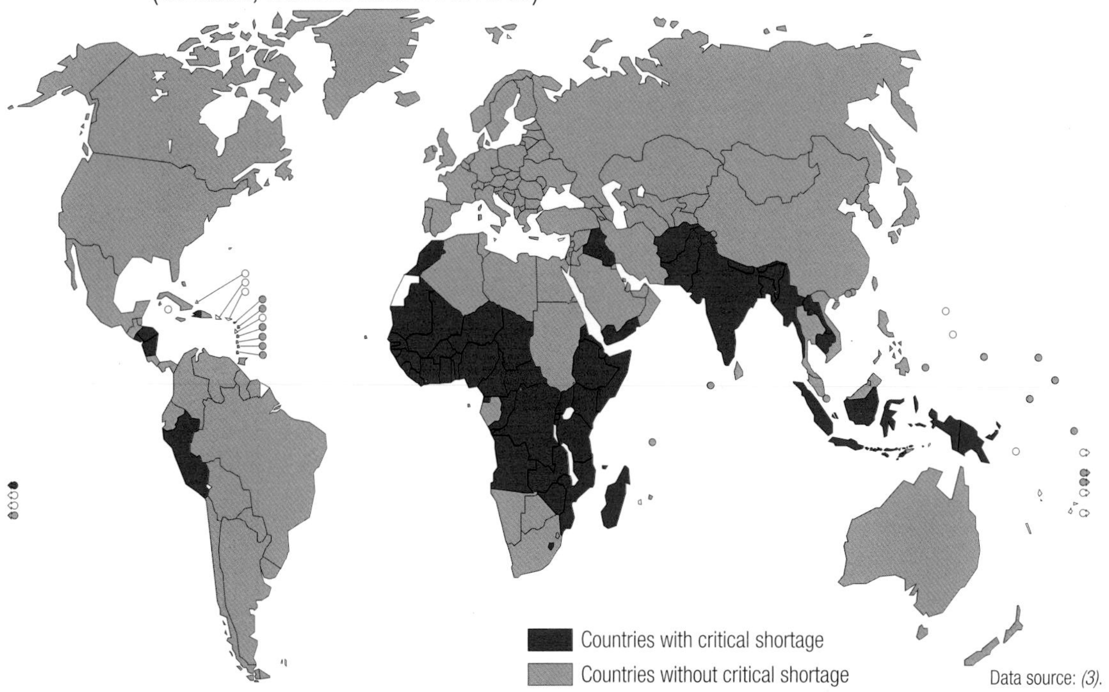

Data source: *(3)*.

method and updated information on the size of the health workforce obtained for this report, the JLI analysis has been repeated for skilled birth attendants (see Figure 1.4). A remarkably similar threshold is found at 2.28 health care professionals per 1000 population, ranging from 2.02 to 2.54 allowing for uncertainty.

The 57 countries that fall below this threshold and which fail to attain the 80% coverage level are defined as having a critical shortage. Thirty-six of them are in sub-Saharan Africa (Figure 1.5). For all these countries to reach the target levels of health worker availability would require an additional 2.4 million professionals globally (Table 1.3). (Based on the upper and lower limits of the threshold, the upper and lower limits of the estimated critical shortage are 3 million and 1.7 million, respectively.) This requirement represents only three types of health service provider. Multiplying the 2.4 million shortage by 1.8, which is the average ratio of total health workers to doctors, nurses and midwives observed in all WHO regions (except Europe, where there are no critical shortages based on these criteria), the global shortage approaches 4.3 million health workers.

In absolute terms, the greatest shortage occurs in South-East Asia, dominated by the needs of Bangladesh, India and Indonesia. The largest relative need exists in sub-Saharan Africa, where an increase of almost 140% is necessary to meet the threshold.

These estimates highlight the critical need for more health workers in order to achieve even modest coverage for essential health interventions in the countries most in need. They are not a substitute for specific country assessments of sufficiency, nor do they detract from the fact that the effect of increasing the number of health

Table 1.3 Estimated critical shortages of doctors, nurses and midwives, by WHO region

| WHO region | Number of countries | | In countries with shortages | | |
|---|---|---|---|---|---|
| | Total | With shortages | Total stock | Estimated shortage | Percentage increase required |
| Africa | 46 | 36 | 590 198 | 817 992 | 139 |
| Americas | 35 | 5 | 93 603 | 37 886 | 40 |
| South-East Asia | 11 | 6 | 2 332 054 | 1 164 001 | 50 |
| Europe | 52 | 0 | NA | NA | NA |
| Eastern Mediterranean | 21 | 7 | 312 613 | 306 031 | 98 |
| Western Pacific | 27 | 3 | 27 260 | 32 560 | 119 |
| World | 192 | 57 | 3 355 728 | 2 358 470 | 70 |

NA, not applicable.
Data source: *(3)*.

workers depends crucially on other determinants such as levels of income and education in the community *(21, 25)*. Furthermore, economic factors also enter the equation: shortfalls based on need can co-exist with unemployment of health workers due to local market conditions (see Chapter 6 for further discussion).

## ADDRESSING THE SHORTAGE – HOW MUCH WILL IT COST?

Making up the shortfall through training requires a significant investment. Assuming very rapid scaling up in which all the training is completed by 2015, the annual training costs range from a low of US$ 1.6 million per country per year to almost US$ 2 billion in a large country like India. The average cost per country of US$ 136 million per year is of the same order of magnitude as the estimated cost of Malawi's Emergency Human Resources Programme (see Chapter 2). Financing it would require health expenditures to increase by US$ 2.80 per person annually in the average country (the range is from US$ 0.40 to just over US$ 11) – an increase of approximately 11% on 2004 levels *(34)*.

The estimate is limited to doctors, nurses and midwives, the occupations for which data on workforce numbers and training costs are most complete, so can be considered a lower limit. In the calculations, the target number of health workers has been adjusted upwards to account for population growth between 2005 and 2015, and student intakes have also been adjusted upwards to account for attrition during and after training. Region-specific training costs that include a capital component have been used where possible, though data are limited and the results should be interpreted with caution.

These estimates also assume that present trends and patterns of training will continue. Other ways of helping to tackle the observed shortages, including those aimed at increasing the productivity and motivation of the current workforce, or changing the skill mix of health workers, are described in subsequent chapters.

The additional annual cost of employing the new doctors, nurses and midwives once training has been fully scaled up is just over US$ 311 million per country in 2004 prices. By 2015, to pay the salaries of the scaled-up workforce would require a minimum increase of US$ 7.50 per person per year in the average country. This can be taken to be a lower limit cost because some level of salary increase is likely to be necessary to retain the additional health workers in the health sector and in the country. The extent of the required increase is difficult to determine, partly because salaries in the deficit countries can be up to 15 times lower than those in countries that are popular destinations for migrants *(32)*. The Millennium Project assumed salaries would need to double if the Millennium Development Goals were to be achieved *(33)*, which would increase the current annual salary cost by US$ 53 billion in the 57 countries. To put this figure into perspective, this represents an increase in the annual global wage bill for health workers of less than 5%. It would also require an increase in annual health spending by 2015 of US$ 20 per person in the average country – an increase of over 75% on 2004 levels.

These figures need to be interpreted with caution, particularly because labour markets for health workers are evolving rapidly as globalization increases. It is very likely, for example, that salaries in some of the countries where shortages were not identified would have to be increased as well, to ensure that their workers did not migrate to some of the deficit countries. This type of effect is difficult to predict, but the numbers reported here clearly show the need for the international community actively to support the process of strengthening human resources for health.

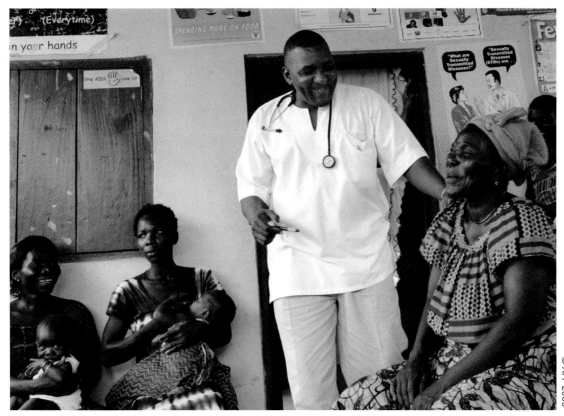

© AFP 2005

**Dr John Awoonor-Williams is the only doctor at Nkwanta District Hospital, Ghana, serving a population of 187 000 in a remote, vast area in the northern part of the Volta Region.**

## CONCLUSION

The global profile presented here shows that there are more than 59 million health workers in the world, distributed unequally between and within countries. They are found predominantly in richer areas where health needs are less severe. Their numbers remain woefully insufficient to meet health needs, with the total shortage being in the order of 4.3 million workers.

The profile also shows how much is not known. Information on skill mix, age profiles, sources of income, geographical location, and other characteristics that are important for policy development is far from complete. One reason for this is the variation between countries in the definitions used to categorize health workers, which makes it difficult to ensure that the same people are being included as part of the health workforce in different settings. WHO is confronting this issue by developing a standard classification of health workers in collaboration with countries and other partners.

The other reason is simply the lack of data. In some countries, information on the total size of the health workforce is not routinely collected, while little is known about certain categories of health workers even in countries with extensive data reporting systems. The lack of reliable, up-to-date information greatly restricts the ability of policy-makers at national and international levels to develop evidence-based strategies to resolve the health workforce crisis, or to develop health systems to serve the needs of disadvantaged populations. Relatively small investments by the global community in this area could well have substantial returns. Chapter 7 returns to this issue and suggests some possible solutions. Meanwhile, Chapter 2 discusses some of the most important challenges that face the global health workforce today.

## REFERENCES

1. Dal Poz MR, Kinfu Y, Dräger S, Kunjumen T, Diallo K. *Counting health workers: definitions, data, methods and global results.* Geneva, World Health Organization, 2006 (background paper for *The world health report 2006;* available at: http://www.who.int/hrh/documents/en/).
2. International Labour Organization. *International Standard Classification of Occupations* (http://www.ilo.org/public/english/bureau/stat/class/isco.htm, accessed 19 January 2006).
3. World Health Organization. *Global Atlas of the Health Workforce* (http://www.who.int/globalatlas/default.asp, accessed 19 January 2006).
4. Zurn P, Vujicic M, Diallo K, Pantoja A, Dal Poz MR, Adams O. Planning for human resources for health: human resources for health and the projection of health outcomes/outputs. *Cahiers de Sociologie et de Démographie médicales*, 2005, 45:107–133.
5. Buchan J, Dal Poz MR. Skill mix in the health care workforce: reviewing the evidence. *Bulletin of the World Health Organization,* 2002, 80:575–580.
6. Dussault G, Adams O, Fournier P. *Planejamento de recursos humanos em saúde [Human resources for health planning].* Translation, adaptation and preface by Dal Poz MR. Rio de Janeiro, Universidade do Estado do Rio de Janeiro, Instituto de Medicina Social, 1997 (Série Estudos em Saúde Coletiva, 158).
7. Lave JR, Lave LB, Leinhardt S. Medical manpower models: need, demand and supply. *Inquiry*, 1975, XII:97–126.
8. Reinhardt UE. Projecting long-term trends in health manpower: methodological problems. In: Culyer AJ, ed. *The economics of health.* Great Yarmouth, Edward Elgar Publishing Ltd, 1991:262–83.

9. McPake B , Asiimwe D, Mwesigye F, Ofumbi M, Streefland P, Turinde A. Coping strategies of health workers in Uganda. In: Ferrinho P, Van Lerberghe W, eds. *Providing health care under adverse conditions: health personnel performance and individual coping strategies.* Antwerp, ITG Press, 2000 (Studies in Health Services Organisation and Policy, 16:131–150).

10. Macq J, Van Lerberghe W. Managing health services in developing countries: moonlighting to serve the public? In: Ferrinho P, Van Lerberghe W, eds. *Providing health care under adverse conditions: health personnel performance and individual coping strategies.* Antwerp, ITG Press, 2000 (Studies in Health Services Organisation and Policy, 16:177–186).

11. Ferrinho P, Van Lerberghe W, Fronteira I, Hipolito F, Biscaia A. Dual practice in the health sector: review of the evidence. *Human Resources for Health*, 2004, 2:14.

12. Gupta N, Diallo K, Zurn P, Dal Poz MR. Assessing human resources for health: what can be learned from labour force surveys? *Human Resources for Health,* 2003, 1:5.

13. Dubois C-A, McKee M, Nolte E. Analysing trends, opportunities and challenges. In: Dubois C-A, McKee M, Nolte E, eds. *Human resources for health in Europe.* Brussels, European Observatory on Health Systems and Policies, 2005.

14. Buerhaus P, Staiger D, Auerbach D. Implications of a rapidly aging registered nurse workforce. *JAMA*, 2000, 283:2948–2954.

15. Buchan J. The "greying" of the United Kingdom nursing workforce: implications for employment policy and practice. *Journal of Advanced Nursing*, 1999, 30:818–826.

16. Hernandez P, Dräger S, Evans DB, Tan-Torres T, Dal Poz MR. Measuring expenditure for the health workforce: challenges and evidence. Geneva, World Health Organization, 2006 (background paper for *The world health report 2006*; available at: http://www.who.int/hrh/documents/en/).

17. Speybroeck N, Ebener S, Sousa A, Paraje G, Evans DB, Prasad A. *Inequality in access to human resources for health: measurement issues.* Geneva, World Health Organization, 2006 (background paper for *The world health report 2006*; available at: http://www.who.int/hrh/documents/en/).

18. *The world health report 2005 – Make every mother and child count.* Geneva, World Health Organization, 2005:200–203.

19. World Health Organization. *Burden of Disease Statistics* (http://www.who.int/healthinfo/bod/en/, accessed 19 January 2006).

20. Prasad A, Tandon A, Sousa A, Ebener S, Evans DB. *Measuring the efficiency of human resources for health in attaining health outcomes across provinces in Viet Nam.* Geneva, World Health Organization, 2006 (background paper for *The world health report 2006*; available at: http://www.who.int/hrh/documents/en/).

21. Sousa A, Tandon A, Prasad A, Dal Poz MR, Evans DB. *Measuring the efficiency of health workers in attaining health outcomes across sub national units in Brazil.* Geneva, World Health Organization, 2006 (background paper for *The world health report 2006*; available at: http://www.who.int/hrh/documents/en/).

22. Population Reference Bureau. *Search Population and Health Data* (http://www.prb. org/datafind/datafinder6.htm, accessed 20 January 2006).
23. Anand S, Bärnighausen T. *Human resources for health and vaccination coverage in developing countries* (unpublished document, Oxford University, 2005).
24. Chen L, Evans T, Anand S, Boufford JI, Brown H, Chowdhury M et al. Human resources for health: overcoming the crisis. *Lancet*, 2004, 364:1984–1990.
25. Speybroeck N, Kinfu Y, Dal Poz MR, Evans DB. *Reassessing the relationship between human resources for health, intervention coverage and health outcomes*. Geneva, World Health Organization, 2006 (background paper for *The world health report 2006*; available at: http://www.who.int/hrh/documents/en/).
26. Tandon A, Sousa A, Prasad A, Evans DB. *Human resources and health outcomes in Brazil and Viet Nam: a comparative perspective*. Geneva, World Health Organization, 2006 (background paper for *The world health report 2006*; available at: http://www.who. int/hrh/documents/en/).
27. Anand S, Bärnighausen T. Human resources and health outcomes: cross-country econometric study. *Lancet,* 2004, 364:1603–1609.
28. Smith O. Human resource requirements for scaling up antiretroviral therapy in low-resource countries (Appendix E). In: Curran J, Debas H, Arya M, Kelley P, Knobler S, Pray L, eds. *Scaling up treatment for the global AIDS pandemic: challenges and opportunities*. Washington, DC, National Academies Press (Board of Global Health), 2004.
29. Kurowski C, Wyss K, Abdulla S, Yémadji N, Mills A. *Human resources for health: requirements and availability in the context of scaling-up priority interventions in low-income countries. Case studies from Tanzania and Chad*. London, London School of Hygiene and Tropical Medicine, 2003 (Working Paper 01/04).
30. UNICEF. *WHO UNICEF Estimates on Immunization Coverage 1980–2004* (http://www. childinfo.org/areas/immunization/database.php, accessed 20 January 2006).
31. United Nations Population Division. *World Population Prospects: the 2004 Revision. Population Database* (http://esa.un.org/unpp, accessed 20 January 2006).
32. Vujicic M, Zurn P, Diallo K, Adams O, Dal Poz MR. The role of wages in the migration of health care professionals from developing countries. *Human Resources for Health*, 2004, 2:3.
33. *Millennium Development Goals needs assessments: country case studies of Bangladesh, Cambodia, Ghana, Tanzania and Uganda*. New York, NY, Millennium Project, 2004 (http://www.unmillenniumproject.org/documents/mp_ccspaper_jan1704.pdf, accessed 23 February 2004).
34. Verboom P, Tan-Torres Edejer T, Evans DB. *The costs of eliminating critical shortages in human resources for health*. Geneva, World Health Organization, 2006 (background paper for *The world health report 2006*; available at: http://www.who.int/hrh/ documents/en/).

responding to u

chapter two

# *gent health needs*

**This chapter identifies some of the most important performance challenges facing health systems and the global health workforce today, examines the ways in which the health workforce is meeting them, and suggests how these responses can be improved. These challenges are, first, to scale up interventions to attain the health-related MDGs; second, to shift successfully to community-based and patient-centred paradigms of care for the treatment of chronic diseases; third, to tackle the problems posed by disasters and outbreaks; and fourth, to preserve health services in conflict and post-conflict states.**

They have been chosen because they provide a reasonable sample of the kinds of challenges that exist in many countries and settings. Each of the four sections of this chapter describes the main characteristics of one performance challenge, and how the health workforce is responding or can more adequately respond.

## HIGH-PRIORITY SERVICES: HUMAN RESOURCES FOR HEALTH AND THE MDGs

It is now widely accepted that the dire shortage of health workers in many places is among the most significant constraints to achieving the three health-related Millennium Development Goals (MDGs): to reduce child mortality, improve maternal health, and combat HIV/AIDS and other diseases, such as tuberculosis and malaria *(1–6)*. Chad and the United Republic of Tanzania, for example, have less than half the workforce they require to meet essential health needs adequately *(5)*. It is not only health service providers who are in short supply – shortfalls exist in all categories of health workers including laboratory technicians, pharmacists, logisticians and managers.

The impressive mobilization of donor funds to achieve the health-related MDGs, and in particular to combat HIV/AIDS, has created a new environment in which a shortage of human resources has replaced finance issues as the most serious obstacle to implementing national treatment plans *(7)*.

Achieving the MDGs will depend on finding effective human resources approaches that can be implemented rapidly *(6)*. But simply training people to deliver disease-specific interventions is unlikely to be sufficient. Such approaches should also consider the larger health systems challenges that are related to the pervasive disadvantages associated with low income. For example, there are huge disparities between income groups in access to facility-based health services (see Figure 2.1).

Systematic thinking in several areas is required to formulate ways of recruiting and retaining health workers to provide the necessary MDG-related health actions (see Box 2.1). More effective human resources efforts need to employ critical evaluation of current behaviours.

### Epidemics of in-service training

The numerous projects and programmes created in response to the MDGs are replete with budget lines to train staff, but lack comprehensive workforce strategies. As a result, a great deal of effort is directed towards running short training courses, often held in hotels in other countries. The aim of most of these courses is to equip health workers or the trainers of health

> " *A shortage of human resources has replaced financial issues as the most serious obstacle to implementing national treatment plans* "

## Figure 2.1 From massive deprivation to marginal exclusion: moving up the coverage ladder

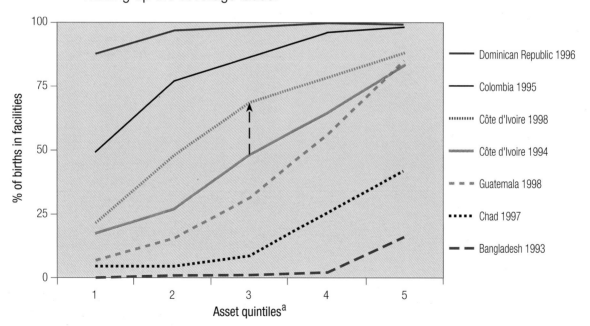

*legend:*
- Dominican Republic 1996
- Colombia 1995
- Côte d'Ivoire 1998
- Côte d'Ivoire 1994
- Guatemala 1998
- Chad 1997
- Bangladesh 1993

*y-axis:* % of births in facilities
*x-axis:* Asset quintiles[a]

[a] Asset quintiles provide an index of socioeconomic status at the household level. They divide populations into five groups (in ascending order of wealth from 1 to 5), using a methodology that combines information on household head characteristics as well as household ownership of certain assets, availability of services, and housing characteristics.

Source *(8)*.

workers with the skills to deliver specific interventions. While trainees may welcome an expense-free trip to a major urban centre, these trips pose significant opportunity costs. Staff are rarely replaced when they travel and often the same staff will attend several courses every year. Furthermore, the courses often have few links with local training institutions, and thereby opportunities are missed to involve faculty members or to contribute to the development of locally-based courses. Evaluations of short-term training in Africa in 2000–2001 led to the strong recommendation that training should be on-site as much as possible and delivered through local institutions *(9)*.

## Overburdened district staff

National programmes to achieve disease-specific MDGs place many parallel demands on district health managers and service providers, such as reading documents, filling forms, writing reports, attending meetings and making field visits. These demands are often imposed by international donors, and can quickly overwhelm limited, underfunded and insufficiently supported district-level staff. Simply keeping up with the reporting requirements of various programmes can occupy between 10% and 20% of a district health manager's time *(10)*.

## Two tiers of salaries

The onslaught of MDG-related programmes is also exerting severe pressure on salaries. In order to attract workers, well-funded programmes that are implemented through nongovernmental mechanisms – notably those focused on HIV/AIDS treatment – often pay salaries that exceed local wages in the public sector. As a result, two tiers of salaried workers are emerging, often within the same institution. This situation creates significant problems. The workers who receive less pay often feel aggrieved, resenting the fact that, for example, as an obstetric nurse they earn less than an HIV nurse. Furthermore, certain critical services may not be carried out if employers are unable to provide competitive salaries to attract and maintain staff.

> " *Two tiers of salaried workers are emerging, often within the same institution. This creates significant problems* "

## Box 2.1 Health workers and the Millennium Development Goals

Several constraints face the health workforce in the delivery of interventions aimed at achieving the health-related Millennium Development Goals. The main problems can be summarized as follows:

- inappropriate or inadequate training, with curricula that are not needs-based;
- poor access to information and knowledge resources;
- inadequate numbers and skills of health workers;
- uneven distribution of workers at different levels of service delivery, from national programme officers through to health facility personnel;
- low morale and motivation;
- unsafe conditions in the workplace;
- poor policies and practices for human resources development (poor career structures, working conditions and remuneration);
- lack of supportive supervision;
- lack of integration of services with the private sector;
- high attrition of health workers, as a consequence of death from the very diseases they work to cure, or because of migration.

Source: *(2)*.

## Strategy 2.1 Scale up workforce planning

> *Workforce expansion requires political leadership, adequate financing and a comprehensive plan*

The enormous shortfall in the human resources needed to provide MDG-related services demands an accelerated expansion of the workforce. Three factors must be present for this kind of expansion to take place – political leadership, adequate financing and a comprehensive plan.

Before necessary reforms can take place, political leaders, donors and governments alike must view the workforce as an investment to be nurtured, and not as a cost to be minimized. Along with strong leadership must come a commitment to devote the necessary funds. This funding must not only cover health service providers, but also the management and support workers who provide crucial services to the front lines of the health system.

The third requirement is a sensible strategy to boost the health workforce, one with short-term as well as longer-term performance goals. The strategy must be based on established human resources needs for priority programmes *(2)* and it must mobilize the institutions involved in both the production and management of the workforce (see Chapters 3 and 4).

These three elements have converged in Malawi, where the Emergency Human Resources Programme has become a top priority for the Ministry of Health (see

## Box 2.2 An emergency programme for human resources in Malawi

Staffing in Malawi's health service is inadequate to maintain a minimum level of health care, and is particularly low even by regional standards. It is also insufficient for the delivery of antiretroviral therapy and other HIV/AIDS-related services in response to demand. Of 27 districts, 15 have fewer than 1.5 nurses per facility, and five districts do not have even one each, while four districts have no doctor at all. HIV/AIDS-related attrition among the workforce compounds the shortage. In addition, up to 800 qualified nurses living in Malawi choose not to work in the health sector.

In April 2004, the Ministry of Health called for action to retain current staff and prevent brain drain as a top priority, highlighting the need to attract back into the system those who had left it and remained in Malawi. The 6-year Emergency Human Resources Programme includes: improving incentives for recruitment and retention of Malawian staff by 52%, gross salary increases for 11 selected professional and technical cadres; external stop-gap recruitment of physicians and nurses; and significant expansion of domestic training capacity. The programme recognizes the need to address a range of non-financial factors affecting retention, including policies for postings and promotions, performance management, regrading, opportunities for training and upgrading of skills, gender issues and quality of housing. Human resources planning and management capacity in the Ministry of Health and at local level is also being strengthened.

The programme, which is supported by the Global Fund to Fight AIDS, Tuberculosis and Malaria, the United Kingdom Department for International Development, the Malawi Government and other donors, is estimated to cost about US$ 278 million. Up to US$ 98 million will support salary top-ups, with a further US$ 35 million for improved staff housing, and US$ 64 million earmarked for expansion of training capacity.

While it is early days, the approach appears to be having a positive impact. By the end of 2005, some 5400 doctors, nurses and other key staff were receiving the salary top-up and there has been a reduction in the outflow of staff from the public sector. Over 700 new health staff have been recruited by the government since July 2004, with interviews for nearly 200 further posts currently taking place. Plans for infrastructure expansion and additional teaching staff for Malawi training schools will increase training capacity by over 50% on average, triple the number of doctors and nearly double the number of registered nurses in training. While more Malawians are being trained, expatriate doctors and nurses will continue to be relied on to fill critical positions.

Source: *(11).*

Box 2.2). With the support of the international community, countries experiencing similar human resources crises should consider developing similar plans.

## Strategy 2.2 Capitalize on synergies across priority programmes

In responding to the specific health challenges of the MDGs, given the urgency and the availability of financing, there is a tendency to plan the workforce around specific diseases or interventions. As mentioned, this sort of planning risks a number of inefficiencies that result mainly from inadequate consideration of the systemic nature of human resources and health services delivery more broadly. Increasingly, this is being recognized and important innovations are emerging.

In many cases, channels for delivering these interventions can be combined to use scarce human resources more efficiently. The term "piggy-backing" has been coined to identify ways in which services can be added to existing delivery vehicles rather than mobilization of workers for separate, single-purpose, community-directed interventions. For example, the WHO Onchocerciasis Control Programme to prevent river blindness in west Africa used community-directed treatment projects to add vitamin A to ivermectin distribution. "Piggy-backing" of other treatment elements is also a deliberate strategy of the WHO Global Programme to Eliminate Lymphatic Filariasis *(12)*.

## Strategy 2.3 Simplify services and delegate appropriately

Greater efficiencies in workforce performance can be achieved by applying two of the cardinal rules for scaling up interventions effectively: simplification and delegation. Simplification often improves staff productivity by allowing more to be done, with greater consistency, and often by less skilled colleagues. Simplifying all basic tasks is the first element of the Global Polio Eradication Initiative, is crucial to the scaling up of oral rehydration therapy in Bangladesh *(13)*, and is a core strategy of the WHO/UNAIDS 3 by 5 Initiative *(14)*. Within the Polio Eradication Initiative, for example, all basic tasks were simplified as a result of strategic decisions, technological innovations and locally appropriate adaptation. All available human resources, from unskilled volunteers to highly skilled workers, both inside and outside the health sector, were considered to be potential "vaccinators" and, if necessary, surveillance officers *(15)*. The WHO/UNAIDS 3 by 5 Initiative has shown that people living with HIV/AIDS can make important contributions across the spectrum of HIV/AIDS prevention and treatment services *(16)*.

In many areas, programmes aimed at integrating skills among providers of primary care for children, adolescents and adults are taking place at the district and primary care level. WHO's Integrated Management of Adolescent and Adult Illness (IMAI) and the HIV adaptation of Integrated Management of Childhood Illness (IMCI-HIV) provide a novel approach to scaling up HIV prevention, care and treatment, as well as tuberculosis care and co-management of TB/HIV/AIDS patients (see Box 2.3). Despite these promising examples, increased efforts will be required to identify pragmatic ways of working across priority programmes.

Simplification facilitates but is not a prerequisite of task delegation. Tasks related to service delivery can often be carried out as or even more efficiently by less senior staff. Task delegation is especially important in resource-constrained settings where skilled staff are in very short supply. The delegation of malaria diagnosis to volunteer health workers using village-based microscopy in Myanmar and the Philippines, for

> *In several southern African countries, death from HIV/AIDS is the largest cause of worker exits from the workforce*

example, has been shown to be reliable and to improve the treatment of malaria, while at the same time raising the morale and self-esteem of workers *(18, 19)*.

Plans to simplify and to delegate tasks require careful assessment of the intended impact. In the 1970s and 1980s, for example, tens of thousands of traditional birth attendants were trained throughout the developing world *(20)* in the hope of improving the survival of mothers in settings where professional midwives were rare. But, after more than three decades of well-meant attempts, there is no convincing evidence that the training strategy has reduced maternal mortality rates *(8)*.

## Strategy 2.4 Secure the health and safety of health workers

In several southern African countries, death from HIV/AIDS is the largest cause of worker exits from the workforce. Those who remain often work in understaffed health facilities that are overburdened with patients (many with HIV/AIDS) and that have inadequate means to treat them. These working conditions, in turn, fuel low morale, burn-out and absenteeism. In light of this fact, efforts are now under way to address occupational health and safety risks through the prevention of needle-stick injuries, post-exposure prophylaxis, and increasing the supplies of protective equipment. More and more countries are making provisions to ensure treatment access to workers who become infected with HIV *(21)*, and in 2005 the International Labour Organization and WHO agreed to joint guidelines designed to help workers involved in the global struggle against HIV/AIDS stay healthy (see Chapter 5).

## PREPARING THE WORKFORCE FOR THE GROWING BURDEN OF CHRONIC DISEASES AND INJURIES

As well as those diseases which form the primary focus of the MDGs, the world is faced with a massive and growing burden of chronic diseases, which are among

## Box 2.3 Task shifting in the health care workforce

More than 25 countries in Africa are now using a set of simplified operational guidelines from WHO's Integrated Management of Adult and Adolescent Illness (IMAI) to train health workers. These guidelines clearly define the tasks required for chronic HIV/AIDS prevention, care, and antiretroviral therapy (ART), as well as tuberculosis care and co-management of TB/HIV/AIDS patients; they allow these interventions to be delivered by nurses, clinical officers, midwives and various cadres of medical assistants, working together in a clinical team in the hospital outpatient facility or in peripheral health centres.

Shifting tasks between health care workers and expanding the clinical team can relieve short-term human resource limitations in settings with low resources. Rapid scaling up involves:

- shifting tasks to the lowest relevant cadre;
- expanding the clinical team by including people living with AIDS;

- placing strong emphasis on patient self-management and community involvement.

Based on this approach, tasks in many health care settings can be shifted from specialized (and therefore scarce) workers to less specialized ones. The most important task shift is to the patients themselves (i.e. self-management). The community can be progressively involved in managing HIV/AIDS care and antiretroviral therapy for such tasks as treatment support, repeat drug prescriptions and simple monitoring.

IMAI training focuses on the needs of the clinical team. The training uses adult participatory training methods that emphasize the acquisition of skills and case practice, rather than just knowledge. It also considers people living with HIV/AIDS as experts in their own illness and as a valuable educational resource to support the training of health workers.

Source: *(17)*.

the world's leading causes of death and disability. Trends indicate that they are likely to become even more important over the next decade *(22)*. The epidemiologic importance of such conditions is matched by their direct and indirect social and economic consequences.

## New paradigms of care require a workforce response

In recent years, the traditional focus on acute, inpatient and sub-specialty care has given way to new paradigms of care emphasizing self-management, and community-based patient-centred pre-hospital care *(23)* (see Figure 2.2). This evolution has been accompanied by a recognition by experts, professional bodies and health workers themselves of both the inadequacies of traditional training and deployment of the workforce, and the imperative for new approaches *(25–29)*.

## Strategy 2.5 Deploy towards a continuum of care

Five core competencies for long-term patient care have been identified: patient-centred care, partnering, quality improvement, information and communication technology, and a public health perspective (see Box 2.4). The challenge is to translate these into practice through the institutions that produce and deploy the health workforce. Changes in the curriculum, new teaching methods, and innovative training models are necessary *(31–33)*.

Decisions surrounding training and recruitment must also reflect the continuum of care and take into account the distribution and type of workers required to meet the health care needs of the population. Provision of community mental health services for example relies heavily on effective education outreach programmes for police officers, religious healers and social workers. Non-professional workers can help meet some of the demand for care as long as they are competent and supervised, and can draw upon professional staff when necessary to deal with complex cases.

## Box 2.4 Core competencies for long-term patient care

**PATIENT-CENTRED CARE**
- Learn how to negotiate individualized care plans with patients, taking into account their needs, values, and preferences.
- Learn how to support patient self-management efforts.
- Learn how to organize and implement group medical visits for patients who share common health problems.

**PARTNERING**
- Work as a member of a multidisciplinary health care team.

**QUALITY IMPROVEMENT**
- Design and participate in health care quality improvement projects.

**INFORMATION AND COMMUNICATION TECHNOLOGY**
- Develop information systems (e.g. patient registries), even if paper-based, to ensure continuity of care and planned follow-up.
- Use available technology and communication systems to exchange patient information with other health care workers and to consult specialists from primary health care.

**PUBLIC HEALTH PERSPECTIVE**
- Work in a community-based setting and conduct community outreach to promote healthy lifestyles, encourage responsible and safe behaviour, and reduce the stigma associated with physical disability and mental illness.
- Learn to think beyond caring for one patient at a time to a "population" perspective.
- Hone skills for clinical prevention.

Source: *(30)*.

Village volunteers are another largely untapped but potentially valuable resource. In Ghana in 1999, for example, the WHO Nations for Mental Health Project launched a three-year pilot project that trained volunteers selected by their communities to identify, refer and follow-up people in their villages who had mental disorders. The government has now adopted the project and it is being extended to other districts *(24)*.

It is important to recognize that the shift to community-based care should not overlook the other end of the continuum, i.e. specialist and sub-specialist care. In many parts of the world, the critical shortage of such specialists is a major constraint to the integrity of the continuum of care concept. The shortages of specialists, such as psychiatrists, in many parts of the world, means that care is often not available. Psychiatrists have a crucial role to play in managing and treating complex cases of mental disorders, in providing ongoing supervision and support to non-specialists working in the mental health field, and in teaching and training other mental health professionals (see Figure 2.3).

The shift from hospital-based to community-based care, and the new emphasis on multidisciplinary and intersectoral approaches, means changing roles for staff as well. These changing roles present challenges for managers, health workers and regulatory agencies. Scope-of-practice regulations, designed to establish minimum standards and protect patients, can become impediments to the pursuit of change. Managers need to engage actively with health workers, listen to their requirements and present the case for service reform and new, evidence-based ways of working. The challenge for health workers is to embrace change as an opportunity for further learning and personal and professional development, given their legitimate concerns related to personal status and income.

Figure 2.2  Optimal mix of mental health services

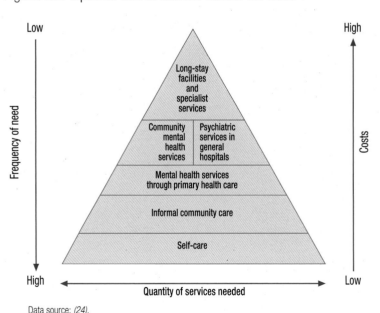

Data source: *(24)*.

## Figure 2.3 Global distribution of psychiatrists

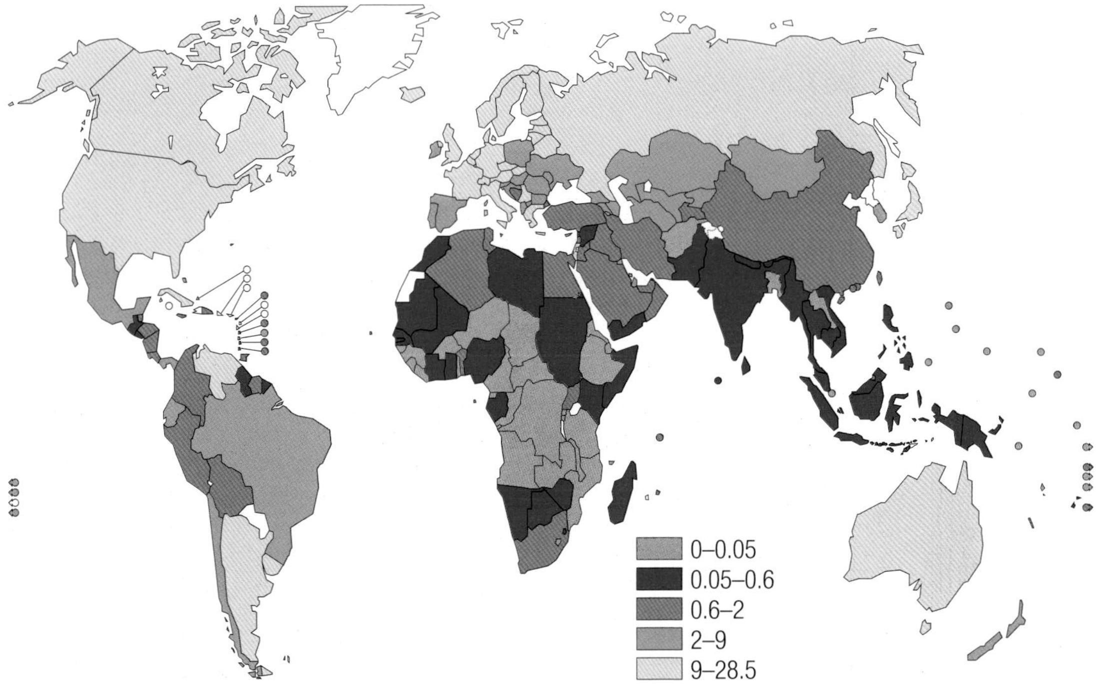

| | |
|---|---|
| 0–0.05 | |
| 0.05–0.6 | |
| 0.6–2 | |
| 2–9 | |
| 9–28.5 | |

Per 100 000 population

Source: *(34)*.

## Strategy 2.6 Foster collaboration

Inherent in the new paradigm of care is a strong emphasis on collaboration and teamwork between health worker and patient. Creating a relationship that values the patient as a partner in his or her own care has been frequently shown to improve health behaviour and clinical outcomes. Extensive evidence shows that interventions designed to promote patients' roles in the prevention and management of chronic diseases can lead to improved outcomes *(31, 35, 36)*. What patients and their families do for themselves on a daily basis, such as engaging in physical activity, eating properly, avoiding tobacco use, sleeping regularly, and adhering to treatment plans, significantly influences their health. Health workers are instrumental in helping patients to initiate new behaviours and to self-manage their conditions more effectively, and thus serious attention must be paid to their communication skills *(33)*.

A team approach is required not only in the management of individuals with chronic conditions but in addressing these public health challenges more broadly. In general, care for chronic diseases is best delivered with a collaborative effort involving public health specialists, policy and service planners, researchers, information technology designers, and support personnel. The multidisciplinary team in mental health includes psychiatrists, psychologists, nurses, general practitioners, occupational therapists and community/social workers who can share their expertise and collaborate with each other *(37)*.

> *Studies show that errors in health care are not only frequent but also leading causes of mortality and morbidity*

## Strategy 2.7 Promote continuous learning for patient safety

As health services for chronic conditions have evolved, so too has their complexity. Although much has improved, the volume of information, the number of medications, and the myriad of providers has led to a number of unintended consequences. There may be, for example, errors related to dosages, misidentification of patients, insanitary or unhygienic practices related to hand washing or equipment, or inadequate follow-up of patients. Studies show that errors in health care are not only frequent but are also leading causes of mortality and morbidity *(33)*.

Although awareness of errors and unsafe practices is an important first step in dealing with the complexities of care provision, there is also a need to develop evidence-based approaches to deal with them more effectively, such as risk management programmes, patient-centred approaches, and patient empowerment *(38)* (see Box 2.5).

## Box 2.5 Patient safety

A growing body of research evidence suggests that unsafe patient care is very common in health care systems globally. No country – rich or poor – can claim to be coping fully with the problem.

Caring for patients involves a complex interplay of people, technology, devices and medicines. Health care workers must make many decisions and judgements on a daily basis, and things can and do go wrong.

Experience in both health care and other high-risk industries shows that errors and mistakes are often provoked by weak systems. Deficiencies in system design can create problems at many levels including the individual clinician, health care team, organization and health care system. Such deficiencies can include a lack of clear protocols for treating patients, lack of knowledge and experience among health care workers, poor supervision of junior staff, fragmented patient information and poor coordination.

A completely risk-free health care environment is probably unattainable. Much can be done, however, to improve the "error wisdom" of front-line staff. In particular, health care workers who are educated and trained to work together well can reduce risks to patients and themselves. Three core knowledge and performance requirements are suggested below.

- Communicate effectively and honestly with patients and their families about the risks of health care interventions, especially when things have gone wrong. Unintended harm to patients is often made worse by the defensive way that many health care organizations respond to patients and their families after a serious event. In some countries, secretiveness on the part of health care organizations is associated with increased litigation.

- Identify risks and hazards in the health care environment and act to reduce their potential to cause patient harm. At its simplest this requires ways in which staff can report hazards and events within the health care organization. Identifying problems should be seen as a source of learning, not blame. Reporting is of little value, however, if no action is taken. Strategies to minimize identified risks and hazards are also vital.

- Work safely as part of a team. Even where human resources are limited, effective teamwork can promote good communication, willingness to share information and effective interpersonal relationships. Effectively transferring information between health care workers is increasingly recognized as an important part of improving patient safety. Problems in teamwork can lead to diagnostic delays and poor management of life-threatening events.

It is vital to ensure that patient safety is a key component of educational curricula, training programmes and induction schemes. Organizations have a responsibility to provide the appropriate systems and support to enable their workforce to learn and apply the skills and knowledge required for patient safety. Strong organizational leadership for patient safety is important.

The WHO World Alliance for Patient Safety is leading the global work on patient safety. Launched in October 2004, the Alliance provides a vehicle for international collaboration and action to coordinate, spread and accelerate improvements in patient safety worldwide. This includes international action on patient safety education and training. More information is available at www.who.int/patientsafety.

Sources: *(39, 40)*.

To improve the quality of long-term care more generally, continuing education in chronic disease management is necessary. Lifelong learning is a cornerstone of continued fitness to practice, and is closely connected to the quality of care and patient safety *(25, 28)*.

## MOBILIZING FOR EMERGENCY NEEDS: NATURAL DISASTERS AND OUTBREAKS

At least 40 countries worldwide are at risk of being affected by severe natural disasters and no country is immune to an outbreak of a highly infectious disease. Sudden catastrophic events can quickly overwhelm local and national health systems, especially those that are already suffering from staff shortages or lack of funds. During disasters, local communities are the first to respond, followed by local and national governments. Because no society has the resources to be prepared adequately at all times, no nation can manage a major disaster or outbreak on its own. Qualified, experienced, and well-prepared international health personnel are usually needed to help (see Box 2.6)

Furthermore, when the immediate priority of humanitarian assistance is to save lives, partnership with, and strengthening of, local institutions is often seen by external actors as an obstacle that delays the delivery of relief. Early investment in national staff is rarely considered a necessary component of an emergency response. Sub-Saharan Africa, the area of the world most severely affected by natural and man-made disasters, is particularly vulnerable in this regard *(42)*. An international emergency response workforce has not yet been organized in a systematic way. As a result, human resource shortages remain a serious constraint to achieving better humanitarian and health outcomes.

### Preparedness plans can help

The loss of life, illness and disease caused by outbreaks and other natural disasters can be reduced if preparedness plans are in place and easily and quickly activated. Emergency preparedness requires the availability of an up-to-date database of the

## Box 2.6 Responding to infectious disease outbreaks – SARS

The WHO Regional Office for the Western Pacific is based in Manila, Philippines. In responding promptly to the SARS threat, it formed an outbreak response and preparedness team. This initially drew on the expertise of WHO staff in the region, but was quickly complemented by professionals in the field of epidemiology, infection control, laboratory diagnosis and public information.

WHO teams of epidemiologists and infection control experts fanned out across the region to China, Hong Kong (China), the Philippines, Singapore and Viet Nam. Infection control equipment, such as masks and gowns, was dispatched from Manila to newly affected countries and to those considered vulnerable to an attack.

The region was fortunate to have a network in place before SARS struck called the Global Outbreak Alert and Response Network, which was established in 2000. This was very important as it provided operational support teams with specific tasks, from coordination through to resource mobilization, including human resources. WHO support to countries consisted of providing technical guidelines, on-site expertise and resource mobilization. It was important that the kind of expertise developed matched the needs in each country. Among the lessons learnt were the need to have one focal point to coordinate partners who share a commitment and common goals, and the need for transparent policies and political commitment at the country level.

Source: *(41)*.

" *The loss of life, illness and disease caused by outbreaks and other natural disasters can be reduced by preparedness* "

actual competencies of health personnel, knowledge about how to communicate risk effectively, and a way of prioritizing training needs, policies and actions to ensure the safety of health personnel.

Comprehensive preparedness plans should include components related to the way the health system needs to react, and those related to preparing the overall workforce response. Three general responses are critical during a disaster or outbreak situation: a "command and control approach", collaboration across sectors, and risk communication. In turn, the plans for health workforce response should include training of appropriate staff, adequate deployment and match of skills, and protection of health workers.

### Strategy 2.8 Take a "command and control" approach

A "command and control" approach to management is critical if resources are to be directed in a timely manner. Coordination and team work are essential but once consensus has been reached, the speed of an intervention can be enhanced if action is triggered in a directive fashion. In such situations, feedback channels must be established so that corrective action can be taken when new situations during an unfolding crisis demand changes in the direction of action. Simple management tools for supportive staff supervision using equally simple indicators facilitate the flow of information in such situations. This approach calls for the integration of existing resources, thus avoiding duplication or unnecessary diversion of human resources. It also requires the mapping of all existing resources including appropriate back-up support and response scenarios in case of loss of resources or sudden increase in demand.

Another essential action that is required in order to control the rapid spread of fear and panic during disease outbreaks is risk communication. This includes conveying information about risks of infection to health workers, lay people and the media, in a way that is transparent, honest, credible and compassionate *(43)*.

### Strategy 2.9 Help remove sector boundaries

An "all out" response to a disaster or outbreak requires the removal of boundaries between health workers in different sectors. Preparing the workforce at all levels of the system and coordinating with other sectors greatly reduces the impact of the emergency. Collaboration with other sectors permits the best use of existing resources, prevents the often observed confusion found during initial intervention periods, and allows rapid implementation of life-saving measures. Planning specific roles and functions for staff in the military, transport and education sectors minimizes confusion and maximizes the input of scarce human resources. Moreover, as the tsunami of December 2004 and the earthquake in South Asia of October 2005 have shown, international support must be mobilized and coordinated.

At international level, the Global Outbreak Alert and Response Network (GOARN)[1] provides an operational framework that links international networks and institutions and keeps the international community alert to the threat of outbreaks and ready to respond.

---

[1] http://www.who.int/csr/outbreaknetwork/en/.

## Strategy 2.10 Train appropriate health staff for emergency response

Mounting immediate and effective responses to disasters and outbreaks as varied as earthquakes, tsunamis, hurricanes, floods, SARS and avian influenza requires an agile workforce with highly specialized skills. These include the ability to carry out rapid diagnosis, surveillance, organization and logistics, containment, communications and emergency surgery, and to create temporary facilities. But emergency preparedness must go beyond identification of skills. Training institutions and programmes must be designated where these skills are generated and updated (see Box 2.7).

A weakness found in many countries is a scarcity of planning and management capacity, both to prepare for emergencies and to deal with them when they happen. Many countries simply do not have enough human resource planners and managers, so new ways must be developed to produce them and to activate them when the need arises. One approach is to give supplementary training on the management of emergencies to managers who already occupy key positions in agencies or organizations likely to be involved in an emergency response. These organizations usually include hospitals, ministries of health, local government, the military, those responsible for transport and communications, civil protection, social welfare and so on. This supplementary training can be conducted by national government or nongovernmental agencies.

Priority should also be given to the development of new cadres focused on emergency planning and management within the various agencies and institutions responsible for emergency management. These new cadres could be developed

## Box 2.7 Thailand's response to epidemics and disasters

Thailand is a middle income country (with a per capita GDP of US$ 2000) that in recent years has been affected by SARS, the tsunami of December 2004 and avian influenza. In the avian influenza epidemic, 60 million chickens were killed and the government paid US$ 120 million to farmers in compensation. A vertical plan for avian influenza was approved by the cabinet in January 2005, for US$ 120 million for three years, with an intensive human resources component. In the recent epidemic, Thailand called on its 800 000 village health volunteers to assist in bird surveillance. These volunteers have existed in Thailand's villages since the era of primary health care. The country also used its network of 100 000 health centres, 750 public hospitals, 95 provincial hospitals and 1330 teams in every district, who were on call 24 hours a day.

Balanced distribution of health workers is of the utmost importance in the rapid response to infectious diseases and disasters. Inequitable distribution leaning towards urban centres makes an effective response difficult: during the tsunami it was possible to recruit from districts around the capital, because health workers were equitably distributed. Incentives are important to facilitate balanced distribution: a newly graduated medical doctor receives US$ 1500 per month to go to the most remote districts, which provides very strong encouragement to serve in such areas.

It is also important to strengthen the limited speciality of "field epidemiologists", as they are the first group to move into disaster areas. Thailand's Field Epidemiology Training Programme (FETP) was launched in 1980 to train epidemiologists with an interest in public health and to improve epidemiological capacity within the Ministry of Public Health. The programme requires three years' training after graduation from medical school. FETP trainees have responded rapidly to 353 health threats to date, and the government has started to double the intake.

Thailand's field epidemiologists were mobilized when the tsunami hit in December 2004. They carried out active disease surveillance in all affected districts. Data were collected from all medical facilities, two shelters for displaced persons, and two forensic identification centres. FETP trainees visited each site daily and collected individual case-report forms that included information on disease syndrome, age, sex and nationality. These teams analysed data and identified events requiring further action. Given the threat of pandemics, governments need to invest now in their human resources, before the epidemics arrive.

Sources: *(44, 45)*.

> *In responding to major natural disasters or disease outbreaks, skilled disaster coordination teams are as essential as a large number of trained volunteers*

through training, capacity assessment exercises, simulations and using emergencies as opportunities for learning by doing. All these actions should be part of a national strategy for capacity development which is attuned to the different risks and levels of preparedness of individual countries.

At the global level, training of interagency and national country teams needs to emphasize the importance of working effectively, efficiently and safely, and according to agreed benchmarks and standards. To that end, WHO and other members of the Inter-Agency Standing Committee are developing a Health Emergency Action Response Network,[1] one component of which is a specialized training course aimed at improving the skills of humanitarian personnel working in the field. The training programme includes the necessary mix of scientific knowledge, technical skills, attitudes, behaviours and field know-how, and familiarity with standard operating procedures and support platforms.

### Strategy 2.11 Develop an emergency deployment strategy for different kinds of health workers

Strategies for the deployment of different types and cadres of health workers with specific roles and functions during a crisis period is an essential component of an emergency preparedness plan. The plan should include a distribution of tasks across the health workforce which matches skills and capacities to anticipated health interventions. Table 2.1 lists the various types of health personnel that were redeployed within Turkey's public health care delivery system during the recent avian influenza outbreak. In addition to ministry of health personnel, those in other sectors must also be mobilized.

In responding to major natural disasters or disease outbreaks, skilled disaster coordination teams are essential, particularly to manage the large number of trained volunteers that are deployed in these situations. Given the scarcity of skilled workers and overwhelming demand, efficient triage is imperative. Transferring simplified tasks and skills to the right members of the workforce and avoiding "de-skilling" of highly qualified staff are essential components of an effective deployment of the health workforce during emergencies.

### Strategy 2.12 Ensure adequate support for front-line workers

Staff dealing with emergencies must be supported with sufficient transport, supplies and communications equipment. These should all be specified in the emergency response plan. In the case of pandemics, providing access to prevention and treatment for the health workforce is a priority *(46)*. Information about infection control measures needs to be made available and taught regularly. In accordance with clear guidelines, medicines or vaccines should be made available to front-line workers.

Emergencies demand extra working hours beyond the call of duty, often leading to physical and mental exhaustion *(21)*. Incentives and rewards, both financial and personal, have to be provided to compensate health workers for their extra efforts. This helps to boost morale and maintain levels of service commitment at the highest level possible. Planning for losses will further enhance preparedness *(47)*.

---

[1] For more information, see http://www.who.int/hac/techguidance/training/hearnet/en.

## Table 2.1 Deployment of state-employed health personnel in response to avian influenza outbreak in Turkey

| Competencies required in an outbreak of avian influenza | MOH (Central) PHS/ GP/N/ NM | District health directorate | | | Secondary and tertiary level health care (hospitals) | | | | Primary level health care (health centres) | | | | | |
|---|---|---|---|---|---|---|---|---|---|---|---|---|---|---|
| | | PHS | GP | N/NM | IDS | Other S | GP | N | PHS | Other S | GP | N/ NM | HO | EHT |
| Operations management | ■ | ■ | | | | | | | ■ | ■ | | | | |
| Surveillance | ■ | ■ | ■ | ■ | ■ | ■ | ■ | ■ | ■ | | ■ | ■ | ■ | ■ |
| Identification of cases | ■ | ■ | ■ | ■ | ■ | ■ | ■ | | ■ | ■ | ■ | ■ | ■ | ■ |
| Verification of cases | * | ■ | ■ | ■ | ■ | ■ | | | ■ | ■ | ■ | ■ | ■ | ■ |
| Isolation of new cases | ■ | ■ | ■ | ■ | ■ | ■ | ■ | ■ | ■ | ■ | ■ | ■ | ■ | ■ |
| Treatment of new cases | | | | | ■ | ** | ** | ■ | | | | | | |
| Quarantine of contacts | ■ | ■ | ■ | ■ | ■ | ■ | ■ | ■ | ■ | | ■ | ■ | ■ | ■ |
| Management of health personnel information | ■ | ■ | ■ | ■ | | | | | | | | | | |
| Risk communication | ■ | | | | | | | | | | | | | |
| Management of media and public information | *** | | | | | | | | | | | | | |
| Veterinary containment (culling chickens) | | | | | | | | | | | | | ■ | ■ |
| Intersectoral issues (transport, tourism) | ■ | ■ | ■ | ■ | | | | | ■ | | ■ | ■ | ■ | ■ |

\* By central national reference laboratories.

\*\* In Turkey only infectious disease specialists have the legal right to prescribe Tamiflu.

\*\*\* Nobody but high-level MOH officials have the authority to speak to the media.

EHT: Environmental health technician: 4 years of high school training with special emphasis on environmental health issues.

GP: General practitioner: graduate of 6 years of medical school with a licence to practice medicine.

HO: Health officer: same as nurse but only high school graduates.

IDS: Infectious disease specialist: medical school graduate with 4–5 years of training.

N: Nurse: 4 years of high school or university training; no difference in employment or job definitions though more college graduates employed in hospitals.

NM: Nurse/midwife: same as nurse but trained more specifically to provide MCH services, including home deliveries.

Other S: Other specialist: internal medicine, pediatrics, etc.: medical school graduate with 4–5 years of training.

PHS: Public health specialist: medical school graduate with 3–4 years of community medicine and public health training.

> *Conflict often causes severe and long-lasting damage to the health workforce*

# WORKING IN CONFLICT AND POST-CONFLICT ENVIRONMENTS

Conflict often causes severe and long-lasting damage to the health workforce. Qualified personnel may be killed or forced to abandon their jobs. In protracted conflicts, a number of destructive tendencies emerge. Civilian workers flee health centres and hospitals in dangerous areas, and those in safer areas become overstaffed. Management systems collapse, working environments deteriorate and professional values decline *(48)*. Health workers desperate to make a living may slide into practices such as taking under-the-table fees or embezzling drugs. In long-lasting conflicts, relief agencies, whose main objective is often to recruit personnel to care for refugees, may compete for the few available health workers. In such situations the local public services are almost invariably the losers *(49)*.

A severe crisis, especially if it is protracted, can radically distort the composition and diminish the competence of the health workforce. "Crash courses" intended to prepare health workers to cope with epidemics of infectious diseases and sexual violence during the acute phase of a crisis are often inadequate. Improvised training tends to continue through the post-conflict reconstruction period, as the complexities of educating health personnel are ignored and hasty initiatives – involving abbreviated courses of study – are taken to fill the gaps of key staff, such as doctors and nurses. Such distortions – which hamper the recovery of the health sector after conflicts have ended, and often demand aggressive, sustained and well-resourced strategies to remedy them – can be minimized through effective stewardship.

## Strategy 2.13 Obtain and maintain strategic information

In the ever-changing environment of complex emergencies, those with stewardship responsibilities in the health sector have to invest from a very early stage in obtaining and updating strategic information on the health workforce. This means finding out how many health workers there are, where they are, and what their capacities are. Such assessments, drawing on quantitative and qualitative information, should include all categories of health workers, whatever their status or qualifications (not just those in the public sector). A frequently made mistake is to launch ambitious and detailed field studies or inventories which take too long to be useful and carry heavy opportunity costs. Efforts to obtain strategic information should be pragmatic, and a stimulus to action. Such information, even if incomplete, can help maintain a human resource focus in wider sectoral plans or initiatives.

## Strategy 2.14 Invest in advanced planning and focused interventions

The establishment of a high-level focal point for human resources for health within the ministry of health – as in Afghanistan, where it was placed at General Directorate level – or within the body which is acting as health authority, can be a useful rallying and reference point *(50)*. Such a move makes it more likely that advance plans for the rehabilitation of human resources will be considered when spending priorities and public expenditure management are reviewed. Mozambique, for example, made human resources for health plans before conflict had ended and was able to introduce corrective measures in a timely manner *(51)*. At the same time, action needs to be focused on and geared towards the specific context. In phases of acute conflict the

protection of human resources will be paramount. Similarly, in times of protracted conflict, repair will be essential, as will be rehabilitation during transition phases.

> ❝*Even in countries in crisis, many professionals work tirelessly and often without salaries*❞

## Strategy 2.15 Protect what works

During acute conflict the focus should be on maintaining and supporting what works. Box 2.8 highlights the importance of protecting health systems and services during conflicts. The workforce must be marshalled to support institutional islands of dependable critical services, particularly medical supply depots and hospitals. Maintaining a number of centres of good clinical and managerial practice is paramount for safeguarding the concept of what a functioning hospital, health centre or operational district really means. Donor funds should be channelled into structures that are still functioning in order to keep them adequately supplied and maintained. This is better than using them hastily to introduce new modes of intervention, such as mobile clinics, or to launch population-wide immunization campaigns. All this works better if it is done with the full involvement of nongovernmental organizations and humanitarian agencies, and with short-term planning horizons such as the 90-day cycle used in Darfur (Sudan) and Liberia.

Even in countries in crisis, there are many professionals working tirelessly at field level, often without salaries. To make progress the first need is cash to get institutions working, to enable those who work in them to feed themselves, and to prevent recourse to levying of user charges or pilfering of supplies. Paying decent wages to local workers is far cheaper than bringing in foreign volunteers.

## Strategy 2.16 Repair and prepare

Protracted conflicts and complex emergencies require the initial focus to be on repair, on getting things working, and not on reform. Offering minimum health services in rural areas requires immediate strengthening of the health care system and the workforce. This is a difficult process to manage and depends partly on identifying incentives (such as monetary or career incentives) to encourage health workers to take positions in less desirable locations.

Keeping a focus on repairing and preparing means:

- redeploying health workers on an area per area or district per district basis (rather than programme per programme), in a pragmatic and flexible fashion;
- providing protection and support to health workers;
- taking early measures to avoid commercialization of the health sector. User charges are inefficient and have perverse effects;
- obtaining the commitment of the donor community and all the other major actors to reach a consensus on human resource planning criteria and standards concerning support for existing networks, salary scales, contracts, and essential drug guidelines.

## Strategy 2.17 Rehabilitate when stability begins

Once a crisis situation has begun to stabilize, the first need is to adopt measures to correct distortions in the labour market. These include the following:

- Establish systems to assess the level of competence of health workers emerging from the crisis, in combination with a review of categories, job descriptions and training programmes that have proliferated during the crisis.

- Establish retraining to fill gaps. Health workers who have received mostly classroom training should receive clinical training, while people who received hands-on training should in turn obtain the classroom background necessary to gain more autonomy.
- Limit further unregulated workforce expansion. If the size of the workforce is too great, freeze recruitment and pre-service training and invest in in-service training. Consideration should be given to whether it is preferable to train additional staff or whether priority should be given to retrain existing staff with limited qualifications.
- Emphasize medical and nursing education quite early in post-conflict situations, to re-establish educational standards, and avoid the mass training of poorly qualified doctors and nurses.
- Continue to redeploy personnel and establish health care networks in the areas that have remained excluded.
- Extend the supply of health services, offer access to all, regardless of ability to pay, and protect against any financial consequences of seeking care.

## CONCLUSION

The challenges highlighted in this chapter illustrate the spectrum of needs to which the health workforce is expected to respond. Viewing these challenges from a workforce perspective helps identify both opportunities and constraints. The specific assessments reveal a tremendous amount of diversity and at the same time a number of commonalities – working across sectors, simplification of tasks, adequate support to health workers.

Importantly, for the theme of this report, the imperative of working together emerges repeatedly. Collaboration across sectors for chronic diseases and emergencies, striking synergies across programmes for the MDGs, and bringing stakeholders together to reach consensus on strategies to protect what works in the context of conflicts makes the case for working together abundantly clear.

## Box 2.8 Protecting health systems and biomedical practice during conflicts

Uses and misuses of biomedical and public health knowledge during time of war or armed conflict are commonplace. Public health and medical crimes such as diverting medical supplies and human resources, abuse and torture, medical killing in the name of science, and eugenics for social goals, have been perpetrated with the complicity of health and medical professionals in countries such as Bosnia and Herzegovina, Cambodia, Nazi Germany and Rwanda. Much more frequent, though, are cases in which health professionals are victims themselves. The attack against Vukovar Hospital on the eve of the war in the former Yugoslavia, in 1991, underscores the extreme vulnerability of health facilities and medical personnel operating in war zones.

Since the Nuremberg Code in 1947 concluded the judgement of the Doctors Trial – the Medical Case of the subsequent Nuremberg Proceedings – and founded bioethics as an independent discipline, dozens of binding treaties, declarations and other texts have drawn up very specific provisions that protect the public and biomedical practitioners from harm (and from doing harm) both in peacetime and in times of conflict. In June 1977, for example, 27 articles, which are known as the "principles of medical neutrality" in times of war, were added to the body of International Humanitarian Law, the Protocols Additional to the Geneva Conventions. The most recent reformulation of aid workers' competencies and responsibilities in times of conflict and man-made disasters appears in the Sphere Handbook, a document that aims to improve the quality and the accountability of the humanitarian system.

The protection of health systems and biomedical practice from harm requires a universal commitment. As prerequisites to such a commitment, formal education curricula for health professionals should gradually incorporate studies in bioethics, human rights and humanitarian law.

Examining each from a workforce perspective reveals important insights not only about needs but also exciting innovations. The efforts to integrate clinical management of adult illness and the shift to competencies arising from the new paradigm of chronic care management represent important innovations in the training and deployment of the workforce. Harnessing and nurturing these insights and innovations should be a primary focus of more systematic planning for the health workforce.

Planning for the health workforce both within these major challenges and across them is a key message that emerges from this chapter. As suggested, in conflict/post-conflict situations, a human resources assessment is an important first step. When shortfalls in the existing total of health workers related to achieving service delivery targets are known, appropriately scaled (as opposed to incremental) responses can be articulated. The findings of such assessments help create a more realistic, broader picture of the needs of the health sector.

These specific analyses, however, point to the need for more comprehensive planning of the workforce along the lines of the entry, stock and exit model (see Overview). The call for new types of skills, workers, better standardization of skills, new programmes and retraining, places significant demands on the health worker training institutions. These are discussed in more depth in Chapter 3. The importance of effective "skills to tasks" management, information on performance, and the use of different management approaches, from delegation to collaboration to command and control, are among the challenges in optimizing the performance of the workforce in situ (see Chapter 4). Finally, the need to ensure the health of the workforce and plan for adequate respite or even demise of individual workers are important dimensions of managing outflows (see Chapter 5).

# REFERENCES

1. Travis P, Bennett S, Haines A, Pang T, Bhutta Z, Hyder A et al. Overcoming health-systems constraints to achieve the Millennium Development Goals. *Lancet,* 2004, 364:900–906.
2. Dreesch N, Dolea C, Dal Poz MR, Goubarev A, Adams O, Aregawi M et al. An approach to estimating human resource requirements to achieve the Millennium Development Goals. *Health Policy and Planning,* 2005, 20:267–276.
3. Chen L, Evans T, Anand S, Boufford JI, Brown H, Chowdhury M et al. Human resources for health: overcoming the crisis. *Lancet*, 2004, 364:1984–1990.
4. The Joint Learning Initiative. *Human resources for health. Overcoming the crisis.* Cambridge, MA, Harvard University Press, 2004.
5. Kurowski C, Wyss K, Abdulla S, Yémadji N, Mills A. *Human resources for health: requirements and availability in the context of scaling-up priority interventions in low-income countries. Case studies from Tanzania and Chad.* London, London School of Hygiene and Tropical Medicine, 2003 (Working Paper 01/04).
6. Haines A, Cassels A. Can the Millennium Development Goals be attained? *BMJ*, 2004, 329:394–397.
7. Kober K, Van Damme W. Scaling up access to antiretroviral treatment in southern Africa: who will do the job? *Lancet,* 2004, 364:103–107.
8. *The world health report 2005 – Make every mother and child count.* Geneva, World Health Organization, 2005.
9. *Evaluation of short-term training activities of technical divisions in the WHO African Region. Final draft.* Brazzaville, World Health Organization Regional Office for Africa, 2004.
10. *Global health partnerships: assessing country consequences.* Bill & Melinda Gates Foundation/McKinsey & Company, 2005.
11. Palmer D. *Human resources for health care study: Malawi's emergency human resources programme.* DFID–Malawi, December 2004.

12. Molyneux D. Lymphatic Filariasis (Elephantiasis) Elimination: a public health success and development opportunity. *Filaria Journal*, 2003, 2:13.
13. Chowdhury AMR, Cash RA. *A simple solution: teaching millions to treat diarrhoea at home*. Dhaka, University Press, 1996.
14. *The world health report 2004 – Changing history*. Geneva, World Health Organization, 2004.
15. Aylward RB, Linkins J. Polio eradication: mobilizing the human resources. *Bulletin of the World Health Organization*, 2005, 83:268–273.
16. *Scaling up HIV/AIDS care: service delivery and human resource perspectives*. Geneva, World Health Organization, 2004 (http://www.who.int/hrh/documents/en/HRH_ART_paper.pdf).
17. Gove S, Celletti F, Seung KJ, Bitalabeho A, Vansson M, Ramzi A et al. *IMAI operational package for integrated management of HIV/AIDS prevention, treatment and care in the health sector*. Paper presented at: 14th International Conference on HIV/AIDS and Sexually Transmitted Infections in Africa, 4–9 December 2005, Abuja, Nigeria.
18. Bell D, Rouel G, Miguel C, Walker J, Cacal L, Saul A. Diagnosis of malaria in a remote area of the Philippines: comparison of techniques and their acceptance by health workers and the community. *Bulletin of the World Health Organization*, 2001, 79:933–941.
19. Cho-Min-Naing, Gatton ML. Performance appraisal of rapid on-site malaria diagnosis (ICT malaria Pf/Pv test) in relation to human resources at village level in Myanmar. *Acta Tropica*, 2002, 81:13–19.
20. Sibley M, Sipe A, Armelagos GJ, Barrett K, Finley EP, Kamat V et al. *Traditional birth attendant training effectiveness: a meta-analysis*. Washington, DC, Academy for Educational Development, 2002 (SARA Project unpublished document).
21. Kinoti S, Tawfik L. *Impact of HIV/AIDS on human resources for health*. Geneva, World Health Organization, 2005 (background paper for *The world health report 2006*; available at: http://www.who.int/hrh/documents/en/).
22. *Preventing chronic diseases: a vital investment*. Geneva, World Health Organization, 2005.
23. *Improving medical education: enhancing the behavioral and social science content of medical school curricula*. Washington, DC, National Academies Press for the Institute of Medicine, 2004.
24. *Human resources and training in mental health. WHO mental health policy and service guidance package*. Geneva, World Health Organization, 2005.
25. O'Neil EH, Pew Health Professions Commission. *Creating health professional practice for a new century*. San Francisco, CA, Pew Health Professions Commission, 1998.
26. *Human resources and national health systems: shaping the agenda for action*. Geneva, World Health Organization, 2002.
27. *Making medical practice and education more relevant to people's needs: the contribution of the family doctor*. Geneva, World Health Organization, 1994.
28. Griner P. The workforce for health: response. In: *2020 vision: health in the 21st century*. Washington, DC, National Academies Press for the Institute of Medicine, 1996:102–107.
29. *Physician concerns: caring for people with chronic conditions*. Baltimore, MD, Partnership for Solutions, 2003 (http://www.partnershipforsolutions.com, accessed 26 January 2006).
30. Pruitt SD, Epping-Jordan JE. Preparing the 21st century global healthcare workforce. *BMJ*, 2005, 330:637–639.
31. Holman H, Lorig K. Patients as partners in managing chronic disease. Partnership as a prerequisite for effective and efficient health care. *BMJ*, 2000, 320:525–527.
32. Clark NM, Gong M. Management of chronic disease by practitioners and patients: are we teaching the wrong things? *BMJ*, 2000, 320:572–575.

33. *Crossing the quality chasm: a new health system for the 21st century.* Institute of Medicine, National Academy Press, Washington, DC, 2001.
34. World Health Organization. *Mental health atlas 2005* (http://www.who.int/mental_ health/evidence/atlas/, accessed 30 January 2006).
35. Lorig KR, Ritter P, Stewart A, Sobel D, Brown B, Bandura A et al. Chronic disease self-management program: 2-year health status and health care utilization outcomes. *Medical Care*, 2001, 39:1217–1223.
36. Fu D, Fu H, McGowan P, Shen YE, Zhu L, Yang H et al. Implementation and quantitative evaluation of chronic disease self-management programme in Shanghai, China: randomized controlled trial. *Bulletin of the World Health Organization*, 2003, 81:174–182.
37. *Pulling together: the future roles and training of mental health staff.* London, The Sainsbury Centre for Mental Health, 1997.
38. Adams O, Dolea C. *Social valuation of the medical profession.* Paper presented at: Congress on health-related professions as a social risk, Albert Schweitzer Centre, Turin, 31 January 2004. Geneva, World Health Organization, 2004.
39. Australian Council for Safety and Quality in Health Care. *National patient safety education framework* (http://www.safetyandquality.org/framework0705.pdf, accessed 30 January 2006).
40. *World alliance for patient safety. Forward programme 2005.* Geneva, World Health Organization, 2005.
41. Nukuro E. *Engaging stakeholders for health workforce issues. Lessons from pandemic influenza outbreak in the Western Pacific Region.* Paper presented at: WHO Forum on Combating the Global Health Workforce Crisis, 26–28 October 2005. Geneva, World Health Organization, 2005.
42. Liese B, Blanchet N, Dussault G. *The human resource crisis in health services in sub-Saharan Africa.* Washington, DC, World Bank, 2003.
43. Covello V, Allen F. *Seven cardinal rules of risk communication.* Washington, DC, United States Environmental Protection Agency, Office of Policy Analysis, 1988.
44. Limpakarnjanarat K, International Emerging Infections Program (IEIP), Thailand, MOPH–US CDC Collaboration. Personal communication, 25 October 2005.
45. Wibulpolprasert S. WHO Forum on Combating the Global Health Workforce Crisis, 26–28 October 2005. Geneva, World Health Organization, 2005 [personal communication].
46. World Health Organization. *Global outbreak alert and response network* (http://www.who. int/csr/outbreaknetwork/en/, accessed 30 January 2006).
47. Wilson N, Baker M, Crampton P, Mansoor O. The potential impact of the next influenza pandemic on a national primary care medical workforce. *Human Resources for Health*, 2005, 3:7.
48. Pavignani E. The impact of complex emergencies on the health workforce. *Health in Emergencies*, 2003, 18:4–6.
49. Van Lerberghe W, Porignon D. Of coping, poaching and the harm they can do. *Health in Emergencies*, 2003, 18:3.
50. Smith JH. *Issues in post-conflict human resources development.* Paper presented at: REACH–Afghanistan, Management Sciences for Health, Geneva, 12 September 2005. Geneva, World Health Organization, 2005.
51. Health service delivery in post-conflict states. High level forum on health MDGs. Paris, 14–15 November 2005 (http://www.hlfhealthmdgs.org/Documents/ HealthServiceDelivery.pdf, accessed 30 January 2006).

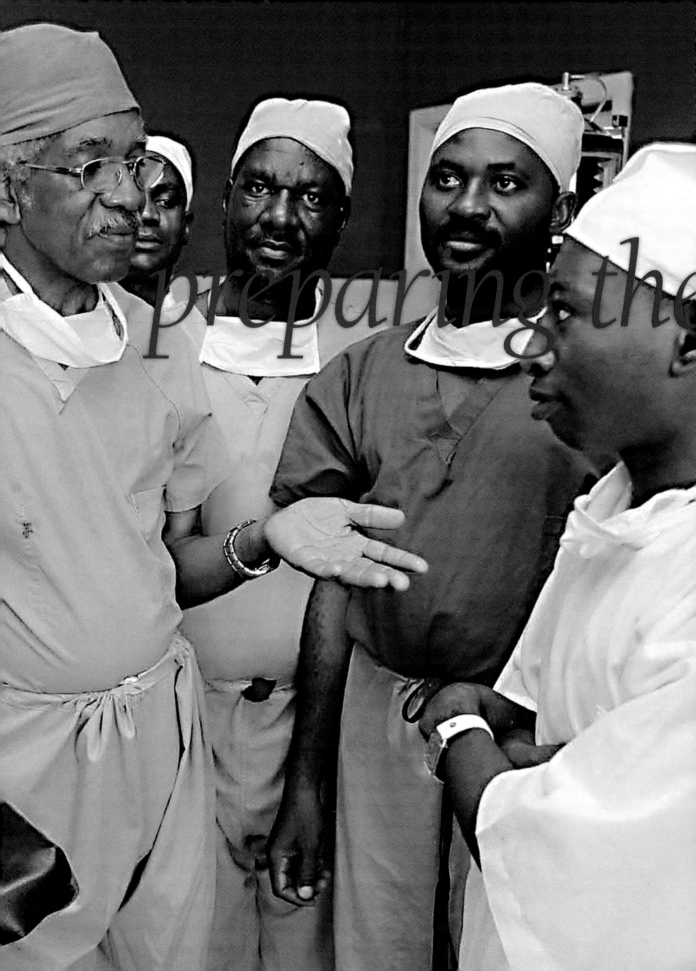

# chapter three
# health workforce

**The previous chapter provided an overview of the enormous challenges facing the health workforce. Chapter 3 and the following two chapters deal with many of these challenges, using the framework of strategies to train, sustain and retain the workforce. This chapter is about preparation: getting it right at the beginning; giving the right training to the right people to create an effective workforce for the delivery of health care. It focuses on the entry of health workers into the workforce and on the health training institutions – schools, universities and training colleges – which provide them with the knowledge and competencies for the jobs they will be required to do.**

## WORKFORCE ENTRY: THE RIGHT MIX

Preparing the health workforce to work towards attainment of its health objectives represents one of the most important challenges and opportunities for health systems. Going beyond the traditional notion of skill mix, this chapter extends the concept of mix to include: how many people are trained (*numbers*); the degree to which they reflect the sociocultural and demographic characteristics of the population (*diversity*); and what tasks the different levels of health workers are trained to do and are capable of performing (*competencies*). Maintaining a reasonable balance in terms of numbers, diversity and competencies of the health workforce requires a thorough understanding of the driving forces and challenges that shape health and education systems as well as labour markets, as depicted in Figure 3.1. This understanding, however imperfect, can be used as a guide to policies and possible actions related to training and recruitment.

Figure 3.1  Getting the mix right: challenges to health workforce production

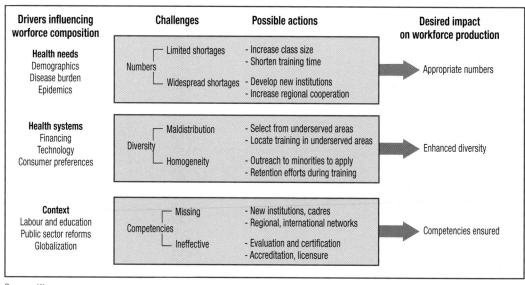

Source: *(1)*.

## The "pipeline" for recruitment

The process that leads to health workers' entry into the workforce can be seen as one by which individuals progress through educational institutions and graduate with specific skills or degrees that facilitate their recruitment by employers to the health workforce (see Figure 3.2). This "pipeline" spans primary, secondary and tertiary education institutions and health services facilities that produce a range of workers from auxiliaries to technicians and professionals. Along the pipeline, criteria for entry to training institutions, attrition while training, and the markets for recruitment determine how many and what types of individuals move forward to become health workers. A focus on health training institutions and the markets for recruitment yields insights on how to manage entries to the health workforce in line with performance objectives.

Figure 3.2  Pipeline to generate and recruit the health workforce

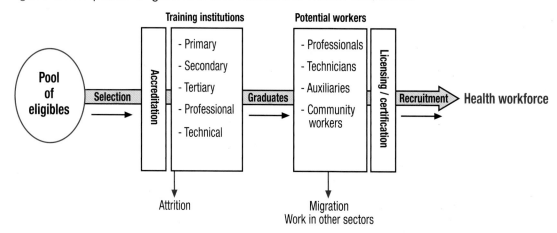

# TRAINING: THE RIGHT INSTITUTIONS TO PRODUCE THE RIGHT WORKERS

The 20th century produced sweeping changes to the health training institutional landscape. Flexner's seminal report in 1910 instilled a scientific approach to medical education that led to the closure of more than half the medical schools in the United States and strengthened public confidence that all doctors would meet similar standards of knowledge, skills and competencies *(2)*. Less than a decade later, demand for the training of field workers for public health campaigns was part of the rationale for the building of schools of public health in China, the United States, Yugoslavia and many other countries *(3)*. As part of a comprehensive plan for the development of essential health services, the Bhore report's recommendations led to an overhaul of India's health training institutions *(4)*. Other major reforms with widespread impact have emphasized new types of workers such as China's "barefoot doctors" *(5, 6)* or new ways of training health workers emphasizing problem solving *(7)*.

The 21st century is bringing new challenges, with many observers expressing concern that the institutional landscape is neither responding to current problems nor preparing for what lies ahead (see Box 3.1). Worldwide, increasing prevalence of chronic diseases, unanticipated disease outbreaks, and the race to meet the Millennium Development Goals (MDGs), place enormous expectations and responsibility on the role of health training institutions, as discussed in Chapter 2. A clearer understanding of the institutional landscape is required, combined with greater support for change, so that health training institutions are more effective in responding to these challenges *(9)*. Health training institutions undertake six key functions: stewardship or institutional governance; provision of educational services; selection and

## Box 3.1 Is the future of academic medicine in jeopardy?

"Academic medicine" is often defined as a triad of research, clinical service, and medical education. It might also be defined as the capacity to study, discover, evaluate, teach, and improve health systems. But many commentators and reports worry that academic medicine is in crisis around the world. The lack of basic infrastructure in lower income countries means that it is floundering, if not absent. Even in high income countries, government investments may be wasted if structural changes, such as creating better and more flexible career paths, are not made. Academic medicine seems to be failing to realize its potential and leadership responsibility, at a time when the disease burden and poverty are increasing.

In response to these concerns, in 2003 the *BMJ*, the *Lancet*, and 40 other partners launched the **International Campaign to Revitalize Academic Medicine** (ICRAM), a global initiative to debate the future of academic medicine which focuses on two issues:

- **Redefining core values of academic medicine.** Even though many institutions state that they promote the goals of scientific excellence, innovation, and patient-oriented care, no consensus on a global vision for academic medicine exists. What impact does introducing commercial activity and corporate models into medical education have? Most medical students and trainees appear to hold strong views on the importance of values such as altruism, collaboration, and shared learning, and on the role of academic medical institutions to provide ethical leadership.
- **Developing a strategy to reform medical training and enhance diversity.** Overcoming significant disincentives for pursuing a career in academic medicine, across regions and settings, is a key point for action. Evidence suggests that even though the intellectual rewards are appealing, the lack of pay parity with clinical colleagues and the uncertainty of funding for research are major drawbacks. Others include absence of a clear career path, the lack of flexible training opportunities, and insufficient mentoring, which further detract from a supportive work environment. These factors are even more salient for women. Despite the fact that mentoring is associated with career advancement and satisfaction, publication in peer-reviewed journals and success with grant applications, it is almost non-existent in academic medical training.

Source: *(8)*.

## Table 3.1 Functions of health educational institutions to generate the health workforce

| | |
|---|---|
| **Governance** | Managing the stock and quality of institutions across education and health sectors |
| **Educational services** | Orienting curriculum content and process towards professional competencies |
| **Selecting staff** | Deploying good quality, well supported and motivated teaching staff or trainers |
| **Financing** | Ensuring adequate levels, fair financing for student access and efficient coordination of sources |
| **Infrastructure and technology** | Developing training sites and learning materials to accommodate diverse student needs |
| **Information and knowledge** | Generating information to inform policy and evaluate health workforce production |

employment of staff members; financing of training; development and maintenance of infrastructure and technology; and generation of information and knowledge. These functions are described in Table 3.1. Together, they make up the system to support the generation of the health workforce and are explored in more detail in the following sections.

### Governance

The specific priorities related to the number, range and quality of health training institutions are: the disciplinary mix of institutions, accreditation to maintain standards, management of the applicant pool, and retention of students through to graduation.

### *Getting the right balance of schools and graduates*

Globally, educational establishments training health workers are heavily tipped towards the production of physicians and nurses: 1691 and 5492, respectively, in contrast to 914 schools of pharmacy, 773 schools of dentistry and 375 schools of public health. The WHO Eastern Mediterranean and South-East Asia regions have remarkably fewer schools of public health (not counting departments within other schools) than other regions (see Table 3.2). In too many countries, unfortunately, data on institutions are lacking or, if available, are not part of a comprehensive strategy

## Table 3.2 Health professional training institutions, by WHO region

| WHO region | Medical | Nursing and midwifery | Dental | Public health | Pharmacy |
|---|---|---|---|---|---|
| Africa | 66 | 288 | 34 | 50 | 57 |
| Americas | 441 | 947 | 252 | 112 | 272 |
| South-East Asia | 295 | 1145 | 133 | 12 | 118 |
| Europe | 412 | 1338 | 247 | 81 | 219 |
| Eastern Mediterranean | 137 | 225 | 35 | 8 | 46 |
| Western Pacific | 340 | 1549 | 72 | 112 | 202 |
| **Total** | **1691** | **5492** | **773** | **375** | **914** |

Source: Mercer H, Dal Poz MR. *Global health professional training capacity* (background paper for *The world health report 2006*; http://www.who.int/hrh/documents/en/).

for the health workforce *(10)*. To be able to respond to shortages or surpluses by implementing such actions as altering class sizes or opening or closing institutions, it is first necessary to evaluate the current capacity to train different types of workers, the relationship between pre-service and in-service training, and the politics of changing the situation. The costs of inaugurating new training institutions may appear high in the short term, yet will need to be compared with the rate of returning foreign-trained graduates.

## Strategy 3.1 Encourage training across the health care spectrum

Widespread shortages of public health and management cadres need to be tackled urgently through new approaches to leadership and feasible strategies. In South-East Asia, a public health initiative is serving as a catalyst for greater regional institutional capacity: in Bangladesh, the innovative nongovernmental organization BRAC has opened a school of public health to foster leadership in improving the health of

## Box 3.2 The public health movement in South-East Asia: regional initiatives and new schools

Countries in South-East Asia have less than 5% of the world's schools of public health, but almost a third of the world's population. Thus, increasing public health training for the health professions is urgently needed in these countries. National, regional and international stakeholders are aligning resources and political will to make this happen with new and innovative approaches to creating schools of public health.

The South-East Asia Public Health Initiative was launched in 2004 with the aim of strengthening public health planning with five goals:
- position public health high on regional and national agendas;
- strengthen public health education;
- enhance technical cooperation on the development of national public health training institutions;
- establish a public health education institutions' network;
- facilitate the definition of an appropriate package of essential public health functions in countries.

In Dhaka, Bangladesh, the BRAC University James P Grant School of Public Health aims to train a cadre of professionals who will improve the health outcomes of populations in disadvantaged areas of the world.
- Its first 25 students are mostly from low income countries – Afghanistan, Bangladesh, India, Kenya, Nepal, Pakistan, the Philippines and Uganda – but also from the United States, and graduated in January 2006.
- Students learn through fieldwork centred around the public health problems of Bangladeshi communities.
- Graduates are expected to become leading public health practitioners, managers, researchers, educators and policy-makers, and the school will run an active placement service.

- Students and teaching staff benefit from a close collaboration with Bangladesh's Centre for Health and Population Research (ICDDR,B). Staff members are drawn from Bangladesh, the region and internationally, which adds to a stimulating environment, as do the prestigious academic partners from around the world.

In India, the newly created Public Health Foundation is mobilizing resources to establish five schools of public health spread across the country in Ahmedabad, Chennai, Hyderabad, New Delhi and Kolkata. The foundation reflects a public–private partnership based on the principles of strengthening existing institutions and enabling multiple stakeholders to work together. These new schools will offer:
- structured, multidisciplinary educational programmes combining standards of excellence comparable to the best institutions in the world and course content relevant to India's needs;
- shorter and longer term training of health and allied professionals drawn from people already engaged in occupations relevant to public health – employed in government, academic institutions or nongovernmental organizations – and people not currently employed who want to pursue a career in public health, such as potential health policy analysts and health managers;
- research on the prioritized health problems of India, including knowledge generation and knowledge translation components.

Sources: *(11, 12)*.

poor and disadvantaged population groups. In India, a new partnership between the Ministry of Health and key players from academia and the private sector, are planning to establish five schools of public health to address national public health priorities (see Box 3.2).

### Accreditation: promoting competence and trust

Accreditation is an essential mechanism not only for assessing institutional performance but, more fundamentally, for securing public trust (see Chapter 6). Conducted primarily by ministries of education or delegated councils, accreditation requires facilities to generate evidence in support of performance objectives related to training. A recent survey of medical schools (13) shows that accreditation programmes are unevenly spread – they exist in three quarters of Eastern Mediterranean countries, just under half of the countries in South-East Asia, and only about a third of African countries. Furthermore, private medical schools are less likely than publicly funded ones to undergo accreditation procedures, a worrying fact in light of their growing role in educating the workforce (see Box 3.3). In relatively poor countries where efforts to scale up the health workforce using workers with less formal training are widespread, ingenuity is required to expand rapidly the effective capacity of training centres, including skills to carry out accreditation and the modest financial resources to sustain it. Efforts are also needed to extend accreditation and quality improvement beyond schools of medicine or nursing to include other faculties such as schools of public health (19).

> " Ingenuity is required to expand training centres' capacity "

### Managing admissions to enhance diversity

Entrance to most training programmes for health professions requires a secondary education. Many countries suffer from inadequate financing at this level, however, and struggle with high secondary school drop-out rates and low enrolment, especially among poorer groups. These factors severely limit the pool of people who can enter education programmes for health careers. The profiles of students entering health professions rarely reflect national profiles of social, linguistic and ethnic diversity, as students are disproportionately admitted from the higher social classes and dominant ethnic groups in society (20, 21).

## Box 3.3 Rapid growth in private education of health professionals

Private universities offering training for health professionals are rapidly increasing in low and middle income countries, reflecting a wider phenomenon of increasing private provision of technical and vocational education.

Recent data from around the world are indicative of this trend:

- In the WHO Eastern Mediterranean Region, between 1980 and 2005, private training institutions increased from 10% to almost 60% of all training institutions.
- In South America, between 1992 and 2000, Argentina, Chile and Peru experienced 60–70% increases in the number of medical schools, which is mainly a reflection of the growth in the private sector.

- In Karnataka State, India, 15 of 19 medical colleges are private.
- In the Philippines: in 2004, 307 of 332 nursing schools, were private institutions.
- In Côte d'Ivoire, 60% of all technical students are enrolled in private schools.
- In the Democratic Republic of the Congo between 2001 and 2003 the number of medical and nursing graduates doubled, largely as a result of a private sector-led increase in the training of health workers.

Sources: (14–18).

## Strategy 3.2 Develop admissions policies to reflect diversities

The growing diversity of patient populations, combined with a growing awareness of the importance of sociocultural and linguistic issues in providing care *(22, 23)*, has brought new attention to imbalances in the admissions processes. Along with admission quotas, other approaches to increase diversity include outreach to those who might not consider health professional training to be an option *(24)*; specialized programmes for under-represented students in secondary schools *(25)*; and expanded selection criteria to offer admission to students with personal attributes that make them well suited to providing health services *(26)*.

### *Retaining students through to graduation*

It is not enough to have the right mix of people entering the educational pipeline – institutions must also carry these trainees to the end of their instruction *(27)*. Very little information from low and middle income countries is available about student attrition rates or the factors that contribute to attrition across institutions, types of training programmes and the sociodemographic profiles of students. The limited evidence available points to as much as 20–30% of the student body not completing courses because of poor academic performance, financial constraints and other personal circumstances including health problems and inadequate housing *(28, 29)*. Retention of nursing students in the United Kingdom and the United States is enhanced through a broad range of activities including academic advice, tutoring for non-native speakers, affordable child care, financial aid, career counselling and guaranteed placement upon successful completion of studies *(30–32)*. Mechanisms designed to boost student retention through to graduation should consider existing policies related to admissions criteria and selection procedures.

## Educational services

The knowledge and skills of different kinds of health workers are determined by what they learn, so the organization and administration of the curriculum can be an important catalyst for change and innovation in health systems. Including a new course in a curriculum provides legitimacy to a subject or approach that can spawn changes leading to new disciplines, departments, schools and types of health workers, with huge impact on the practice of health care. Over the last 40 years, for example, clinical epidemiology has moved from the margins of medicine to lead the evidence-based transformation of health and health care *(33)*.

## Strategy 3.3 Ensure quality and responsive curricula

In preparing the workforce, the curriculum is expected to meet standards that are often defined as core competencies. For example, all cardiologists must be able to read an electrocardiogram, while all public health specialists must understand an odds ratio. Beyond guaranteeing this core, the curriculum must also be responsive to the changing state of knowledge in health and the needs and demands emerging from health systems, including consumers' expectations. For example, growing recognition of powerful social forces that determine health and access to services has given rise to new courses on social status, globalization, public health ethics and cultural competency *(34–41)*.

Aligning what is being taught to what is appropriate – given the needs of specific constituencies or populations – demands careful attention. A standard curriculum for nurses reflecting the realities of health care in a tertiary care setting may not develop the requisite competencies to respond to the needs of indigenous populations in remote areas. Likewise, the core competencies for a Masters in Public Health (MPH) in Europe may be expected to differ from what is required of an MPH in Africa. A recent study found that less than half of all training institutions in several African countries covered immunization adequately *(42)*, despite declining national immunization coverage rates. Many recommendations for change in curricula emerging from consensus panels and commissions are insufficiently sensitive to the challenge of implementation. New courses cannot find their way into the programme if faculty skills, key learning materials or institutional supports are not available.

Curricular decisions require more than just simple changes on paper, as their implications may challenge professional boundaries, hierarchies, responsibilities, and remunerated services. Changes in content – which constitute one dimension of orienting skills, numbers and diversity more generally – require broad participation not only by faculty members but also by professional organizations, regulatory bodies and patient groups *(43, 44)*. Engagement of these groups with their different interests may limit the scope and speed of decisions *(45)* but is essential to the legitimacy of curriculum change. The nature of curricular development is usually to acquire new content without being able to shed the old *(46)*. This one-way movement has led to overloaded curricula, often resulting in dilution of their focus and insufficient depth in the treatment of the subjects they cover.

> " *The workforce refrain in this report – train, sustain and retain – extends to teachers* "

### Acquiring competencies to learn

In recognition of the rapid growth and rate of change of knowledge, and the dynamics of the workplace, there is increasing acceptance that training programmes cannot teach people everything they will need to know. The ability to acquire new skills and knowledge that prepare for lifelong learning is itself a core competency that curricula must nurture. In response, educational processes have been moving away from didactic teaching and towards student-centred and problem-based learning, with greater emphasis on "know how" rather than "know all" *(47)*. Students and their teachers express satisfaction with this shift, and faculty members enjoy teaching using problem-based learning *(48, 49)*.

Early exposure to clinical practice or public health service promotes competence by teaching students how to integrate and apply knowledge in practice settings, learn from role models, and experience interdisciplinary and team approaches to the provision of health services *(50, 51)*. Recent evaluations of this method, referred to as practice-based or apprentice learning, have demonstrated an increase in empathy towards people with illnesses, greater self-confidence and professional identity among students, and effective learning from the tacit knowledge of experienced practitioners *(52–54)*. An example of patient-focused practice in a school of pharmacy is given in Box 3.4.

### Workforce of teachers

The workforce refrain of this report – train, sustain and retain – extends to teachers and faculty members in health professional education institutions. A lack of flexible training opportunities, insufficient mentoring, and career advancement difficulties for women when the "feminization" of medicine is increasing are among the key findings of the international campaign described in Box 3.1. Although published evidence is scarce, the challenges faced by other trainers of health workers are not unlike those in academic medical faculties.

Typically, academic training centres have a three-part mission: teaching, research and service delivery. These three aspects should ideally receive equal attention and institutional resources, with staff being encouraged to contribute to each. The reality is that incentives are often heavily weighted in favour of research and service delivery, to the detriment of teaching.

In parallel, the imperative to generate income to support overhead costs through service delivery or research leaves education and teaching as the poor relations *(59)*. In South-East Asia, the trend towards following money is steering teaching towards more lucrative areas of specialty medicine, potentially decreasing the capacity of the health workforce to respond to basic public health needs *(60)*.

Understanding what motivates teachers and supporting them in ways that help increase motivation is important. A study in Australia, for example, found that clinical supervisors rated personal satisfaction as the main motivating factor to teach, followed by the opportunity to attract students to their own area of specialty *(61)*. Personal acknowledgment by the school through faculty appointments, subsidized continuing education, and access to information were other incentives to pursue

## Box 3.4 Practice-based teaching, problem-based learning, and patient-focused practice all go together

It is crucial to encourage health professionals to undertake lifelong learning and develop relevant workplace competencies that can adapt to diverse challenges and populations. New trends in education aim to improve the health of the public by implementing this idea in training methods; this involves integrating three approaches and yields greater improvements in skills, attitudes and behaviours of health professionals than programmes that do not employ this integration *(55)*.

**Practice-based teaching** aims to:
- bridge the gap between academia and practice;
- benefit students, schools, agencies and communities;
- involve and develop critical thinking and problem-solving skills;
- be interdisciplinary, multidisciplinary and multidimensional;
- develop learning partnerships among academic staff, practitioners and students, to educate teachers, practitioners and researchers;
- incorporate experiential education, including critical reflection, observation and learning by doing *(56)*.

**Problem-based learning** complements practice-based teaching through:
- identifying the problem;
- exploring pre-existing knowledge;
- generating hypotheses and possible mechanisms;
- identifying learning issues and objectives;
- self study and group learning;
- re-evaluation and application of new knowledge to the problem;
- assessment and reflection on learning *(57)*.

**Patient-focused practice:**
- integrates teaching and learning with clinical practice;
- shares experiences of illness, disease and recovery with patients;
- understands varying needs for care;
- observes and participates in the ways in which different service providers work together to meet the needs of patients.

**Training pharmacy students: the Clinical Partners Programme at the Ohio State University College of Pharmacy** provides an active learning environment, offers a patient-focused model based on pharmaceutical care principles, and is an arena for applied research in pharmacy practice. Integration with clinical practice is undertaken at an early stage and sustained, with students attached to specific patients – called "longitudinal patients" – whom they follow through all stages of care. The programme offers multiple services and competency development, including anticoagulation management, diabetes self-management, cholesterol management, hepatitis C education, herbal product and dietary supplement consultations, medication management, smoking cessation, and wellness *(58)*.

teaching. In contrast, reluctance to teach was based on lack of rewards, perceived emphasis on research for promotions with little value placed on teaching, lack of teaching skills, the competitive agendas of clinical service and research, perceived inappropriateness of curriculum design, and heavy administrative load resulting from large classes.

Despite these disincentives, a strong commitment to teaching and mentoring has been observed among health professionals in many countries *(62)*. Twinning arrangements and long-term partnerships between academic medical centres in high income countries with universities and health facilities in low income countries, such as on HIV/AIDS care, have the potential to strengthen faculty development and enrich curricula and teaching materials *(63–66)*. Similarly, the appearance of networks of health training institutions – with virtual links – promises additional opportunities to share teaching resources *(67)*. An international foundation with the specific aim of supporting the development of an academic medical faculty is described in Box 3.5. Sharing experience of these and similar innovative arrangements gives the opportunity of evaluating what does and does not work.

## Strategy 3.4 Encourage and support teaching excellence

The critical role of teaching staff in preparing the health workforce justifies a much more comprehensive strategy to support teaching excellence. Key components might include: more credible career tracks for teaching; career advancement for women faculty members, particularly in academic medicine; good material and technical support; reasonable remuneration; constructive feedback and evaluation; access to mentoring; training opportunities to improve teaching; and awards for teaching as well as innovation in curriculum content.

## Financing

At present there are no normative guidelines on the amount of money that should be invested in generating the health workforce. Although there are scattered studies on the costs of training specific types of health workers *(68)*, in most countries there are no comprehensive data on the amounts countries and development agencies invest in pre-service and in-service training of the health workforce. Despite this evidence gap, it is clear that the level of financing and the way in which it is disbursed to health training institutions have important implications for the size, skills and diversity of the health workforce.

## Box 3.5  Faculty development programmes: training trainers in professional health education

One goal of the **Foundation for Advancement of International Medical Education and Research** (FAIMER) is to create a global network of medical educators to develop and exchange information and ideas to improve education. It offers a two-year, part-time fellowship programme designed for international medical school educators. The first year consists of two residential sessions in the USA, and an intersession curriculum innovation project at the participant's home institution. The second year, completed from the Fellow's home country, involves mentoring an entering Fellow and active engagement in an Internet discussion group. The programme is designed to teach education methods and leadership skills, as well as to develop strong professional bonds with other medical educators around the world. FAIMER's educational programmes currently focus on serving medical educators and institutions in South Asia, sub-Saharan Africa and South America. The goal is to establish regional networks of educators who can develop such programmes locally. For more information, see http://www.ecfmg.org/faimer.

## Box 3.6 From in-service to pre-service training: Integrated Management of Childhood Illness (IMCI)

Integrated Management of Childhood Illness (IMCI) was developed in the mid-1990s by WHO and other partners as a prevention and treatment strategy to ensure the health and well-being of children aged under five years around the world. The IMCI strategy consists of improving the case management skills of health workers, health systems generally, and family and community health practices *(71)*. It supports the training of physicians, nurses and other health workers to provide integrated care *(72)*.

**In-service training** broadens existing health workers' skill sets primarily via an 11-day clinical training block with lectures, active teaching methods and accompanying practical aids all ideally catered to the specific type of health professional and the extent of their previous training.

**Pre-service training** is a more recent addition to IMCI, and aims to introduce these same core skills much earlier to health workers, as a core training module within health education curricula.

**Benefits of pre-service over in-service training**. The benefits of diverting more limited funds from *in-service* to *pre-service* training programmes are numerous, based on the shared experiences of health education institutions in all six WHO regions: Bolivia, Ecuador, Egypt, Ethiopia, Indonesia, Moldova, Morocco, Nepal, the Philippines, United Republic of Tanzania, Uzbekistan, Viet Nam and many other countries are involved in this exercise *(73–76)*. Key lessons learnt include the following:

- Funding for *in-service* IMCI training is difficult to secure from national and/or district health budgets, and the standard 11-day training presents substantial personnel time diverted from patient care, particularly for resource-constrained health facilities.

- Given limited trainers – as in-service trainers are more expensive yet often have high rates of turnover and attrition – *pre-service* training might lower costs and increase returns to investment by leveraging both limited training resources and captive student audiences.
- Even if instituted only for medical students, *pre-service* training would infuse future doctors with core IMCI principles to integrate eventually into their own practices, that of their peers and that of other cadres of health workers, since doctors are often responsible for training nurses, paramedics, and other auxiliary health workers.
- The *IMCI model chapter for textbooks* (see figure), developed by WHO and UNICEF *(77)*, facilitates the process of introducing IMCI content into locally authored and edited health training textbooks.

### The Integrated Case Management Process

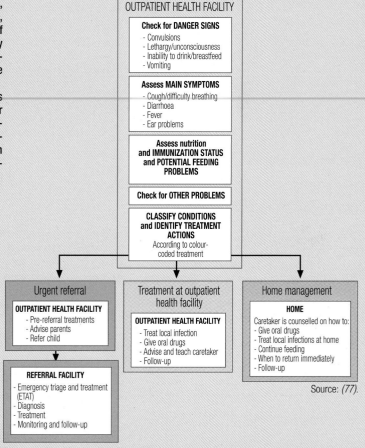

Source: *(77)*.

Drawing on the pipeline model of the ways in which health workers are recruited (Figure 3.2), the pool of applicants for health training is contingent more broadly on the level of financing of education. In poorer countries, very low enrolment rates for secondary and tertiary school attendance reflect inadequate financing of education *(69)* and may limit the overall size and socioeconomic diversity of the applicant pool, or compromise preparedness. In these contexts, improved financing of primary and secondary education is essential to increase the supply of health workers *(70)*.

The significant training costs associated with scaling up the health workforce, identified in Chapter 1, suggest that major increases in the funding of health training are critically needed in countries with severe health worker shortages. Higher levels of financing are required to increase training capacity (more institutions or expanded enrolment) and to improve quality with better infrastructure and highly motivated teachers. Redirecting some resources currently spent on in-service training to pre-service training would tap an important source of financing for resource-strapped establishments. Innovative efforts to integrate training for priority programmes into the curricula of health training institutions are demonstrating that this works (see Box 3.6). Achieving large increases in levels of financing and better coordination across sectors requires political commitment, donor support and negotiation with finance, education and other ministries (see Chapter 7).

Attaining the desired diversity of the workforce is linked, in part, to the way health training is financed. Private sector health training institutions are increasing in number worldwide (see Box 3.3). The decline in public sector subsidies of health training institutions raises concerns that students who are less well-off may avoid considering health care as an occupation, cluster in programmes where the training is less costly, take on paid work while training (at the expense of the acquisition of skills and knowledge), or find their career choices limited by indebtedness. Provision of fee exemptions, scholarships and loans are among the mechanisms to preserve access to training *(78)*.

## Infrastructure and technology

The construction, repair and maintenance of buildings, special laboratories and other field sites, along with the acquisition of learning materials, are among the infrastructure requirements of health training institutions. Insufficiencies in infrastructure may place a significant constraint on the numbers of students who can be taught effectively and limit expansion of training, even for basic services *(79)*. A recent survey of psychiatric training infrastructure in 120 countries found that about 70 countries had grossly inadequate facilities *(80)*. Given the expense involved in building and maintaining health training institutions for very small countries such as small island states, regional training facilities offer a more affordable option to build up national capacities and leadership (see Box 3.7).

The physical location of training facilities can influence considerably the diversity profile of staff and students. Health training institutions are most often located in urban areas, and recognition of this urban bias has led to increasing efforts to build them in rural areas or create effective virtual links using information communication technologies *(81, 82)*.

## Box 3.7 Regionalization of training for health professionals: University of the South Pacific and the University of the West Indies

By working together, small island nations provide better access to education and training, build their own capacity and national leadership, promote values appropriate for the region, and become globally competitive. Regional institutions spanning large geographical areas need well-developed distance learning programmes, with flexible schedules to accommodate students needs. Advanced communication technologies are also required to reach students. Two successful examples of regional collaboration and integration in education offer a potential model for the education of health professionals in other areas of the world.

**University of the South Pacific (USP).** Established in 1968, USP spreads across 33 million square kilometres of ocean, an area more than three times the size of Europe. The university is jointly owned by the governments of 12 island countries: the Cook Islands, Fiji, Kiribati, the Marshall Islands, Nauru, Niue, Samoa, the Solomon Islands, Tokelau,

Tonga, Tuvalu and Vanuatu. It has campuses in all the 12 member countries and the main campus, Laucala, is in Fiji. Although there is no faculty for health sciences, there are faculties for arts and law; business and economics; islands and oceans; and science and technology.

**University of the West Indies (UWI).** Established in 1948 as a College of the University of London, UWI is a regional training institution that gained full university status in 1962, with a current student population of 11 000. One of four different faculties, Medical Sciences offers a wide range of undergraduate, graduate and postgraduate programmes. Critical to the success of the university is the fact that graduates all return to their respective countries and work in the health sector as care providers, managers or policy-makers. One prime minister and four ministers of health in the region are graduates of the Faculty of Medical Sciences.

### Sixteen countries support and benefit from the University of the West Indies

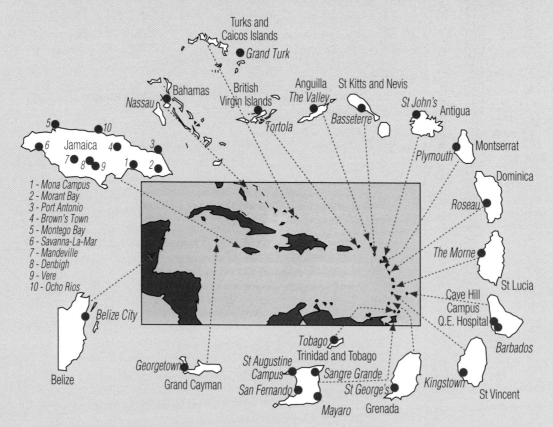

### Strategy 3.5 Find innovative ways to access teaching expertise and materials

Access to textbooks and other quality teaching materials represents an important challenge and can be tackled in a number of ways. The PALTEX programme in Latin American and Caribbean countries screens for quality and offers volume discounts for a wide range of textbooks and basic diagnostic tools to over 600 institutions *(83)*. Information and communication technologies are being used in remote and resource-poor settings to access expertise in the faculty and diffuse training materials more effectively. The Health InterNetwork Access to Research Initiative (HINARI), set up by WHO with the committed involvement of major publishers, enables academic and research institutions, government offices and teaching hospitals, particularly in low income countries, to gain access to one of the world's largest collections of biomedical and health literature. Over 3200 full-text journals and other resources are now available free to health institutions in 69 countries, and for very low cost in a further 44 countries *(84)*.

### Information for policy-making

Countering the dearth of information about the provision of educational and training services, students, programmes and graduates is a major priority. Analysis of the literature databases over the last 30 years reveals that the overwhelming focus of enquiry has been on education evaluation, teaching methods and the curriculum (see Box 3.8). Few of the countries with the most acute health worker shortages routinely collect and report data on the number of graduates, or even the number of training facilities for health professionals *(87)*. Even fewer countries break this information down subnationally in terms of the reach of different institutions, or by various socioeconomic attributes of students and graduates. Although important for description and comparison with normative standards, from a planning perspective numbers alone are just a start.

### Strategy 3.6 Evaluate institutional performance, policy options and actions

To inform policy and decision-making related to health worker training, information about current and prospective performance is required. For example, an analysis from the Canadian province of Nova Scotia indicates that demand for physician services will grow faster than supply over the next 15 years if current policies on training remain unchanged *(88)*. To evaluate the performance of health training institutions, a national strategy to strengthen workforce data generation and synthesis is needed. These national data should be coupled with cross-national information on the costs and effectiveness of different ways of training and recruiting health workers, such as through observatories on human resources for health (see Chapters 6 and 7).

## RETHINKING RECRUITMENT: GATEWAY TO THE WORKFORCE

Recruitment represents entry into the formal health workforce. It is thus a critical function whose performance has to be managed at the levels of both the system and individual employers. Five performance outcomes are relevant to assess recruitment: numbers, competencies, background (diversity), location, and time.

## Box 3.8  The evidence base to enhance performance of health educational institutions

Figure (a) below shows that roughly 90% of all research articles on topics addressing health workforce training, indexed in PubMed between 1970 and 2004, focused on educational measurement, teaching methods or curriculum issues. The level of research on other topics that may provide important insights on enhancing skills, diversity and numbers – such as fellowships and scholarships, school admissions and student drop-outs – has remained marginal. More research on appropriate topics should be conducted in low income countries *(85)* and included within research syntheses.

The range of health educational institutions represented in research is too narrow. Figure (b) below shows that of all research articles indexed in PubMed on health professional schools for the same period, 55% concerned medical schools, 17% nursing schools and only 2% public health schools. Despite huge shortages in the health workforce across different classes of workers, each year research addressing health educational institutions remains heavily skewed towards medical schools, without significant increases in the number of articles addressing dental, nursing, veterinarian, public health, pharmacy or other health occupation schools. Similar findings are noted from the analysis of regional databases of scientific literature *(86)*.

(a) Research articles on topics addressing health workforce training[1]

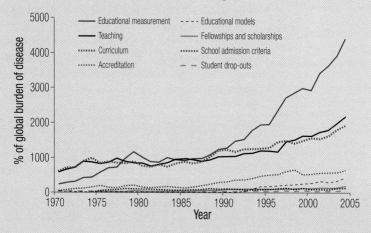

(b) Research articles on health professional schools[1]

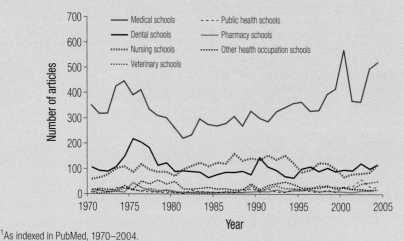

[1]As indexed in PubMed, 1970–2004.

- **Numbers** recruited should reflect not only current needs and demands but also the extent of underemployment or low productivity (see Chapter 4) and attrition (see Chapter 5).
- **Competencies**, the skills and experience of recruits, should reflect both the products of the educational pipeline and non-technical qualities (e.g. compassion and motivation) required for effective health services delivery.
- The **background** of health workers recruited and their positioning in the right **location** must be compatible with the sociocultural and linguistic profiles of the population being served.
- Recruitment must be **time** sensitive as in the case of the rapid mobilization of workers to deal with responses to humanitarian emergencies and disease outbreaks.

### Imperfect labour markets

To a large degree, recruitment performance outcomes reflect the context of the broader labour market. Employers, on the demand side of the market, delineate the types and conditions of employment, while the workers, on the supply side, contribute their skills and their individual preferences about how and where to work. Market equilibrium is reached once labour demand equals supply of workers. Market equilibrium can coexist, however, with urban over-supply and rural scarcity of health workers as well as underserved population subgroups.

A more complex picture is illustrated in Figure 3.3: that labour supply reflects the outcome of demand for education, whereas labour demand reflects the outcome of demand for health services mediated through employers and financing mechanisms.

Figure 3.3 Relationship of education, labour and health services markets with human resources

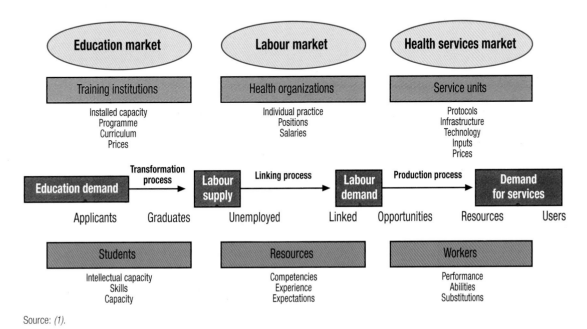

Source: (1).

This more realistic situation reflects values, priorities, constraints and competition across different sectors, institutional actors and individuals. Prospective students often consider how quickly they are able to pay off educational debts and work in a desirable location. Based on a study from Colombia, the minimum working time needed to pay off debt incurred during pre-service training is shown in Figure 3.4 for two different health workers *(1)*. At the same time, many governments pursue numbers-based recruitment strategies reflecting broader reforms, such as overall downsizing of the public sector or structural adjustment, rather than specific health

**Figure 3.4  Projected time to recuperate student investments in education, Colombia, 2000**

a) Non-specialist physicians

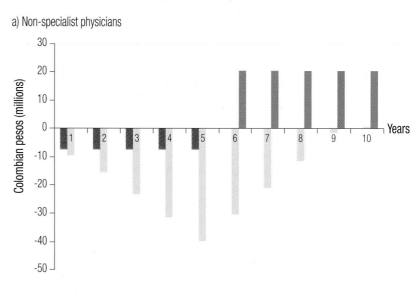

b) Physiotherapists

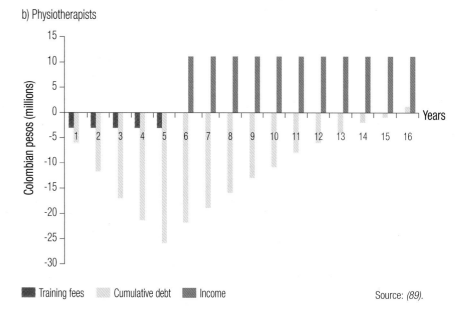

Training fees    Cumulative debt    Income

Source: *(89)*.

priorities *(89)*. Standardized government wage and work conditions, which rarely accommodate health worker needs, also limit the public sector to hire and retain workers in the health labour market.

In low income countries where trained health service providers are scarce, the public sector often competes to recruit workers with the private sector, international nongovernmental organizations and other donors, and multilateral entities offering attractive local or international employment packages. Dr Elizabeth Madraa, manager of Uganda's AIDS Control Programme, laments, "We keep training them and they go to NGOs or abroad, where they can get better money; then we have to train [more people] again." *(90)*. Recruitment agencies, contracted by large employers, further fuel this exodus. These imperfections necessitate strong leadership and actions that push forward health goals. The magnitude of health workforce migration and the unregulated practices of recruitment agencies have resulted, for example, in a growing number of ethical recruitment guidelines (see Chapter 5).

### Strategy 3.7 Improve recruitment performance

Actions on several fronts can enhance recruitment performance. These relate to increasing information, striving towards greater efficiency, managing incentives for self-employed workers and increasing equity in the coverage of health services, and are expanded below.

*"Actions on several fronts can enhance recruitment performance"*

*Information*. Recruitment needs, demands and performance are often not articulated well through the existing planning processes or survey instruments. Furthermore, poor recruitment capacity impedes efforts to scale up activities, respond rapidly or develop new cadres. Essential data inputs for recruitment management include vacancy rates and trends, gaps or surpluses in worker supply relative to regional demand, and performance metrics such as time taken to hire individuals or fill vacant posts. Gauging workers' perceptions of employers (see Chapter 4 on magnet institutions) provides the basis for recruiters to respond more appropriately to prospective employees' concerns.

*Efficiency*. The consequences of institutional inefficiency abound: sluggish bureaucracies encourage prospective recruits to withhold applications, quit prior to starting work or simply succumb to the low morale pervading many public health services; failure to define or establish posts for rural health workers has led new recruits to saturate urban areas *(91)*; and non-transparent, politically motivated appointments supplant the best recruits. To improve recruitment efficiency, bureaucracies must hire qualified human resources personnel who must be supported to manage recruitment according to best practices. Merit-based recruitment is a good example of best practice that is strongly correlated with the quality and integrity of government institutions. Complex issues such as the appropriate degree of centralization or decentralization of recruitment procedures, as in government-run health services, require context-specific analysis of costs, benefits and the political realities concerning the overall management of government-run health services across central, district and local levels *(92–94)*.

*Management of self-recruitment*. In many settings, health workers are not formally recruited by an employer but set up their own practice, i.e. are self-employed. Licensure, certification and registration of health workers as well as professional associations can help to manage and ensure competence of the self-employed health workforce. If these regulatory capacities are lacking or weak, then public trust may

be eroded (see Chapter 6). In Bangladesh, for example, the risk of neonatal mortality was found to be six times higher when mothers consulted self-employed health workers with no recognized qualifications, rather than health workers possessing recognized qualifications *(95)*. Where government reimburses self-employed health workers it can exercise influence over their numbers and locations as an important mechanism to achieve better balance between types of workers (for example generalists or specialists), where they work, and whom they serve.

*Recruitment to areas of need.* Recruitment represents an ideal opportunity to place workers where they are needed. Around the world, affluent urban areas are magnets for health workers, leaving urban slums and remote rural areas relatively underserved. Compulsory service or bonding arrangements following publicly subsidized education are widespread but are rarely evaluated *(96)*. There is growing evidence to suggest that local recruitment is a strong predictor of long-term staff retention *(97)*, thus highlighting the importance of training opportunities for people from rural and remote communities. Identifying respected members of such communities who are suitable for training and acceptable to the population, as in Pakistan (see Box 3.9), meets health service needs, training objectives, and diversity selection.

## CONCLUSION

This chapter has reviewed issues associated with generating and recruiting the health workforce. The policy questions that have been discussed here – related to training, health workers' competencies, and labour markets – lead naturally to questions about the management of the existing health workers, the subject of Chapter 4.

## Box 3.9  Pakistan's Lady Health Workers: selection and development of new cadres

Created in 1994 to improve health care access in rural communities and urban slums, Pakistan's National Programme for Family Planning and Primary Health Care has relied heavily on the performance of its 80 000 Lady Health Workers who provide basic health care to nearly 70% of the country's population *(98)*. The stringent selection criteria used include the requirement that they come from the community they will serve, be at least 18 years old, have successfully completed a middle school education and be recommended by the residents of their community as a good candidate. Married women are given preference. They receive 15 months of training (three months full time, 12 months part time), and study basics of primary health care and hygiene, community organization, interpersonal communication, data collection and health management information systems. Once installed, they report to a supervisor weekly.

Training is aligned to practice: they treat minor ailments and make referrals for more serious conditions, record the community's vital statistics, conduct basic health education, provide contraception to couples and serve as a liaison between their communities and the formal health system, helping coordinate such services as immunization and anaemia control, and provide antenatal and postnatal care to mothers. Recent research shows a clear connection between the presence of Lady Health Workers and improved community health *(99–100)*. Independent evaluations note that after Lady Health Worker cadres were introduced, substantial increases were documented in childhood vaccination rates, child growth monitoring, use of contraception and antenatal services, provision of iron tablets to pregnant women and in lowering rates of childhood diarrhoea *(101)*.

**Key lessons:**
- It is important to develop strategies to meet health workforce objectives with a spectrum of health workers.
- Combining appropriate recruitment, simplification of tasks, training and supervision can lead to efficient and effective new cadres.

# REFERENCES

1. Ruiz F, Camacho S, Jurado C, Matallana M, O'Meara G, Eslava J et al. *Human resources in health in Colombia: balance, competencies and perspectives.* Bogotá, Ministry of Health, Cendex, Pontificia Universidad Javeriana, and Fundación Cultural de Artes Gráficas, Javegraf, 2001.
2. Flexner A. *Medical education in the United States and Canada. A report to the Carnegie Foundation for the Advancement of Teaching.* New York, NY, Carnegie Foundation, 1910 (Bulletin No. 4).
3. *Welch-Rose report on schools of public health.* New York, NY, Rockefeller Foundation, 1915.
4. *Report of the Health Survey and Development Committee.* Delhi, Government of India, Manager of Publications, 1946 (Chairman: Bhore).
5. Chang K. Health work serving the peasants. *Chinese Medical Journal*, 1966, 85:143–144.
6. The orientation of the revolution in medical education as seen in the growth of "barefoot doctors": report of an investigation from Shanghai. *China's Medicine*, 1968, 10:574–581.
7. Neufeld VR, Woodward CA, MacLeod SM. The McMaster MD program: a case study of renewal in medical education. *Academic Medicine*, 1989, 64:423–432.
8. International campaign to revitalise academic medicine (ICRAM) (www.bmj.com/academicmedicine, accessed 13 February 2006).
9. Kachur DK, Krajic K. Structures and trends in health profession education in Europe. In: Dubois C-A, McKee M, Nolte E, eds. *Human resources for health in Europe.* Brussels, European Observatory on Health Systems and Policies, 2005:79-97
10. Huddart J, Picazo OF, Duale S. *The health sector human resource crisis in Africa: an issues paper.* Washington, DC, United States Agency for International Development, Bureau for Africa, Office of Sustainable Development, 2003.
11. *South-East Asia public health initiative 2004–2008.* New Delhi, World Health Organization Regional Office for South-East Asia, 2004 (document SEA-HSD-278).
12. Reddy SK. Establishing schools of public health in India. In: Matlin S, ed. *Global forum update on research for health.* London, Pro-Brook, 2005:149–153.
13. *Survey of medical education accreditation capacity at national level, as part of the Strategic Partnership to Improve Medical Education.* Copenhagen, World Health Organization and World Federation for Medical Education, 2004.
14. Bansai RK. Private medical education takes off in India. *Lancet*, 2003, 361:1748–1749.
15. Kingma M. *Nurses on the move: migration and the global health care economy.* Ithica, NY, ILR Press, 2006.
16. Homedes N, Ugalde A. Human resources: the Cinderella of health sector reform in Latin America. *Human Resources for Health*, 2005, 3:1.
17. Van Lerberghe W, Essengue MS, Lokonga J-P. Les stratégies de réforme du secteur de la santé en RDC [Reform strategies for the health sector in the DRC]. Geneva, World Health Organization, 2005.
18. Verspoor A, Mattimire A, Watt P. A chance to learn: knowledge and finance for education in sub-Saharan Africa. Washington, DC, The World Bank, 2001 (http://www.worldbank.org).
19. Bury JA, Gliber M. *Quality improvement and accreditation of training programmes in public health.* Lyon, Fondation Mérieux and Association of Schools of Public Health in the European Region, 2001.
20. McLachlan JC. Outreach is better than selection for increasing diversity. *Medical Education*, 2005, 39:872–875.
21. *Recreating health professional practice for a new century – The fourth report of the PEW Health Professions Commission.* San Francisco, CA, The Pew Health Professions Commission, 1998.
22. Heaton T, Forste R, Hoffman J, Flake D. Cross-national variation in family influences on child health. *Social Science and Medicine*, 2005, 60:97–108.
23. Day RD, Gavazzi S, Acock A. Compelling family processes. In: Thornton A, ed. *The well-being of children and families: research and data needs.* Ann Arbor, MI, The University of Michigan Press, 2001:103–126.
24. Ara T (chair), Affirmative Action Committee. *Education in the professions: affirmative action and diversity in professions education.* San Diego, CA, American Educational Research Association, 2004.

25. Fincher RM, Sykes-Brown W, Allen-Noble R. Health science learning academy: a successful "pipeline" educational program for high school students. *Academic Medicine*, 2002, 77:737–738.

26. Howe A, Campion P, Searle J, Smith H. New perspectives–approaches to medical education at four new UK medical schools. *British Medical Journal*, 2004, 329:327-31.

27. Simpson KH, Budd K. Medical student attrition: a 10-year survey in one medical school. *Medical Education*, 1996, 30:172–178.

28. *Human resources for health, strategic plan, 2006–2010*. Lusaka, Ministry of Health of the Republic of Zambia, 2005.

29. Huda N, Agha S. Attrition in medical college: experience at Ziauddin Medical University in Pakistan. *Education for Health*, 2004, 17:232–235.

30. Holt M. Student retention practices in Associate Degree, entry-level dental hygiene programs. *Journal of Dental Hygiene*, 2005, 79:1–13.

31. Continuing concern at student nurse attrition rates in Northern Ireland [press release]. Royal College of Nursing (http://www.rcn.org.uk/news/display.php?ID=1136, accessed 7 February 2006).

32. Jalili-Grenier F, Chase M. Retention of nursing students with English as a second language. *Journal of Advanced Nursing*, 1997, 25:199–203.

33. Daly J. *Evidence-based medicine and the search for a science of clinical care*. New York, NY, University of California Press and Milbank Memorial Fund, 2005.

34. Singh-Manoux A, Marmot MG, Adler NE. Does subjective social status predict health and change in health status better than objective status? *Psychosomatic Medicine*, 2005, 67:855–861.

35. Melchior M, Goldberg M, Krieger N, Kawachi I, Menvielle G, Zins M et al. Occupational class, occupational mobility and cancer incidence among middle-aged men and women: a prospective study of the French GAZEL cohort. *Cancer Causes and Control*, 2005, 16:515–524.

36. Slovensky DJ, Paustian PE. Preparing for diversity management strategies: teaching tactics for an undergraduate healthcare management program. *Journal of Health Administration Education*, 2005, 22:189–199.

37. Reynolds PP, Kamei RK, Sundquist J, Khanna N, Palmer EJ, Palmer T. Using the PRACTICE mnemonic to apply cultural competency to genetics in medical education and patient care. *Academic Medicine*, 2005, 80:1107–1113.

38. Smith R, Woodward D, Acharya A, Beaglehole R, Drager N. Communicable disease control: a "Global Public Good Perspective". *Health Policy and Planning*, 2004, 19:271–278.

39. Beauchamp D, Steinbock B. *Public health ethics – New ethics for the public's health*. New York, NY, Oxford University Press, 1999.

40. Banerji D. *Poverty, class and health culture in India*. Prachi Prakashan, New Delhi, 1982.

41. Laurell AC. El estudio social del proceso salud-enfermedad en América Latina [Latin American social study on health disease process]. *Cuadernos médicos-sociales*, 1986, 37:3–18.

42. Mutabaruka E, Nshimirimana D, Goilav C, Meheus A. EIP training needs assessment in 12 African countries, 2002–2004. *Communicable Diseases Bulletin for the African Region*, 2005, 3:1–4.

43. Jones RB, Hampshire AJ, Tweddle S, Moult B, Hill A. The clinician's role in meeting patient information needs: suggested learning outcomes. *Medical Education*, 2001, 35:565–571.

44. Matillon Y, LeBoeuf D, Maisonneuve H. Defining and assessing the competence of health care professionals. A survey of 148 organizations. *Presse Médicale*, 2005, 34:1703–1709.

45. Buchan J. A certain ratio? The policy implications of minimum staffing ratios in nursing. *Journal of Health Services Research and Policy*, 2005, 10:239–244.

46. Jamshidi HR, Cook DA. Some thoughts on medical education in the twenty-first century. *Medical Teaching*, 2003, 25:229–238.

47. Jones R, Higgs R, de Angelis C, Prideaux D. Changing face of medical curricula. *Lancet*, 2001, 357:699–703.

48. Butler R, Inman D, Lobb D. Problem-based learning and the medical school: another case of the emperor's new clothes? *Advances in Physiology Education*, 2005, 29:194–196.

49. Dolmans DH, De Grave W, Wolfhagen IH, van der Vleuten CP. Problem-based learning: future challenges for educational practice and research. *Medical Education*, 2005, 39:732–741.

50. *Critical challenges: revitalizing the health professions for the twenty-first century – The third report of the PEW Health Professions Commission.* San Francisco, CA, The Pew Health Professions Commission, 1995.

51. *Duties of a doctor.* London, General Medical Council, 1993.

52. Littlewood S, Ypinazar V, Margolis SA, Scherpbier A, Spencer J, Dornan T. Early practical experience and the social responsiveness of clinical education: systematic review. *BMJ*, 2005, 331:387–391.

53. Dornan T. Osler, Flexner, apprenticeship and "the new medical education". *Journal of the Royal Society of Medicine*, 2005, 98:91–95.

54. Sturmberg JP, Reid S, Khadra MH. A longitudinal, patient-centred, integrated curriculum: facilitating community-based education in a rural clinical school. *Education for Health: Change in Learning and Practice*, 2002, 15:294–304.

55. Coomarasamy A, Khan KS. What is the evidence that postgraduate teaching in evidence-based medicine changes anything? A systematic review. *BMJ*, 2004, 329:1017–1021.

56. Atchison C, Boatright DT, Merrigan D, Quill BE, Whittaker C. *Demonstrating excellence in practice-based teaching for public health.* United States Department of Health and Human Resources, Health Resources and Services Administration, Bureau of Health Professionals, 2004 (http://www.asph.org/UserFiles/ASPH_10_2004.pdf, accessed 8 February 2006).

57. Walsh A. *The tutor in problem-based learning: a novice's guide.* Hamilton, McMaster University, 2005.

58. Mehta BH, Rodis JL, Nahata NC, Bennett MS. Advancing patient care through innovative practice: the Clinical Partners Program. *American Journal of Health System Pharmacy*, 2005, 62:2501–2507.

59. Gerbert B, Showstack J, Chapman S, Schroeder S. The changing dynamics of graduate medical education: Implications for decision-making. *Western Journal of Medicine*, 1987, 146:368–373.

60. PLoS Medicine editors. Improving health by investing in medical education, *PLoS Medicine*, 2005, 2:e424.

61. Dahlstrom J, Dorai-Raj A, McGill D, Owen C, Tymms K, Watson DA. What motivates senior clinicians to teach medical students? *BMC Medical Education*, 2005, 5:27.

62. Macq J, Van Lerberghe W. Managing health services in developing countries: moonlighting to serve the public? In: Ferrinho P, Van Lerberghe W, eds. *Providing health care under adverse conditions: health personnel performance and individual coping strategies.* Antwerp, ITG Press, 2000 (Studies in Health Services Organisation and Policy, 16:177–186).

63. *Strengthening health systems: promoting an integrated response for chronic care.* The Tropical Health and Education Trust (THET) (http://www.thet.org, accessed 13 February 2006).

64. Hern MJ, Vaughn G, Mason D, Weitkamp T. Creating an international nursing practice and education workplace. *Journal of Pediatric Nursing*, 2005, 20:34–44.

65. Ozgediz D, Roayaie K, Debas H, Schecter W, Farmer D. Surgery in developing countries: essential training in residency. *Archives of Surgery*, 2005, 140:795–800.

66. Wright S, Cloonan P, Leonhardy K, Wright G. An international programme in nursing and midwifery: building capacity for the new millennium. *International Nursing Review*, 2005, 52:18–23.

67. L'Institut de Santé Publique, d'Épidémiologie et de Développement (ISPED) (http://ead.isped.u-bordeaux2.fr, accessed 13 February 2006).

68. *Literature review on the costs of education of human resources for health.* Geneva, World Health Organization, 2003 (Department of Human Resources for Health working paper).

69. *Global education digest 2004: comparing education statistics across the world.* Montreal, UNESCO, Institute for Statistics, 2004.

70. Bhargava A. The AIDS epidemic and health care infrastructure inadequacies in Africa: a socioeconomic perspective. *Journal of Acquired Immune Deficiency Syndromes*, 2005, 40:41–42.

71. Naimoli JF, Rowe AK, Lyaghfouri A, Larbi R, Lamrani LA. Effect of the Integrated Management of Childhood Illness strategy on health care quality in Morocco. *International Journal for Quality in Health Care*, 2006, 18 (published electronically in advance of print publication).

72. *Integrated Management of Childhood Illness (IMCI)*. World Health Organization, Bangladesh (http://www.whoban.org/imci.html, accessed 8 February 2006).

73. *Pre-service training for the Integrated Management of Childhood Illness (IMCI): report of an informal consultation*. Geneva, World Health Organization, 1998 (http://www.who.int/child-adolescent-health/New_Publications/IMCI/Reports/Report-Informal_Consultation_1998.htm).

74. *Report of an intercountry training workshop on IMCI pre-service training*. Geneva, World Health Organization, 1999 (http://www.who.int/child-adolescent-health/New_Publications/IMCI/Reports/Report-Intercountry_Workshop_1999.htm, accessed 13 February 2006).

75. *IMCI pre-service training review and planning meeting*. Harare, World Health Organization Regional Office for Africa, Integrated Management of Childhood Illness (IMCI) Unit, 2002 (http://www.afro.who.int/imci/reports/pre-service_training_review_report.pdf, accessed 8 February 2006).

76. *IMCI pre-service training*. Cairo, World Health Organization Regional Office for the Eastern Mediterranean, Child and Adolescent Health and Development, 2004 (http://www.emro.who.int/cah/PreServiceEducation-IMCI.htm, accessed 8 February 2006).

77. *IMCI (Integrated Management of Childhood Illness) model chapter for textbooks*. Geneva, World Health Organization and United Nations Children's Fund, 2001 (http://www.who.int/child-adolescent-health/New_Publications/IMCI/WHO_FCH_CAH_00.40/WHO_FCH_CAH_00.40.pdf, accessed 8 February 2006).

78. Pechura CM. Programs of the Robert Wood Johnson Foundation to develop minority medical careers. *American Journal of the Medical Sciences*, 2001, 322:290–292.

79. Muula A, Mfutso-Bengo J, Makoza J, Chatipwa E. The ethics of developed nations recruiting nurses from developing countries: the case of Malawi. *Nursing Ethics*, 2003, 10:433–438.

80. *Atlas of psychiatric education and training across the world*. Geneva, World Health Organization and World Psychiatric Association, 2005.

81. Snadden D, Bates J. Expanding undergraduate medical education in British Columbia: a distributed campus model. *Canadian Medical Association Journal*, 2005, 173:589–590.

82. Wang L. A comparison of metropolitan and rural medical schools in China: which schools provide rural physicians? *Australian Journal of Rural Health*, 2002, 10:94-98.

83. Programa Ampliado de Libros de Texto y Materiales de Instrucción (PALTEX) [The Expanded Textbook and Instructional Materials Programme (PALTEX)]. Washington, DC, Pan American Health Organization and Pan American Health and Education Foundation, 2005 (http://www.pahef.org/pahef/pages/paltex, accessed 13 February 2006).

84. Aronson B. Improving online access to medical information for low-income countries. *New England Journal of Medicine*, 2004, 350:966–968.

85. Paraje G, Sadana R, Karam G. Public health. Increasing international gaps in health-related publications. *Science*, 2005, 308:959–960.

86. Nogueira RP. Trends and perspectives in health personnel research in the Americas. *Educación Médica y Salud*, 1985, 19:25–47.

87. *Tracking human resources and wage bill management in the health sector: a study to identify bottlenecks and constraints in the production, recruitment and management of health workers and funds for the wage bill in the public health services*. Kampala, African Medical and Research Foundation and Ministry of Health, 2005.

88. Basu K, Gupta A. Un modèle prévisionnel de l'offre et de la demande de médecins dans la province canadienne de la Nouvelle-écosse [A physician demand and supply forecast model for Nova Scotia]. *Cahiers de sociologie et de démographie médicales*, 2005, 45:255–286.

89. Joint Learning Initiative (JLI). Human resources for health, 2004: health human resources demand and management: strategies to confront crisis. Report of the working group on demand. Boston, MA, Global Health Trust, 2004 (http://www.globalhealthtrust.org/doc/WG3Report.pdf, accessed 8 February 2006).

90. Uganda leads way in innovative HIV/AIDS treatment. *Bulletin of the World Health Organization*, 2005, 83: 244–245 (http://www.who.int/bulletin/volumes/83/4/infocus0405/en/index.html, accessed 13 February 2006).

91. Egger D, Mouyokani J, Adzodo KMR. *Renforcement de la gestion sanitaire au Togo: Quelles leçons peut-on en tirer? [Strengthening management in Togo: what can be learnt?]*. Geneva, HDS/OMH, World Health Organization, 2005.

92. Ssengooba F. *Human resources for health in decentralized Uganda: developments and implications for health systems research*. Paper presented at: Global Forum for Health Research 9, Mumbai, India, 12–16 September 2005.

93. Bossert T, Beauvais J, Bowser D. *Decentralization of health systems: preliminary review of four country case studies*. Bethesda, MD, Partnerships for Health Reform, Abt Associates Inc., 2000 (Major Applied Research 6, Technical Report 1; http://www.localgovernance.org/documents/aid_healthdecentralization.pdf).

94. Seshamani V, Mwikisa CN, Odegaard K, eds. *Zambia's health reforms: selected papers 1995–2000*. Lund, Swedish Institute for Health Economics and University of Zambia, Department of Economics, 2002.

95. Mercer A, Mobarak HK, Haseen F, Lira Huq N, Uddin N, Larson C. *Level and determinants of neonatal mortality in rural areas of Bangladesh served by a large NGO Programme*. Dhaka, ICDDR,B Centre for Health and Population Research, Bangladesh Population and Health Consortium, 2005.

96. Reid S. Community service for health professionals. In: *South African health review 2002*. Durban, Health Systems Trust, 2002 (Chapter 8:135–160; http://www.hst.org.za/uploads/files/chapter8.pdf).

97. de Vries E, Reid S. Do South African medical students of rural origin return to rural practice? *South African Medical Journal*, 2003, 93:789–793.

98. National Programme for Family Planning and Primary Health Care, Lady Health Workers, Ministry of Health, Government of Pakistan (www.phc.gov.pk/template.php?id=27, accessed 13 February 2006).

99. Jokhio HR, Winter HR, Cheng KK. An intervention involving traditional birth attendants and perinatal and maternal mortality in Pakistan. *New England Journal of Medicine*, 2005, 352:2091–2099.

100. Douthwaite M, Ward P. Increasing contraceptive use in rural Pakistan: an evaluation of the Lady Health Worker Programme. *Health Policy and Planning*, 2005, 2:117–123.

101. *Evaluation of the Prime Minister's Lady Health Worker Programme*. Oxford, Oxford Policy Management, 2002 (http://www.opml.co.uk/social_policy/health/cn1064_lhw.html, accessed 8 February 2006).

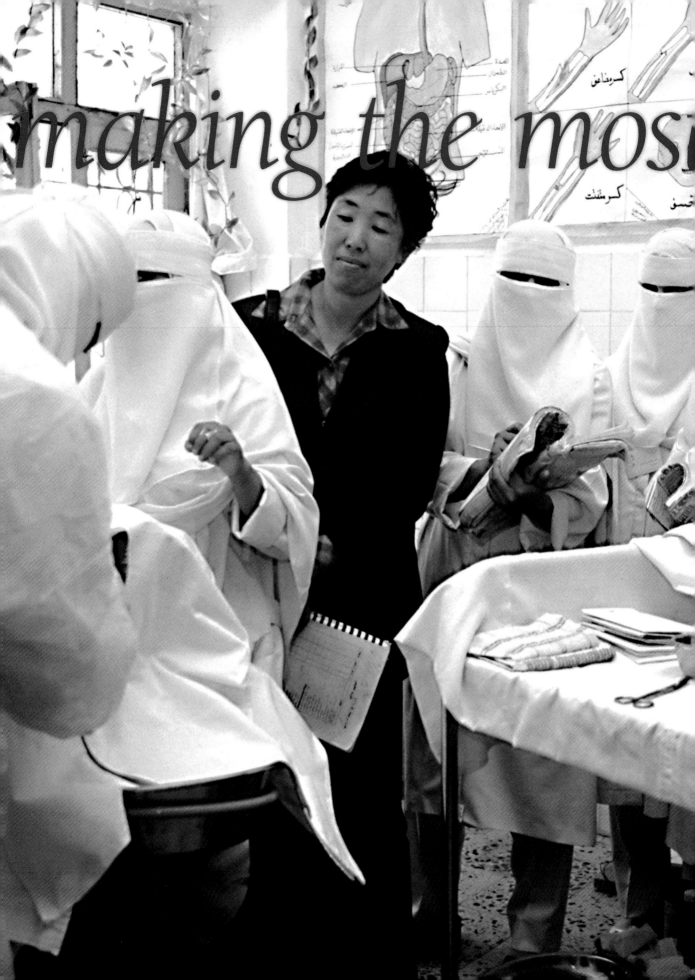

# of existing health workers chapter four

**A country's health workforce is made up of health workers who are at many different stages of their working lives; they work in many different organizations and under changing conditions and pressures. Whatever the circumstances, an effective workforce strategy has to focus on three core challenges: improving recruitment, helping the existing workforce to perform better, and slowing the rate at which workers leave the health workforce. This chapter explores the second of these challenges: optimizing the performance of current workers.**

Strategies to boost worker performance are critical for four reasons:

- They will be likely to show results sooner than strategies to increase numbers.
- The possibilities of increasing the supply of health workers will always be limited.
- A motivated and productive workforce will encourage recruitment and retention.
- Governments have an obligation to society to ensure that limited human and financial resources are used as fairly and as efficiently as possible.

This chapter outlines four dimensions of workforce performance: availability, competence, responsiveness and productivity, and reviews the levers available to improve these different dimensions. Many ways of improving performance exist, some aimed at individual health workers and some directed at the organizations in which they work.

## WHAT IS A WELL-PERFORMING HEALTH WORKFORCE?

Health workforce performance is critical because it has an immediate impact on health service delivery and ultimately on population health. A well-performing workforce is one that works in ways that are responsive, fair and efficient to achieve the best health outcomes possible, given available resources and circumstances.

## Table 4.1 Dimensions of health workforce performance

| Dimension | Description |
| --- | --- |
| Availability | Availability in terms of space and time: encompasses distribution and attendance of existing workers |
| Competence | Encompasses the combination of technical knowledge, skills and behaviours |
| Responsiveness | People are treated decently, regardless of whether or not their health improves or who they are |
| Productivity | Producing the maximum effective health services and health outcomes possible given the existing stock of health workers; reducing waste of staff time or skills |

Evaluations of health workforce performance by the extent to which it contributes to the desired improvement in population health leave no doubt that performance can vary widely. Box 4.1 provides one illustration of how health workers use available financial resources to very different effect on infant mortality, even after controlling for education and poverty in the population. Examining performance this way reveals areas where a workforce is performing well and areas where improvements should be possible, but this method does not explain why performance varies or what can be done about it.

## Box 4.1 Infant mortality and health worker density, Viet Nam

Infant mortality rates were examined in relation to the density of health service providers in 1999. Average results across the provinces are represented by the black points in the figure below. Many provinces, denoted by the red points, do better than expected for their health worker densities – they lie below the black line – while others do less well. More detailed analysis reveals that this is explained, in part, by differences in financial resource availability, measured in terms of health expenditure per capita. An indicator was derived of the efficiency with which health workers in each province use the available financial resources to reduce mortality, controlling for education and poverty. Efficiency ranges from 40% to 99%, raising the question of why health workers in some provinces seem to perform better than in others *(1, 2)*.

Infant mortality rate and per capita density of health professionals, by province, Viet Nam

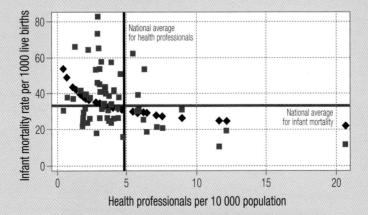

◆ Expected provincial infant mortality rate given available resources (from model).

■ Observed provincial infant mortality rate.

Another approach is to look at four dimensions of workforce performance that are believed to contribute to the achievement of better service delivery and health (see Table 4.1). Looking at the problem this way can help in selecting areas for action.

This simple outline sets the scope for any health workforce strategy and provides a framework for assessing whether or not it is having its desired effects. This framework moves beyond the traditional focus on inputs (having the right number of staff, in the right place, at the right time, with the right skills, and the right support to work *(3))* to consider workforce outputs and outcomes.

What is known about the various dimensions of health workforce performance shown in Table 4.1? Chapter 1 has already outlined what is known about workforce ***availability***, across and within countries. This chapter describes efforts to capture some of the other dimensions more systematically. For all of them data are scarce, especially in lower income countries. However, if countries are to track whether workforce policies are having their desired effects, some metrics of performance are needed. Studies of ***productivity*** in the health sector have been conducted in both rich and poor countries *(4)*. A recent study estimated the potential gains in productivity of existing staff in two African countries could be as much as 35% and 26%, respectively *(5)*. Efforts, ranging from the simple to the sophisticated, are under way to assess the extent to which health workers are ***competent*** *(6–9)*, and

Figure 4.1  Patients' perception of respectful treatment at health facilities in 19 countries

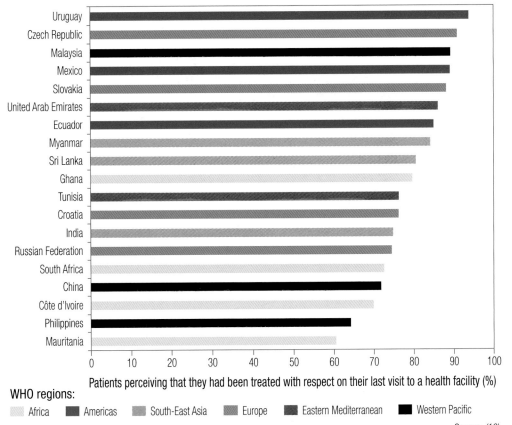

Source: *(10)*.

exhibit aspects of ***responsiveness*** such as respect towards the people they see. Figure 4.1 illustrates results from a survey in 19 countries, which found that the proportion of patients who thought they were treated with respect when they visited health facilities varied from 60% to 90%.

For each dimension of health workforce performance, important differences between health workers may be seen, and policy responses should bear these in mind. Box 4.2 provides one example.

It is difficult to measure and monitor performance and all too easy to manipulate data *(15)*. Many human resource and staffing indicators are routinely collected only in systems with relatively sophisticated information infrastructure. More work is needed to establish which existing indicators could best capture the four dimensions of workforce performance, but Table 4.2 illustrates some possibilities. These four dimensions are a consequence of factors such as staff turnover and motivation. Indicators of the determinants of performance, such as supervision visits and workplace safety, may also be worth measuring.

Many people view feedback on performance not just as a necessity for policy, but also as a powerful tool to influence the behaviour of health workers and organizations if linked to rewards and sanctions. The uses of performance monitoring are discussed later in this chapter.

## WHAT DETERMINES HOW HEALTH WORKERS PERFORM?

To understand why health workers perform differently, it is useful to consider the factors known to influence their work. For many years it was assumed that poor health worker performance was primarily caused by a lack of knowledge and skills. In recent years this perception has changed, and three broad groups of factors are now recognized.

■ *Characteristics of the population being served:* it is simpler to increase immunization coverage or adherence to treatment for tuberculosis or HIV infection where the population understands the benefits and has the motivation and resources to seek services.

■ *Characteristics of health workers themselves,* including their own sociocultural background, knowledge, experience and motivation.

## Box 4.2  Differences in performance of male and female health service providers

Male and female health workers sometimes approach their work and interact with patients in different ways. A recent study in Brazil found that women spent longer in consultation with each child under five years of age (an additional minute, on average) than their male counterparts, even adjusting for other determinants of time inputs such as patient loads. The difference was more pronounced for providers trained in the Integrated Management of Childhood Illness protocols, suggesting that the influence of training might also differ according to the sex of the practitioner *(11)*.

In the United States, women were more likely to undergo screening with Pap smears and mammograms if they were seen by female physicians, and this was more evident with internists and family doctors than with specialist obstetricians and gynaecologists *(12)*. Female patients, especially those seeking gynaecological and obstetric advice, reported greater satisfaction with female than male physicians *(13, 14)*.

Taken together, these findings suggest that certain aspects of the care rendered by women health workers can, in specific circumstances, be more responsive to the needs of patients than the care provided by male physicians. These differences could be important for the development of the health workforce, but need to be better understood.

■ *Characteristics of the health system,* and the wider environment, that determine the conditions under which health workers work. These include the inputs available to them to do their jobs, how the health system is organized, how the workers are paid, supervised and managed, and factors such as their personal safety.

These elements are interconnected. For example, motivation (the level of effort and desire to perform well) is considered by many to be crucial to performance. Motivation is determined both by factors internal to health workers and by factors in their work and social environment *(17).*

Table 4.2 Human resource indicators to assess health workforce performance

| Dimension | Possible indicators |
|---|---|
| Availability | Staff ratios |
| | Absence rates |
| | Waiting time |
| Competence | Individual: prescribing practices |
| | Institutional: readmission rates; live births; cross-infections |
| Responsiveness | Patient satisfaction; assessment of responsiveness |
| Productivity | Occupied beds; outpatient visits; interventions delivered per worker or facility |

Source: *(16).*

## WHAT INFLUENCES HEALTH WORKERS' PERFORMANCE?

Leverage can be applied to stimulate better performance from both individuals and the health workforce as a whole. The main levers available to support performance include a group that are *job related*; those related to the *support systems* that all workers need to do their jobs; and levers that shape and create an *enabling work environment.* It is rare to find a direct relationship between one specific lever and a desired change. Collectively, they make up a checklist of options for policy-makers to consider, from which various instruments have to be selected and combined to meet specific health workforce challenges.

Figure 4.2 summarizes some of the key levers that exist and the characteristics of the workforce that they can collectively influence. Some of these instruments have been found to be relatively easy to implement, others are more complex. Some offer the prospect of relatively early results, others are much longer term. Some are low cost, others are expensive. Some are not exactly policy levers but affect productivity – paying a heating bill, for example, so that a facility is warm enough for staff and patients to use. All of these levers need to be set within a vision for the workforce over the medium to long term. Improvements in workforce performance and productivity usually result from a bundle of linked interventions, rather than uncoordinated or single ones *(18).*

Selecting the right instruments to use and judging when and where to use them, require not just knowledge

Figure 4.2 Levers to influence the four dimensions of health workforce performance

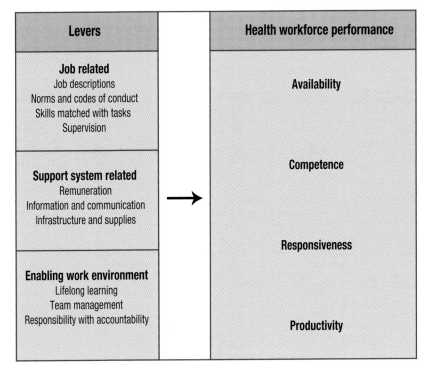

of the instruments themselves, but also an understanding of other important issues that can influence how well the levers work, such as the structure, culture and institutional capacity of the organization concerned, and wider social values and expectations. Action to encourage better performance and productivity can be directed at the individual, team, organization or overall system level *(19)*. Some of these instruments can be introduced within an existing health system by managers of local facilities or services. Others require decisions by higher level authorities or by other sectors – especially if they involve structural change. While it is pragmatic for managers to focus first on one or two things that they can directly influence and that can be changed more easily, there are times when this is inadequate for any substantial improvement in workforce performance and a more comprehensive set of managerial and organizational changes may need to be considered.

The next three sections of the chapter summarize current knowledge about the effectiveness of different levers. For each, four issues of concern to decision-makers are considered: the robustness of the knowledge base, what is known about ease of implementation, the cost, and the time frame for effects to take place. Hard evidence of what works is still limited, but this is no excuse for inaction, given the workforce crisis that is facing many countries. At the same time, this lack of evidence makes two things essential: careful monitoring of trends and effects to allow course corrections as needed, and a much greater effort to evaluate and share findings within and across countries.

### *Job-specific levers*

One set of instruments that influences personnel performance is specific to individual jobs or occupations. These levers include clear job descriptions, professional norms and codes of conduct, the proper matching of skills to the tasks in hand, and supervision *(20–22)*.

## Strategy 4.1 Develop clear job descriptions

Job descriptions that clearly set out objectives, responsibilities, authority and lines of accountability are consistently associated with improved achievement of work goals, for all sorts of worker *(23)*. Moreover, moves to develop clear job descriptions can produce quite rapid effects. A programme jointly undertaken by WHO and the Ministry of Health in Indonesia has demonstrated that establishment of clear job descriptions, along with better in-service training and clearer standards, can enhance job satisfaction and compliance with standards among nurses and midwives (see Box 4.3). Health workers in many countries still lack proper job descriptions, so this strategy has widespread potential.

## Strategy 4.2 Support norms and codes of conduct

The performance of health workers, in terms of both competence and responsiveness, is also influenced by their sense of professional identity, vocation and work ethic. There are many instances of health workers continuing to provide care despite difficult and sometimes dangerous working conditions. Some ways of sustaining or, where necessary, creating values, standards and aspirations are outlined below.

The notion of "professionalism" and vocation in health has a long history. Almost every doctor and patient has heard of the Hippocratic Oath, which is the longest surviving ethical code of conduct. It is still sworn by many medical graduates. Health workers are expected to conduct themselves with integrity, selflessly to apply technical know-how and to put the interests of the patient above their own *(30, 31)*. Professional codes of conduct are often instilled through unwritten channels and take time to develop, but can become a significant source of internal motivation.

One of the functions of professional associations is to foster this sense of valued professional identity and hence responsibility and higher morale *(32)*. For more "modern" professions, such as management, professional associations are relatively new (for example, the European Health Management Association has existed for only 25 years) and still do not exist in many countries. Creating professional associations may be a desirable long-term strategy, but they take time to establish. The creation of associations for more informal providers such as drug-sellers has also been tried as a means of bringing their activities more into line with accepted good practice.

> *"The performance of health workers is influenced by their sense of professional identity, vocation and work ethic"*

In very poor countries, coping strategies by health workers to deal with difficult living conditions may become so prevalent that maintenance of professional ethos is threatened. Box 4.3 explains how health workers in two countries perceive the problem.

Many employers are now introducing explicit written codes of conduct for all their employees, stating, for example, that they should arrive at work on time, treat patients with dignity and respect, and provide them with full information. The effectiveness of such codes has not been documented (and is usually only one aspect of a larger package of managerial interventions) but logic suggests that their effectiveness will depend on the extent to which they are communicated and enforced.

More formal instruments are also used to steer the behaviour of health workers in a desired direction. For example, a government might introduce a regulation that no private practice by public sector health workers is allowed during working hours in public facilities. To have the desired effect, such rules and regulations need to be well publicized, and action taken when they are broken. Licensing and accreditation are other tools to promote standards of care of existing workers and the institutions to which they belong. The effectiveness of formal regulations is often limited because the institutional capacity to enforce them is just not there. This problem is discussed further in Chapter 6.

## Strategy 4.3 Match skills to tasks

In rich and poor countries alike and in all types of facilities, numerous examples exist of ways in which the skills of individual health workers or the skill mix within the workforce as a whole are being inefficiently used. Common reasons for this include the following:

- Tasks do not match an individual worker's skills – for example, skilled nurses doing clerical tasks because there are no ward clerks. The opposite also occurs: for example, due to skill shortages, management tasks being carried out by scarce medical personnel, who have no specific expertise in these areas; or untrained personnel carrying out skilled tasks such as birth delivery and other interventions *(33, 34)*.
- Certain tasks consume an excessive amount of time, such as hosting missions and reporting.
- Workers are not always at work at the times when the workload is highest, i.e. when their skills would be most productive.

Some examples of skill mismatches are given in Box 4.3.

Often countries with the scarcest human resources have the greatest demands made on their health workers' time by external agencies. This problem concerns senior policy-makers, managers and clinical staff. The Paris Declaration on aid effectiveness has a set of principles for harmonization and alignment with partner countries' systems and procedures that has been endorsed by ministers and development institutions *(35)*. Many health agencies and partnerships are now examining how to put these principles into practice *(36)*. External agencies have a golden opportunity to free up some time for health workers, for example by harmonizing review missions and training courses or by aligning overlapping reporting demands.

Shift patterns and time flexibility could provide another way to increase worker productivity. This strategy could potentially achieve a better match between staffing levels and workload at limited cost, but there are virtually no evaluations from developing countries *(18)*.

Finally, skill delegation or task shifting is another way to increase overall workforce productivity that has received much attention. Most actual experience comes from substitution of physicians by nurses, and from English-speaking countries *(37)*. Chapter 2 provides examples of instances where skill delegation is being adopted.

## Box 4.3 Job-related challenges to improving health worker performance

**Develop clear job descriptions: Indonesia**
In 2000, a survey of 856 nurses and midwives in five provinces found that 47.4% nurses and midwives did not have written job descriptions, 39.8% were engaged in work other than nursing care or midwifery and 70.9% had not received in-service training for the past three years. A Clinical Performance Development Management System was developed: it created clear job descriptions that outlined responsibilities and accountability, provided in-service training consisting primarily of reflective case discussions, and put in place a performance monitoring system. Staff benefiting from the programme reported that the job descriptions, together with standards of operations and procedures, had given them greater confidence about their roles and responsibilities. The participating hospitals also reported that the programme helped to ensure quality and facilitate hospital accreditation *(24)*.

**Maintaining professional values: tensions and suggested solutions from Cape Verde and Mozambique**
A study of how health workers perceive the difficulty of maintaining professional values found that they experience a conflict between their self-image of what it means to be an honest civil servant who wants to do a decent job, and the realities of life that make them betray that image. For example, misuse of access to pharmaceuticals has become a key element in the coping strategies that some health personnel employ to boost their income. The authors conclude that this ambiguity indicates that the opportunity to intervene still exists, and that this should be sooner rather than later before practices become too entrenched. Respondents' suggestions to change the situation included:

improved and tighter management of stock, improved working conditions, informing the population about such practices, and appeals to people's personal and professional values *(25)*.

**Match skills to tasks: examples of mismatches**
A study in the United Republic of Tanzania estimated that 40–50% of a district medical officer's time was being spent on report writing and 20% on hosting missions *(26)*. In Uganda, district managers estimated that they spend 70–80% of their time on planning, reporting and training workshops. This left little time for implementation of activities *(27)*. A survey of hospitals in Washington, DC, United States, showed that for every hour of patient care in an emergency care department there was one hour of paperwork *(28)*.

**Exercise supportive supervision: Ghana**
In quasi-government hospitals, the supervisors' role was the linchpin of performance enhancement: keener pressure and their perceived knowledge of technical processes kept service providers on their toes, with the supervisor themselves feeling more direct pressure to ensure good performance/outputs (for example, to retain their position, financial incentives and other benefits). In the public hospitals studied, supervisors seemed to have less authority and performance emphasis seemed to be placed on behaviours such as obedience, punctuality and respectfulness rather than on performance of technical tasks. Systems for reorientation of supervisors and for formal performance appraisal of productivity of supervisors rather than directly on service providers may be useful *(29)*.

In some cases, professional resistance and the need for changes in legislation can delay implementation.

## Strategy 4.4 Exercise supportive supervision

Supervision, especially coupled with audit and feedback to staff, has been consistently found to improve the performance of many types of health workers, from providers to managers *(21, 38)*. While the intent to supervise is almost universal, it often proves difficult to put into practice and becomes the first casualty in the list of priorities for busy and resource-constrained managers. Supervision often becomes more difficult but even more important in health systems that are decentralizing. Ministry central managers, for example, may be perceived as no longer having the authority to supervise districts, or their posts may have been transferred.

> *Supervision that is supportive and helps to solve specific problems can improve performance, job satisfaction and motivation*

When it does take place, the *nature* of the supervision is important. If supervisory visits become sterile administrative events, or are seen as fault-finding and punitive, they have little positive effect and may have negative effects. In contrast, supervision that is supportive, educational and consistent and helps to solve specific problems, can improve performance, job satisfaction and motivation. Good supervision made a difference in staff motivation and performance between public hospitals and autonomous quasi-government hospitals in Ghana (see Box 4.3).

Strategies to improve supervision tend to neglect three groups, all of whom perform better with supervision. The first of these groups consists of supervisors themselves; the second consists of lay health care providers, be they families or community health workers with more formal roles, who often work alone; and last but not least are private providers, who in many low income countries receive virtually no supervision at all. The challenge is to find ways to oversee performance that will be accepted by independent, self-employed practitioners. Supervision is one element in various strategies being explored to engage private and informal providers in the delivery of commodities and services. In the example of social franchising projects, franchisees such as drug sellers obtain certain benefits, for example subsidized supplies, and in return accept – among other things – to be supervised by the franchiser *(39)*.

### Basic support systems

Every health worker needs some key supports to perform his or her job: remuneration, information, and infrastructure, including equipment and supplies. This section does not provide a comprehensive review of the systems that deliver these supports, but focuses on features that have particular relevance to enhancing health workforce performance.

## Strategy 4.5 Ensure appropriate remuneration

Three aspects of remuneration influence the behaviour of health workers: the level and regularity of pay, the way people are paid, and other incentives.

Health workers must be paid reasonably for the work they do. They need to receive a living wage; they also need to believe that the wage is commensurate with their responsibilities and that it is fair when compared with others in the same or equivalent jobs.

## Box 4.4 Differences in salaries between countries, professions, sectors and sexes

### (a) Cross-country comparisons of annual salaries of physicians and nurses

Doctors and nurses in poor countries earn less than their counterparts in most high income countries, even after accounting for differences in the purchasing power of earnings, so substantial financial incentives exist for them to emigrate. In figure (a), annual salaries are plotted against GDP per capita in international dollars. Available data usually concern doctors and nurses only.

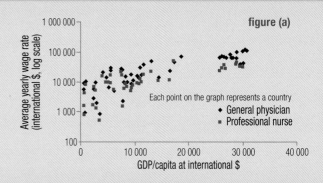

figure (a)

Each point on the graph represents a country
◆ General physician
■ Professional nurse

Average yearly wage rate (international $, log scale)

GDP/capita at international $

### (b) Salary differentials between comparable professions

Differentials in the salaries of health professionals also vary within countries. Salaries can be compared between equivalent professions, public and private sectors, and men and women doing the same job. For countries with available data, the monthly salary of a teacher is typically 1–1.5 times the salary of a nurse (see figure (b)) though in Costa Rica, Estonia and the United States nurses reportedly earn more than teachers. Engineers are paid more than doctors, sometimes substantially more, in most low income countries, for example Bolivia, Côte d'Ivoire and Honduras. In general, this balance is different in countries with incomes per capita above US$ 10 000 (as in Australia, Slovakia and the United States), so that here doctors are paid more on average.

### (c) Comparisons of salaries between the public and private sectors

Such comparisons are sparse. Certainly not all private sector workers are necessarily highly paid: for example, one study found that around 14% (Latvia) and 50% (Georgia) of private sector health workers were paid at or below the minimum wage.

### (d) Ratio of wages (PPP US$), men to women

Likewise, few data are available on differences in earnings between men and women. Figure (c) illustrates salary differentials by sex in four OECD countries: in three of them there seems to be parity across the five occupations studied. The most rigorous cross-country study available suggests that the small differences that exist can be explained by differences in the number of hours worked, type of speciality and seniority. This general finding could well hide considerable variation across countries.

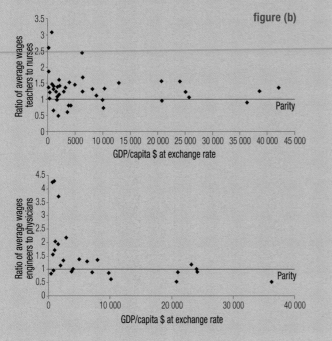

figure (b)

Ratio of average wages teachers to nurses

GDP/capita $ at exchange rate

Parity

Ratio of average wages engineers to physicians

GDP/capita $ at exchange rate

Parity

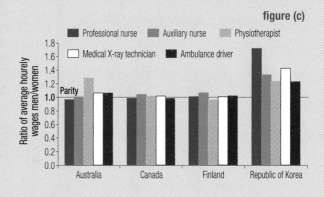

figure (c)

■ Professional nurse    ■ Auxiliary nurse    ▨ Physiotherapist
□ Medical X-ray technician    ■ Ambulance driver

Ratio of average hourly wages men/women

Parity

Australia    Canada    Finland    Republic of Korea

Sources: *(44–49)*. Data from most recent year available.

Underpayment and a sense of unfair differences stunt productivity and performance *(40)*. Public sector health workers have developed many coping strategies to deal with salaries that are unrealistically low, or intermittent: dual or multiemployment, absences and ghost workers; informal payments; referring patients to the private sector; and migration to better labour markets *(25, 41–43)*.

*Raising salaries* in the public sector can be difficult and costly. In some cases ministries of finance set public expenditure ceilings; salary levels may be set for all civil servants by public service commissions, who consider it unfair or unwise to raise salaries in one sector alone, or simply lack the ability to do so. Furthermore, for some particularly skilled and scarce health workers, the public sector may simply be unable to match salaries offered by the private sector or that are found overseas. Not all private sector workers are highly paid, however; in some countries, a significant proportion of workers in the private sector are paid at or below the minimum wage *(44)*. Various comparisons of salaries are described in Box 4.4.

So what can be done? Despite the difficulties, a number of low income countries have dramatically increased the pay of public health workers in recent years. In the United Republic of Tanzania, for example, the Selective Accelerated Salary Enhancement scheme provided an opportunity for ministries to raise levels of remuneration for high priority groups *(15)*. In Uganda, salaries were increased in 2004 for all health workers following a job evaluation exercise across the whole public service, which used a standard set of criteria (such as length of training, cost of errors, and working hours) to rank jobs and set their associated salary scales. As a consequence, the salaries of the lowest level nurse almost doubled and became equivalent to that of a new university graduate *(42)*. Given the cost of salaries, there has recently been increasing acceptance by external agencies that salary support will be needed in very low income countries for the medium term (see Box 2.2).

Some countries have made efforts to remove health workers from the civil service pay structure, to allow for more freedom in the setting of pay and conditions of service. Zambia tried this approach but it was resisted by professional groups and eventually lost momentum. In Ghana, tax-collectors and bank employees have been successfully de-linked from the civil service, but health workers have not *(15)*.

Unpaid salaries present a problem in many countries, from eastern Europe to Africa *(50)*, and may provoke absenteeism. Salaries sometimes remain unpaid because human resources management and payroll systems are not working properly. There is no hard evidence on the effects of investing in functioning administrative systems. However, bolstering this essential ingredient for workforce management may be easier to act on than other more politically charged workforce reforms, need not be costly, and could provide relatively quick and significant results. A second cause of unpaid salaries is lack of funds. In Chad, donor funds have been successfully used to guarantee timely payment for health workers who were previously experiencing delays of 4–7 months *(50)*.

*The way people are paid* makes a major difference to what they deliver. Individual health workers, and the facilities in which they work, can be paid in many different ways. For each, pay may be time-based (salaries or fixed budgets), service-based (fee for service) or population-based (per capita payments or block contracts) *(51)*. Both facility-based and individual payment mechanisms can

> " *Unpaid salaries present a problem in many countries, from eastern Europe to Africa* "

influence how individuals perform. Experience shows that salaries and fixed budgets lead to providers reducing the number of patients seen and services provided, whereas fee-for-service payments encourage incentives for providers to see more cases; offer more services, and deliver more expensive services. Each payment mechanism also has different administrative implications, from simple to more complex *(52)*. Optimal payment systems induce providers to give high-quality, effective treatment while promoting a rational allocation of resources *(40)*.

Middle and upper income countries, including Australia, Hungary, the United Kingdom, and the United States, have been moving away from input-based budgets and salaries towards performance-related pay based on outputs and outcomes *(53–55)*. Mixed provider payment systems have become more common to balance the different incentives each mechanism creates. Robinson's study of physician organizations in the United States found that approximately a quarter of physicians were paid on a purely retrospective basis (fee-for-service), another quarter on a purely prospective basis (capitation, non-productivity-based salary) and about half on a mix of the two *(48)*. Some evidence suggests that performance-related pay can lead to improvements in the quality of care provided *(56, 57)*.

The idea of introducing performance-related pay in lower income countries has gained popularity recently, for the same reasons that this approach is used in richer countries. However, experience remains very limited. In most lower income countries the majority of public health workers still receive salaries together with allowances unrelated to performance, whereas in the private sector the fee-for-service system is more prevalent. The limited introduction of this mechanism may stem in part from the fact that payment methods with stronger incentives for quality, consumer satisfaction, equity or efficiency tend to have higher administrative costs and require greater administrative capacity *(52)*.

The use of **other sources of income**, such as allowances, to increase job attractiveness – whether in general or only in underserved areas – exists in virtually all countries. Types of supplementary pay and allowances valued by health workers include: contract-signing bonuses; reimbursement of job-related expenses such as uniforms and petrol; education, accommodation, transport or child care subsidies;

## Box 4.5 Incentives to enhance health workers' performance

**Thailand.** In the 1990s, payment reforms to improve the availability of health workers in rural areas included: supplements to doctors in eight priority specialties and services who worked in rural areas; non-private practice compensation for doctors, dentists and pharmacists; monthly salary supplements to doctors, pharmacists, dentists and nurses in district hospitals and health centres; and overtime and night shift payments. These supplements were combined with other non-financial incentives. Over time, the availability of health workers in rural areas has improved *(64)*.

**Mali.** In 1986, the Ministry of Health introduced a strategy, which continues today, to encourage newly graduated doctors to serve in rural areas. Doctors are contracted to work in underserved areas to deliver the minimum health package stipulated in the National Health Policy, either as

part of a public health centre which has no doctor, or as a private practitioner. The two sectors have different payment mechanisms but similar non-financial benefits: public sector doctors receive a salary plus a share of facility revenue; private doctors are paid on a fee-for-service basis but the fee level is based on local ability to pay. All participants receive some initial training, plus accommodation, equipment and transport if needed. In addition, all are expected to join the Medical Association and be part of a peer learning network. By 2004, 80 doctors (from Mali's estimated total medical stock of 529) had joined this scheme and were working in rural areas, where some had been for over five years. An assessment in 2001 found that service coverage in rural facilities with a doctor was higher than in those without *(65)*.

health insurance; access to loans (e.g. subsidized mortgages); per diem payments while on training courses; allowances for working in remote areas or out of hours (overtime and night shifts); and specific service output incentives (e.g. for immunization) *(58)*.

Doctors and nurses are often the main beneficiaries of income supplements. In the United States, tuition reimbursement or contract-signing bonuses are commonly used to attract nurses. In Jamaica, health insurance, paid vacation and transport are often offered to nurses *(59)*; while benefits in Botswana include housing, car loans and medical aid *(60)*.

How well these measures work depends on how they are designed and implemented and what other incentives are in place. Objectives and target groups need to be defined, and in some cases incentives must be negotiated with unions; they must also be viewed as fair. Over time they may come to be seen as entitlements rather than incentives, and their effects may change *(61)*. Well-intentioned incentives can have unintended, perverse effects *(58, 62)*. In Ghana, for example, the additional duty hour allowance introduced for doctors and nurses was resented by nurses, because of the perceived or real disparities in the gains, and is thought to have contributed to the increased migration of nurses *(63)*.

***Packages of incentives*** are often required to balance the different effects of individual financial (and non-financial) incentives. In Thailand, for example, efforts to improve the availability of doctors in rural areas have involved several types of additional payment, as well as educational, infrastructure and social strategies *(32)* (see Box 4.5 for two examples). Studies of "magnet institutions" – those which are successful in recruiting, retaining and motivating nursing staff – in the United Kingdom and the United States, found that critical factors include good human resources management and quality of care *(66)*. These are discussed further later in the chapter. All incentives require regular monitoring and adjustment to changing "push and pull" factors: Thailand has employed different tools at different times to improve and maintain the availability of health workers in rural areas.

No discussion of remuneration would be complete without acknowledging that in many countries, in all continents, informal payments provide a major source of income for health workers and thus exert major influences on behaviour towards their clients *(42, 67)*. There is no easy way to address the problem of informal payments but there are encouraging examples. In Cameroon, the government introduced a scheme that is now in place in all larger health facilities. It included: having a single point of payment for patients at the facility; clearly displaying the fees and the rules about payment to patients, and telling them where to report any transgressions; using the fees to give bonuses to health workers, but excluding them from the bonus scheme if they break the rules, and publishing names of those receiving bonuses and those removed from the scheme. A key factor in the success of this scheme has been a strong facility manager who enforces the rules fairly *(43)*.

The above points concerning remuneration of health workers can be summed up as follows:

■ Secure the minimum: a living wage that arrives on time!
■ When it comes to worker performance, pay matters. External agencies could help to improve worker performance in low income countries by providing salary support for the medium term.

> *Doctors and nurses are often the main beneficiaries of income supplements*

■ A mix of payment systems and incentives should be used where possible. If institutional capacity is limited, caution should be exercised in adopting approaches with complex administrative requirements.

■ Salary increases alone are not enough to change performance. These must be combined with other strategies to create significant change.

■ Any incentives or remuneration policies must always be monitored and adapted over time to ensure that they produce the desired outcomes.

## Strategy 4.6 Ensure adequate information and communication

A well-known adage states that you manage what you measure. Evidence shows that having information does help health workers to do their jobs better, as long as certain provisos are met: the information must be relevant to the job and available when needed, and workers must have a degree of confidence in the information's quality and understand what it is "saying" *(21, 68)*. Health workers at different levels need different sorts of information from many sources: medical records, facility activity reports, financial accounts, health workforce inventories and payrolls, population-based survey data and scientific literature, to name just a few. A well-functioning national information system is a key ingredient to improving workforce performance.

Any specific efforts to improve ***overall workforce*** productivity need to be based on reliable data about workforce level, distribution and skill mix, coupled with information on the factors thought to be constraining better health worker performance and intelligence on potential policy options.

In some instances, ***individual provider*** productivity has been improved with communication technologies that help health workers to deliver services. There is a growing amount of evidence to suggest that these technologies can lead to productivity gains in the health workforce by improving the way workers provide clinical and public health services. Examples are given in Box 4.6.

Many organizational, legal, infrastructural, social and financial barriers to the widespread use of modern information and communication technology remain, especially

## Box 4.6 Using modern communication technology to improve data, services and productivity

In well-off countries, health workers increasingly use modern communication technology to provide care, and studies have demonstrated increases in their productivity as a result. The use of telephones to remind high-risk individuals about influenza immunization *(69)* and mammography among managed health care plan members resulted in a significant increase in uptake of these preventive interventions, without any other apparent changes in the workforce *(70)*. Computer-generated telephone reminders have also been effective in improving medication adherence and blood pressure control in hypertension patients *(71)*.

There is evidence that computer-based patient records can improve patient care, outcomes and costs. Computerized reminder systems to alert health care staff to repeat tests have reduced the number of patients subjected to unnecessary repeat testing, while automatic systems communicating critical laboratory results reduced the time for

getting appropriate treatment when compared with the existing paging systems *(72–74)*. The need for chronic care of HIV/AIDS patients has triggered an exploration of models for resource-poor settings, which are being piloted in a number of low income countries.

Handheld computers are powerful data collection tools, providing rapid access to information needed to prevent or respond to disease outbreaks. They can furnish data at the point of need, even in the absence of Internet or telephone connectivity. For example, a Red Cross survey team gathering data for measles immunization in Ghana using such devices processed 10 times more questionnaires than usual, and returned results to the Ministry of Health with unprecedented ease and speed. For more information, see http://www.satellife.org/ictinhealth.php.

in low income settings *(75)*. In some cases, these technologies may be viewed as magic bullets to solve problems that need quite different solutions. Nevertheless, it will be important to keep a critical but open mind to their potential: the explosion in the use of mobile telephones in low income countries shows how quickly a new technology can be adopted in countries where traditional communication infrastructure is weak or unaffordable. Simple communication methods such as newsletters and helplines also have a role to play in improving access to information.

### Strategy 4.7 Improve infrastructure and supplies

No matter how motivated and skilled health workers are, they cannot do their jobs properly in facilities that lack clean water, adequate lighting, heating, vehicles, drugs, working equipment and other supplies *(76–78)*. Two examples illustrate the consequences. In Niger, nurses at health centres were reported to be reluctant to refer patients to district hospitals because only three of the 33 hospitals provided surgical care, most of them could not give blood transfusions or oxygen, and laboratory and X-ray facilities were rudimentary *(79)*. In Kyrgyzstan, health professionals in primary care providing diabetes care said that their job was hampered by a lack of testing strips, machines to measure blood sugar, weak laboratories and irregular supplies of insulin *(77)*. Drugs being out of stock is a familiar problem to many health workers (see Table 4.3).

Hard evidence for the performance benefits of improving basic infrastructure and supplies is very thin *(81)* but it seems highly likely that such improvements – once in place – could create significant, almost immediate gains. For example, paying a utility bill so that the electricity or heating is turned on again may make a quicker difference to productivity than any more specific performance management tool. Costs are likely to be variable: some would be unique outlays and some recurring. A simple and obvious, but sometimes overlooked, way to determine the actions that will create the largest and most immediate improvements is to ask the health workers themselves.

The physical work environment also needs to be safe, and health workers themselves need to be provided with health care when sick. Aspects of safety are discussed in Chapter 5.

Functioning support systems require consideration of the management and support workers discussed in Chapter 1, such as store managers, accounts clerks, information officers, equipment technicians, hospital administrators and personnel and

> *When looking for ways to improve performance, we have found nothing works so well as talking to health workers themselves. Their ideas are just amazing. They will tell you what to do*
> **Director of human resources in Africa**

### Table 4.3 Pharmaceutical situations in public health facilities in Africa and South-East Asia

| Indicator | Africa[a] | South-East Asia[a] |
|---|---|---|
| Average number of days during which key medicines were out of stock in the preceding year | 25 | 19 |
| Percentage of facilities meeting basic conservation conditions required to maintain medicine quality | 75% | 75% |
| Percentage of dispensed medicines adequately labelled | 71% | 87% |

[a]Median, seven countries in each region.

Source: *(80)*.

procurement managers. These workers are often neglected in workforce discussions, but are critical to scaling up service delivery.

### An enabling work environment

Three general types of levers can be used to promote an enabling work environment. Most involve the managerial culture and organizational arrangements within which health care providers work. They are grouped as follows: lifelong learning, team management and team working, and responsibility with accountability

### Strategy 4.8 Promote lifelong learning

Health workers require up-to-date knowledge to perform well, as has been mentioned in Chapter 3. Rapid increases in knowledge and changing health systems make this need even more essential today. This is a field full of experimentation, but some clear and straightforward messages have emerged.

Individual needs vary widely. Basic workers with only weeks of pre-service training have different learning needs from doctors or nurses with a decade or more of education and experience. Nurses in rural Switzerland clearly deal with very different everyday challenges than those in rural Malawi. Nevertheless, some common principles underlie any strong approach to professional development. Table 4.4 summarizes some individual and workplace-wide approaches.

Formal one-off, off-site training courses have a poor track record for changing the actual practice of health workers. In-service training is most likely to change worker behaviour when it is interactive, based on real-life problems and coupled with continuing, intermittent support.

To illustrate this fact, although the use of oral rehydration salts for childhood diarrhoea greatly increased in the 1980s and 1990s, after more than 2000 training courses on case management and supervision from 1988 to 1993 in over 120 countries, the median percentage of children correctly rehydrated by health workers (from 22 surveys) was only 20% (21). Simple, low-cost approaches that follow the principles of interactive, realistic training with adequate continuing support can be very effective (38). These lessons have been translated into the more encompassing, long-term concept of continuous professional development or lifelong learning. Con-

## Box 4.7 What sort of training works best?

If performance change is the goal, exclusively didactic approaches, conferences and activities without any practice have little or no role to play (83, 84). Evidence suggests that there is more probability of knowledge and skills transfer into practice when the training course is interactive with as much hands-on real-life experience as possible. Interactive courses improve prescribing or dispensing behaviour (85–88), improve specific clinical skills (89–90) and positively effect health care utilization while promoting favourable patient responses (91). Active learning opportunities, sequenced learning, after-training support, reminders and multifaceted activities are effective (92, 93). Distance education is shown to increase knowledge (94), knowledge-seeking behaviour (95), self-confidence (96) and positive attitudes in three studies, though no effect on behaviour change was observed. When a videoconference-type training session was compared with in-class face-to-face training, there was no difference in knowledge accumulation (97). The most convincing evidence for distance education is a study which shows that a 10-month distance education course, supported with 1–2 contacts by tutors, caused a significant increase in correct assessment of diarrhoea cases (98).

## Table 4.4 Approaches to professional development and performance

| Training | Individual | Team or organization-based |
|---|---|---|
| **Intermittent** | Training courses | Retreats |
| **Continuous** | Continuous professional development | Wide array of approaches with similar principles but many different labels, e.g. total quality management, tools and techniques |
| **Distance learning** | Web-based training and access to literature | Teleconferencing, collaborating workspaces, other web-based groupware |

tinuous professional development can be simply defined as a "systematic, ongoing, cyclical process of self-directed learning" for individuals. Such an approach goes beyond training to include, for example, career paths, feedback from others, mentoring and secondment (82). Distance education in its various forms also deserves further exploration, given the geographical distribution of the many health professionals in need of continuous professional development. Box 4.7 presents some of the options for educational opportunities.

Experience clearly shows that simply disseminating guidelines is ineffective. If guidelines are passively distributed, few people read them, even if they are followed by reminder visits (99–104). When guidelines are distributed during a training course, however, and supported by peer groups to discuss the content and to provide audit and feedback to participants or associated with subsequent supervisory visits, they are significantly more likely to be implemented (105–107).

In recent years, attention has shifted to multifaceted packages of iterative, on-the-job support, with an emphasis on ways to encourage translation of new knowledge

## Box 4.8 Quality assurance, supervision and monitoring in Uganda

Since 1994 Uganda's Ministry of Health has engaged in vigorous quality assurance, supervision and monitoring of districts and sub-districts through the following approaches:
- creation of a Quality Assurance Department;
- development and dissemination of standards and guidelines;
- initial workshops to assist administrators, political leaders and clinical staff with identifying and solving common service-related problems;
- support visits by multidisciplinary teams;
- quarterly supervisory visits with routine monitoring (of finance and planning, for example) and one special focus area such as malaria or child health;
- supervision that is supportive, non-punitive, and exercised in an atmosphere of trust;
- verbal feedback and summary reports with key issues highlighted and action plans agreed on.

The programme includes routine monitoring of indicators at national and district levels, and benchmarking of progress towards the achievement of the national strategic plan. Public service providers and nongovernmental organizations are monitored, but not the private sector.

To provide incentives for improvement, Uganda's Ministry of Health has put in place an award system called the Yellow Star Programme. District health facilities complying fully with the 35 standards considered the best indicators for overall management now receive a plaque in the form of a five-pointed yellow star, along with official recognition and publicity. Forty-seven districts now participate.

Uganda's efforts have resulted in better coordination between health services and local administrators and political leaders. The 2003/4 health sector review found that some districts are performing much better than others, and that unexpectedly, poor and rural districts are not necessarily poor performers. In interviews conducted across Uganda, the view was widely expressed that good performance stems at least in part from good management, especially in a supportive political environment (112).

into changed practices. Such approaches can be judged in many ways, including the quality of services and productivity. Recently, a wide array of programmes has emerged with different labels, degrees of complexity, tools and techniques, but mostly following a similar set of principles. Some focus on individuals and others on organization-wide or team-based approaches – where the team may be a work unit of mixed staff or a group of professionals, such as managers, who share the same responsibilities in different places.

Teamwork and processes such as joint development of guidelines and peer review can be moderately successful in improving health worker performance. The observed benefits of teamwork include improved staff well-being (108, 109) and better quality of care (110). Evidence of the effectiveness of organization-wide approaches to achieve sustained improvements in services is limited. For example, in the United Kingdom and the United States, total quality management approaches have shown mixed results (111). Many forms of quality improvement projects have taken place in low income countries with successes reported (see Box 4.8) – but rigorous evaluations are few (21). Ultimately, of course, the most suitable approach depends on the specific needs and objectives of the workforce.

## Strategy 4.9 Establish effective team management

Along with the shift in approaches to professional development has come a rising recognition that important gaps exist in the scope of the current response. Over the years most attention has focused on knowledge and skills for clinical services, rather than on more generic skills needed to make health systems work, such as management, accounting, procurement and logistics. Some "softer" managerial skills such as team building and negotiation have also received little attention. As a result, many low income countries receiving large amounts of additional funds to scale up services rapidly are facing some basic skill deficits in such areas as simple accounting, drug stock and store management, and basic personnel management. Health system reorganizations may also create a need for new skills. This has been the case in Kyrgyzstan (see Box 4.9), while health reforms in Chile and the United Kingdom increased the need for skilled managers (113, 114).

People respond positively to a host of non-financial incentives that can be collectively captured under the rubric of good management or leadership, terms which are often used interchangeably (116). Whether called management or leadership, these skills benefit health workers at every level of a health system. Limited but positive evidence suggests that the factors listed below may improve individual or organizational

## Box 4.9 Changing tasks and therefore skill needs

In Kyrgyzstan, funds used to be allocated to facilities based on bed and staff numbers. Reforms introduced in 1997 have changed the system from this passive budgeting approach to one relying on active or strategic purchasing of personal health care services. A new agency, the Mandatory Health Insurance Fund (MHIF), pays inpatient facilities on a per case basis and primary care practices by capitation. The hospital payment reforms have involved completely new processes of information management, financial management, and quality control to ensure that contracted providers are paid and that the services provided are appropriate and of good quality. A critical new function performed by the MHIF is utilization review which involves checking claims to protect against fraud while contributing to quality improvement. This has led to the need for a new set of skills: in computer programming, data processing, analysis of clinical data, and the ability to discuss and negotiate with providers on the basis of those analyses (113).

performance (*56, 117–123*). Health workers are more motivated to perform well when their organization and managers:

- provide a clear sense of vision and mission;
- make people feel recognized and valued whatever their job;
- listen to staff and increase their participation in decisions – they often have solutions;
- encourage teamwork, mentoring and coaching;
- encourage innovation and appropriate independence;
- create a culture of benchmarking and comparison;
- provide career structures and opportunities for promotion that are transparent and fair;
- give feedback on, and reward, good performance – even with token benefits;
- use available sanctions for poor performance in ways that are fair and consistent.

> " *These evaluations are a source of motivation for us; if we get a good grade we make even greater efforts to keep our rank or to go even further* "
>
> **Public sector manager, Benin**

Good managers reward their staff. Some examples of non-financial rewards that may be used are: tea during night duty, holidays and days off, flexible working hours, access to and support for training and education, sabbaticals, study leave, and planned career breaks. Some examples of management and leadership are mentioned in Box 4.10.

The introduction of performance appraisal systems, such as Zambia's Performance Improvement Review system and Malawi's Performance Contract scheme, are becoming more common. How effective is performance audit and feedback (*126*)? There are many examples of successful projects, but large-scale evidence that such schemes improve service quality, productivity or health outcomes is still scarce (*15*). A major review of experience with audit and feedback in high income countries concluded that these tools can be effective in improving professional practice but their effect is small to moderate (*127*). Assessment of facility performance is also becoming more common, but experience is still scarce in low income settings.

## Box 4.10 The importance of management and leadership

**South Africa.** Nurses working in maternal health services were asked about the most important characteristics of the workplace and presented with 16 theoretical workplace profiles. The most significant finding was that good management (e.g. clearly defined responsibilities, supportive attitude when mistakes are made, rewarding ability and not length of service) outranked salary as a preference, unless the remuneration was dramatically higher. These results reinforce other research demonstrating the effect of good management on employment choices and job satisfaction among health workers *(124)*.

**Leadership for Change programme.** The International Council of Nurses (ICN) has set up a programme to develop nurses as effective leaders and managers in a constantly changing health environment. The Leadership for Change methodology and key strategic goals are designed to assist them at a country or organizational level to participate effectively in health policy development and decision-making, become effective leaders and managers in nursing and health services, prepare future nurse managers and leaders for key positions, and influence changes in nursing curricula so that future nurses are prepared appropriately.

Nurses in more than 50 low and middle income countries have gained the knowledge, skills and strategies they need to take leadership roles in nursing and health systems, build partnerships, and improve health care through participation in this programme. Evaluations indicate that graduates are involved in a range of nursing leadership roles, with an increase in nurse leaders' influence, ability to build sustainable partnerships, and ability to develop new models of nursing to improve quality of patient care *(125)*.

As for implementation, introduction of the changes mentioned here is not necessarily costly, but neither is it necessarily straightforward. For example, a study on performance management of district health managers in nine Latin American countries found that teamwork was difficult to introduce into a health system that promotes hierarchical structure and favours an authoritative management style *(128)*.

### Strategy 4.10 Combine responsibility with accountability

Giving local managers at least some freedom in the allocation of funds can make a big difference to staff and facility performance, as these managers can then quickly deal with local problems unknown to higher level managers *(129)*. Mechanisms to hold health workers accountable for their actions are another way to improve productivity and performance *(130)*.

Services can be organized in many different ways, but managers cannot manage them properly if they are not given at least some control over money and staff.

Three consistent findings have been identified across different health systems.

■ Decentralization is under way in many countries. However, though local managers are often being given more responsibility for service delivery, they are not always being given the greater authority over money and staff required to enable them to fulfil these new responsibilities.

■ There are often few functioning mechanisms to assure accountability in the use of money, recruitment of staff or quality of services provided.

■ Confused lines of reporting are common, especially during periods of reorganization. This not only reduces accountability and thereby blunts its use as a lever for improving staff performance, but can reduce staff motivation.

The general public also has a role to play in holding health workers accountable for their actions *(130)*. Publicizing what patients should expect from their providers is cheap and easy to do and has been done with good results regarding patients' rights and user fee schedules in both low and high income countries *(131)*. In Uganda, for example, health district performance is ranked and the results are published in the press. Formal mechanisms for handling allegations of provider misconduct can also be effective but have proved difficult to use successfully in practice in low income settings *(132)*.

## HOW ARE LEVERS LINKED TO THE FOUR DIMENSIONS OF HEALTH WORKFORCE PERFORMANCE?

The framework at the start of this chapter listed four desired dimensions of health workforce performance: availability, competence, responsiveness and productivity. Rigorous evidence is limited, but Table 4.5 provides an overview of which levers appear to have the greatest effect on each of these dimensions. The results will naturally be influenced by local context.

### Availability

The levers thought to be most effective at increasing the availability of existing staff are those related to salaries and payment mechanisms, together with the materials to "do the job" and a degree of independence allowed to individual health workers to manage their work – whether in the management and deployment of staff for managers, or in clinical decisions for health care providers. Job descriptions and codes of conduct may also help, by providing clarity and the sense of professionalism which often appears to sustain health workers in difficult conditions.

Table 4.5 An aid to thinking through potential effects of levers on health workforce performance

| | Levers | Dimensions of health workforce performance | | | |
|---|---|---|---|---|---|
| | | Availability | Competence | Responsiveness | Productivity |
| 1 | Job descriptions | + | + | + | + |
| 2 | Norms and codes of conduct | ++ | + | ++ | + / ++ |
| 3 | Match skills to tasks | + | + | + | +++ |
| 4 | Supportive supervision | + | +++ | ++ | ++ |
| 5(a) | Salary levels | +++ | + | + | ++ |
| 5(b) | Payment mechanisms | ++ / −− | + / − | + / − | +++ / −−− |
| 6 | Information and communication | 0 | ++ | + | ++ |
| 7 | Infrastructure and supplies | ++ | 0 | + | ++ |
| 8 | Lifelong learning | + | +++ | + | + |
| 9 | Teamwork and management | + | + | ++ | +++ |
| 10 | Responsibility with accountability | ++ | + | ++ | +++ |

Key:
+ = positive effect; − = negative effect.
+ = some effect; ++ = significant effect; +++ = substantial effect.
Payment mechanisms: the effects will depend on the mechanism used.

## Competence

The levers that seem to have the greatest influence on health workforce competence (here encompassing technical knowledge, skills and behaviours) are supervision coupled with audit and feedback and lifelong learning. It is important to note, however, that it is the *way* in which these levers are applied that is crucial: sterile, fault-finding visits have no effect, whereas supportive supervision (together with audit and feedback) consistently has moderate to large benefits. An institutional approach that fosters the culture and practice of lifelong learning is more effective in changing practice than stand-alone, off-site training courses.

## Responsiveness

Responsiveness refers to the goal that people should be treated decently regardless of whether or not their health improves, and irrespective of who they are. As with the other dimensions of performance, no single lever alone is sufficient but the following appear to have the most significant effect: norms and codes of conduct; supervision; and basic amenities, such as privacy during consultations. Team-based interventions that make health workers feel valued and permitted to innovate can also boost responsiveness.

## Productivity

Many levers have the potential to improve productivity but three stand out. Strategies to redress skill mismatches could reap huge productivity gains. Adjusting the way that health workers are paid, improved teamwork, and responsibility with accountability also offer potentially large benefits.

Table 4.6 Health workforce performance: provisional assessment of implementation and effects of levers

| Levers | Implementation and effects | | | | |
| | Evidence base | Ease of implementation | Relative cost | Potential effect | Timing of impact[1] |
| | 1 = theory<br>2 = anecdote, example<br>3 = some formal studies<br>4 = strong evidence | 1 = easy<br>2 = moderate<br>3 = difficult | 1 = low<br>2 = medium<br>3 = high | 1 = small<br>2=moderate<br>3 = large | 1 = near term<br>2 = medium term<br>3 = long term |
| **Job-specific levers** | | | | | |
| **Job descriptions** | 2 | 1 | 1 | 2 | 1 |
| **Norms and codes of conduct** | 2 | 2 | 1 | 2 | 2,3 |
| **Matching skills to tasks** | 1 | 1,2,3* | 1,2 | 3 | 1 |
| **Supportive supervision** | 3 | 2 | 1,2 | 2,3 | 1 |
| **Basic support systems** | | | | | |
| **Remuneration (salary levels)** | 2 | 2,3 | 3 | 2 | 1 |
| **Remuneration (payment mechanisms)** | 3 | 2,3* | 2 | 3 | 2 |
| **Information and communication** | 2 | 2 | 2 | 2 | 1,2,3* |
| **Infrastructure and supplies** | 2 | 2 | 2,3* | 3 | 1 |
| **Enabling work environment** | | | | | |
| **Lifelong learning** | 3 | 1 | 1 | 2 | 1 |
| **Team management** | 3 | 1,2,3* | 1 | 2 | 1 |
| **Responsibility with accountability** | 3 | 1,2,3* | 2 | 3 | 1 |

[1]Once implemented.
*Depends on cause of problem, specific interventions introduced.

## CONCLUSION

This chapter has described the levers that can influence workforce performance. Table 4.6 summarizes what is known about implementation of the measures proposed here. An inevitable tension exists between the perspectives and goals of individuals and the organizations to which they belong. Organizations have to perform well and deploy their staff to the greatest advantage, while also providing places for individuals to thrive. This tension must be continually monitored and managed. Moreover, managing any change is a subtle and often difficult process, for several reasons. Changes may be needed at several levels. Legal and regulatory frameworks may need to be changed, which can be complex and slow. Resources are often needed to support change. Probably most importantly, local stakeholders must be brought "on board" as they can facilitate or equally effectively block a reform that has been carefully negotiated at central level *(78)*. However difficult, without changes to support improved performance of existing health workers, any recruitment and retention strategies will have limited effect. Retention is discussed in the next chapter.

## REFERENCES

1. Prasad A, Tandon A, Sousa A, Ebener S, Evans DB. Measuring the efficiency of human resources for health in attaining health outcomes across provinces in Viet Nam (background paper for *The World health report 2006*, available at http://www.who.int/hrh/documents/en/).

2. Viet Nam census 1999. In: *Human development report 2001*. New York, NY, United Nations Development Programme, 2001.

3. Hall TL, Mejia A. *Health manpower planning: principles, methods, issues*. Geneva, World Health Organization, 1978.

4. Pantoja A. *What is productivity and how can we measure it?* Geneva, World Health Organization, 2003 (working paper).

5. Kurowski C, Wyss K, Abdulla S, Yémadji N, Mills A. *Human resources for health: requirements and availability in the context of scaling-up priority interventions in low-income countries. Case studies from Tanzania and Chad.* London, London School of Hygiene and Tropical Medicine, 2003 (working paper 01/04).

6. Figueroa-Munoz J, Palmer K, Dal Poz MR, Blanc L, Bergström K, Raviglione M. The health workforce crisis in TB control: a report from high-burden countries. *Human Resources for Health*, 2005, 3:2 (http://www.human-resources-health.com/content/3/1/2, accessed 17 February 2006).

7. Gupta N, Diallo K, Zurn P, Dal Poz MR. Assessing human resources for health: what can be learned from labour force surveys? *Human Resources for Health*, 2003, 1:5.

8. Violato C, Lockyer J, Fidler H. Multisource feedback: a method of assessing surgical practice. *BMJ*, 2003, 326546–548.

9. Groveman HD, Ganiats TG, Klauber MR, Holden MG. Computer-assisted assessment of family physicians' knowledge about cancer screening guidelines [Health Care Delivery]. *The Western Journal of Medicine*, 1985, 143:541–544.

10. Early release data from the World Health Survey (http://www.who.int/healthinfo/survey/whscurrent/en/index.html) 2002.

11. Adam T, Amorim DG, Edwards SJ, Amaral JA , Evans DB. Capacity constraints to the adoption of new interventions: consultation time and the Integrated Management of Childhood Illness in Brazil. *Health Policy and Planning*, 2005, 20 (Suppl. 1):i49–i57.

12. Lurie N, Slater J, McGovern P, Ekstrum J, Quam L, Margolis K. Preventive services for women: does the sex of the physician matter? *New England Journal of Medicine*, 1993, 329:478–482.

13. Comstock LM, Hooper EM, Goodwin JM, Goodwin JS. Physician behaviors that correlate with patient satisfaction. *Journal of Medical Education*, 1982, 57:105–112.

14. Lieberman PB, Sledge WH, Matthews DA. Effect of patient gender on evaluation of intern performance. *Archives of Internal Medicine*, 1989, 149:1825–1829.

15. *Health workforce challenges: lessons from country experiences.* Abuja, High-Level Forum on the Health Millennium Development Goals, 2004 (http://www.hlfhealthmdgs. org/Documents/HealthWorkforceChallenges-Final.pdf, accessed 17 February 2006).
16. Hornby P, Forte P. *Human resource indicators to monitor health service performance.* Keele, Keele University, Centre for Health Planning and Management, 2002.
17. Bennett S, Franco LM. *Public sector health worker motivation and health sector reform: a conceptual framework.* Bethesda, MD, Abt Associates Inc. for Partnerships for Health Reform Project, 1999 (Major Applied Research 5, Technical Paper 1).
18. Buchan J. *Increasing the productivity of an existing 'stock' of health workers:* Unpublished review for United Kingdom Department for International Development, 2005.
19. Ferlie EB, Shortell SM. Improving the quality of health care. *The Milbank Quarterly,* 2001, 79:281–315.
20. Dieleman M, Cuong PV, Anh LV, Martineau T. Identifying factors for job motivation of rural health workers in North Viet Nam. *Human Resources for Health,* 2003,1:10.
21. Rowe AK, de Savigny D, Lanata CF, Victora CG. How can we achieve and maintain high-quality performance of health workers in low-resource settings? *Lancet,* 2005, 366:1026–1035.
22. Mathauer I, Imhoff I. Staff motivation in Africa: The role of non-financial incentives and quality management tools. Eschborn, Germany Agency for Technical Cooperation (GTZ), 2005 (draft).
23. Franco LM, Bennett S, Kanfer, R. Health sector reform and public sector health worker motivation: A conceptual framework, 2002, *Social Science and Medicine,* 54,1255–1266.
24. Dolea C, Zurn P. Mission to evaluate the project of Clinical Professional Development and Management System (CPDMS) for nurses and midwives in hospitals and health centers in Indonesia. World Health Organization, Geneva, 2004.
25. Ferrinho P, Omar MC, De Jesus Fernández M, Blaise P, Bugalho AM, Van Lerberghe W. Pilfering for survival: how health workers use access to drugs as a coping strategy. *Human Resources for Health, 2004, 2*:4.
26. *Global health partnerships: assessing country consequences.* Bill & Melinda Gates Foundation/McKinsey & Company, 2005.
27. Omaswa F, World Health Organization, personal communication.
28. Briley T, Hutson T. *Who will care for you? Washington hospitals face a personnel crisis.* Seattle, WA, Washington State Hospital Association, 2002.
29. Dovlo D, Sagoe K, Ntow S, Wellington E. Ghana case study: staff performance management. In: *Reforming health systems.* 1998 (research report, http://www.liv. ac.uk/lstm/research/documents/ghana.pdf, accessed 17 February 2006).
30. Blumenthal D. Doctors in a wired world: can professionalism survive connectivity? *The Milbank Quarterly,* 2002, 80:525–546.
31. Miettinen OS. Ideas and ideals in medicine: fruits of reason or props of power? *Journal of Evaluation in Clinical Practice,* 1999, 5:107–116.
32. Wibulpolprasert S, Pengpaibon P. Integrated strategies to tackle inequitable distribution of doctors in Thailand: four decades of experience. *Human Resources for Health,* 2003, 1:12.
33. Peduzzi M, Anselmi ML. Os pressupostos, o desenho e os resultados da pesquisa de Avaliação do impacto do PROFAE na qualidade dos serviços de saúde [The assumptions, design and results of the impact evaluation of PROFAE on the quality of the health services]. In: Lima de Castro J, ed. *PROFAE – Educação profissional em saúde e cidadania [PROFAE - Health professional education and citizenship].* Brasilia, Ministry of Health, 2002:149–163.
34. Jaffré, Y, Olivier de Sardan, J-P. *Une médecine inhospitalière: les difficiles relations entre soignants et soignés dans cinq capitales d'Afrique de l'Ouest [Inhospitable medicine: difficult relations between carers and cared for in five West African capital cities].* Paris, Karthala, 2003.
35. *Paris declaration on aid effectiveness: ownership, harmonisation, alignment, results and mutual accountability.* Paris, High Level Forum, 2005:1–13.
36. *Best practice principles for global health partnership activities at country level.* Paris, High Level Forum, 2005 (Working group on global health partnerships: Report:1–28).

37. Buchan J, Hinton L. *Skill mix and new roles in health: what does the evidence base tell us?* Geneva, World Health Organization, 2005 (background paper for *The world health repot 2006*; available at http://www.who.int/hrh/documents/en).

38. Egger D, Travis P, Dovlo D, Hawken L. *Strengthening management in low-income countries.* Geneva, World Health Organization, 2005 (WHO/EIP/health systems/2005.1).

39. *Private sector participation in health.* London, Institute for Health Sector Development, 2004.

40. Langenbrunner JC, Orosz E, Kutzin J, Wiley MM. Purchasing and paying providers. In: Figueras J, Robinson R, Jakubowski E, eds. *Purchasing to improve health systems performance.* Brussels, European Observatory on Health Systems and Policies, 2005: 236–264.

41. Macq J, Van Lerberghe W. Managing health services in developing countries: moonlighting to serve the public? In: Ferrinho P, Van Lerberghe W. *Providing health care under adverse conditions: health personnel performance and individual coping strategies.* Antwerp, ITG Press, 2000 (Studies in Health Services Organisation and Policy, 16:177–186).

42. McPake B, Asiimwe D, Mwesigye F, Ofumbi M, Ortenblad L, Streefland P, Turinde A. Informal economic activities of public health workers in Uganda: implications for quality and accessibility of care. *Social Science and Medicine*, 1999, 49: 849–865.

43. Ambegaokar M, Ongolo-Zogo P, Aly T, Betsi E, Fouda J, Mubudu L, McPake B. *Incentives and penalties: results of research into the drafting of district contracts.* MSP-DROS/PASS-UE/LSHTM-HPU, Yaoundé, 2005.

44. Afford CW. *Failing health services.* Geneva, International Labour Organization/Population Services International, 2001.

45. Dräger S, Dal Poz MR, Evans D. *Health workers wages: an overview from selected countries.* Geneva, World Health Organization, 2006 (background paper for *The world health report 2006;* available at: http://www.who.int/hrh/documents/en/).

46. ILO occupational wages around the world (oww) database, 1999–2002. Geneva, International Labour Organization, 2005 (http://www.nber.org/oww/).

47. OECD Health Data National Correspondents. *Remuneration of doctors and nurses: progress and next steps on data collection.* Paris, Organisation for Economic Co-operation and Development, 2005.

48. Robinson JC, Shortell SM, Rui Li, Casalino LP, Rundall T. The alignment and blending of payment incentives within physician organizations. *Health Services Research*, 2004, 39:1589–1606.

49. Zhang L, Harvard University, personal communication.

50. Zachariah R, Lange L, D'Altilia J. Financing advances on salaries of health workers in Chad: an example of a feasible strategy to sustain the Bamako Initiative. *Health Policy and Planning,* 2001, 16:332–333.

51. Ensor T, Langenbrunner J. Financing health care. In: Healy J, McKee M, eds. *Health care in Central Asia.* Buckingham, Open University Press, 2002.

52. Wouters, A. *Alternative provider payment methods: incentives for improving health care delivery. Primer for policymakers.* Bethesda, MD. PHR, Abt Associates, Inc. 1998.

53. Marsden D. The role of performance-related pay in renegotiating the "effort bargain": the case of the British public service. *Industrial and Labor Relations Review*, 2004, 57:350–370.

54. Isaac J. Performance-related pay: the importance of fairness. *Journal of Industrial Relations*, 2001, 43:111–123.

55. Gosden T, Forland F, Kristiansen IS, Sutton M, Leese B, Giuffrida A et al. Impact of payment method on behaviour of primary care physicians: a systematic review. *Journal of Health Services Research and Policy*, 2001, 6:44–55.

56. Beaulieu, D, Horrigan DR. Putting smart money to work for quality improvement. *Health Services Research,* 2005, 40:1318–1334.

57. Rosenthal M, Frank R, Li Z, Epstein AM. Early experience with pay-for-performance. *Journal of the American Medical Association*, 2005, 294:1788–1793.

58. Arrowsmith J, French S, Gilman M, Richardson R. Performance-related pay in health care. Review Article. *Journal of Health Services and Research Policy*, 2001, 6:114–119.

59. Zurn P, Dal Poz MR, Stilwell B, Adams O. Imbalance in the health workforce. *Human Resources for Health*, 2004, 2:13.

60. *Workshop on attracting and retaining health workers in east, central and southern Africa.* Johannesburg, Commonwealth Secretariat and South Africa Department of Health, 2003.

61. Rosenthal MB, Fernandopulle R, Song HR, Landon B. Paying for quality: providers' incentives for quality improvement. *Health Affairs*, 2004, 23:127–141.

62. Dudley RA. Pay for performance research: what clinicians and policy makers need to know. *JAMA*, 2005, 294:1821–1823.

63. Buchan J, Dovlo D. *International recruitment of health workers to the UK: a report for DFID.* 2004 (http://www.dfidhealthrc.org/Shared/publications/reports/int_rec/int-rec-main.pdf).

64. Nityarumphong S, Srivanichankorn S, Pongsupap Y. Strategies to respond to manpower needs in rural Thailand. In: Ferrinho P, Van Lerberghe W, eds. *Providing health care under adverse conditions: health personnel performance and individual coping strategies.* Antwerp, ITG Press, 2000 (Studies in Health Services Organisation and Policy, 16:55–72).

65. Desplats D, Koné Y, Razakarison C. Pour une médicine générale communautaire en première ligne [For front-line community-based general practitioners]. *Médecine Tropicale*, 2004. 64:539–544.

66. Buchan J, Ball J, Rafferty AM. *A lasting attraction? The "magnet" accreditation of Rochdale Infirmary.* Report commissioned by the Department of Health, 2003.

67. Gaal P, McKee M. Fee for service or donation? Hungarian perspectives on informal payment for health care. *Social Science and Medicine,* 2005, 60:1445-1457.

68. De Savigny D, Kasale H, Mbuya C, Reid G. Fixing health systems. Ottawa: International Development Research centre, 2004.

69. Brimberry R. Vaccination of high-risk patients for influenza: a comparison of telephone and mail reminder methods. *Journal of Family Practice*, 1988, 26:397–400.

70. Davis NA, Nash E, Bailey C, Lewis MJ, Rimer BK, Koplan JP. Evaluation of three methods for improved mammography rates in a managed care plan. *American Journal of Preventive Medicine*, 1997, 13:298–302.

71. Friedman RH, Kazis LE, Jette A, Smith MB, Stollerman J, Torgerson J et al. A telecommunications system for monitoring and counseling patients with hypertension: impact on medication adherence and blood pressure control. *American Journal of Hypertension*, 1996, 4:285–292.

72. *Transforming health care through information technology.* Report of the US President's Information Technology and Advisory Committee, 2001.

73. Bates DW, Kuperman GJ, Rittenberg E, Teich JM, Fiskio J, Ma'luf N et al. A randomized trial of a computer-based intervention to reduce utilization of redundant laboratory tests. *American Journal of Medicine*, 1999, 106:144–150.

74. Kuperman GJ, Teich JM, Tanasijevic MJ, Ma'Luf N, Rittenberg E, Jha A et al. Improving response to critical laboratory results with automation: Results of a randomized controlled trial. *Journal of the American Medical Informatics Association*, 1999, 6:512–522.

75. Tanriverdi H, Iacono CS. Diffusion of telemedicine: a knowledge barrier perspective. *Telemedicine Journal*, 1999. 5:223–244.

76. Stekelenburg J, Kyanamina SS, Wolfers I. Poor performance of community health workers in Kalabo District, Zambia. *Health Policy*, 2003, 65:109–118.

77. Hopkinson B, Balabanova D, McKee M, Kutzin J. The human perspective on health-care reform: coping with diabetes in Kyrgyzstan *International Journal of Health Planning and Management,* 2004, 19:43–61

78. Rese A, Balabanova D, Danishevski K, McKee M, Sheaff R. Implementing general practice in Russia: getting beyond the first steps. *BMJ* 2005; 331; 204-207.

79. Bossyns P, Van Lerberghe W. The weakest link: competence and prestige as constraints to referral by isolated nurses in rural Niger. *Human Resources for Health*, 2004, 2:1 (http://www.human-resources-health.com/content/2/1/1).

80. *Survey of public health facilities using WHO Operational Package for Monitoring and Assessing Country Pharmaceutical Situations, 2001–2003.* Carried out by ministries of health, universities and nongovernmental organizations with the support of WHO Department of Technical Cooperation for Essential Drugs and Traditional Medicine.

81. Kelly P. Local problems, local solutions: improving tuberculosis control at district level in Malawi. *Bulletin of the World Health Organization*, 2001, 79:111–117.

82. *Developing through partnership – Continuous professional development portfolio for healthcare managers*. London, Institute of Healthcare Management, 2004.

83. Davis DA, Thomson MA, Oxman AD, Haynes RB. Changing physician performance. A systematic review of the effect of continuing medical education strategies. *JAMA*, 1995, 274:700–705.

84. Davis D, O'Brien MA, Freemantle N, Wolf FM, Mazmanian P, Taylor-Vaisey A. Impact of formal continuing medical education: do conferences, workshops, rounds, and other traditional continuing education activities change physician behavior or health care outcomes? *JAMA*, 1999, 282:867–874.

85. Hadiyono JE, Suryawati S, Danu SS, Sunartono, Santoso B. Interactional group discussion: results of a controlled trial using a behavioral intervention to reduce the use of injections in public health facilities. *Social Science and Medicine*, 1996, 42:1177–1183.

86. Ratanajamit C, Chongsuvivatwong V, Geater AF. A randomized controlled educational intervention on emergency contraception among drugstore personnel in southern Thailand. *Journal of American Medical Womens Associations*, 2002, 57:196–199, 207.

87. Herbert CP, Wright JM, Maclure M, Wakefield J, Dormuth C, Brett-MacLean P et al. Better Prescribing Project: a randomized controlled trial of the impact of case-based educational modules and personal prescribing feedback on prescribing for hypertension in primary care. *Family Practice,* 2004, 21:575–581.

88. Garcia P, Hughes J, Carcamo C, Holmes KK. Training pharmacy workers in recognition, management, and prevention of STDs: district-randomized controlled trial. *Bulletin of the World Health Organization*, 2003, 81:806–814.

89. Gormley GJ, Steele WK, Stevenson M, McKane R, Ryans I, Cairns AP et al. A randomised study of two training programmes for general practitioners in the techniques of shoulder injection. *Annals of Rheumatic Diseases*, 2003, 62:1006–1009.

90. Roberts I, Allsop P, Dickinson M, Curry P, Eastwick-Field P, Eyre G. Airway management training using the laryngeal mask airway: a comparison of two different training programmes. *Resuscitation,* 1997, 33:211–214.

91. Clark NM, Gong M, Schork MA, Evans D, Roloff D, Hurwitz M et al. Impact of education for physicians on patient outcomes. *Pediatrics*, 1998, 101:831–836.

92. Kaner EF, Lock CA, McAvoy BR, Heather N, Gilvarry E. A RCT of three training and support strategies to encourage implementation of screening and brief alcohol intervention by general practitioners. *British Journal of General Practitioners*, 1999, 49:699–703.

93. Figueiras A, Sastre I, Tato F, Rodriguez C, Lado E, Caamano F et al. One-to-one versus group sessions to improve prescription in primary care: a pragmatic randomized controlled trial. *Medical Care*, 2001, 39:158–167.

94. Stewart M, Marshall JN, Ostbye T, Feightner JW, Brown JB, Harris S et al. Effectiveness of case-based on-line learning of evidence-based practice guidelines. *Family Medicine*, 2005, 37:131–138.

95. Abdolrasulnia M, Collins BC, Casebeer L, Wall T, Spettell C, Ray MN et al. Using email reminders to engage physicians in an Internet-based CME intervention. *BMC Medical Education*, 2004, 4:17.

96. Harris JM Jr, Kutob RM, Surprenant ZJ, Maiuro RD, Delate TA. Can Internet-based education improve physician confidence in dealing with domestic violence? *Family Medicine*, 2002, 34:287–292.

97. Van Boxell P, Anderson K, Regnard C. The effectiveness of palliative care education delivered by videoconferencing compared with face-to-face delivery. *Palliative Medicine*, 2003, 17:344–358.

98. Flores R, Robles J, Burkhalter BR. Distance education with tutoring improves diarrhea case management in Guatemala. *International Journal of Quality in Health Care*, 2002, 14(Suppl. 1):47–56.

99. Hunskaar S, Hannestad YS, Backe B, Matheson I. Direct mailing of consensus recommendations did not alter GPs' knowledge and prescription of oestrogen in the menopause. *Scandinavian Journal of Primary Health Care*, 1996, 14:203–208.

100. Butzlaff M, Vollmar HC, Floer B, Koneczny N, Isfort J, Lange S. Learning with computerized guidelines in general practice?: A randomized controlled trial. *Family Practice*, 2004, 21:183–188.

101. Watson MC, Bond CM, Grimshaw JM, Mollison J, Ludbrook A, Walker AE. Educational strategies to promote evidence-based community pharmacy practice: a cluster randomized controlled trial (RCT). *Family Practice*, 2002, 19:529–536.

102. Kim CS, Kristopaitis RJ, Stone E, Pelter M, Sandhu M, Weingarten SR. Physician education and report cards: do they make the grade? Results from a randomized controlled trial. *American Journal of Medicine*, 1999, 107:556–560.

103. Hall L, Eccles M, Barton R, Steen N, Campbell M. Is untargeted outreach visiting in primary care effective? A pragmatic randomized controlled trial. *Journal of Public Health Medicine*, 2001, 23:109–113.

104. Watson M, Gunnell D, Peters T, Brookes S, Sharp D. Guidelines and educational outreach visits from community pharmacists to improve prescribing in general practice: a randomised controlled trial. *Health Services Research and Policy*, 2001, 6:207–213.

105. Veninga CC, Lagerlov P, Wahlstrom R, Muskova M, Denig P, Berkhof J et al. Evaluating an educational intervention to improve the treatment of asthma in four European countries. Drug Education Project Group. *American Journal of Respiratory and Critical Care Medicine*, 1999, 160:1254–1262.

106. Onion CW, Bartzokas CA. Changing attitudes to infection management in primary care: a controlled trial of active versus passive guideline implementation strategies. *Family Practice*, 1998, 15:99–104.

107. Trap B, Todd CH, Moore H, Laing R. The impact of supervision on stock management and adherence to treatment guidelines: a randomized controlled trial. *Health Policy and Planning*, 2001, 16:273–280.

108. Howie JG, Hopton JL, Heaney DJ, Porter AM. Attitudes to medical care, the organization of work and stress among general practitioners. *British Journal of General Practice,* 1992, 42:181–195.

109. Borrill CS, Carletta J, Carter AJ, Dawson JF, Garrod S, Rees A, et al. *The effectiveness of healthcare teams in the National Health Service.* Final report submitted to the Department of Health, 2000.

110. Kekki P. *Teamwork in primary health care.* Geneva, World Health Organization, 1990.

111. Ham C, Kipping R, McLeod H. Redesigning work processes in health care: lessons from the National Health Service. *The Milbank Quarterly*, 2003, 81:415–439.

112. Egger D, Ollier L. *Strengthening Management in Uganda: What can be learned?* Country case study report. Geneva, World Health Organization, 2005 (WHO/SPO/OMH).

113. Jakab M, Kutzin J, Chakraborty S, O'Dougherty S, Temirov A, Manjieva E. *Evaluating the Manas Health Sector Reform (1996-2005): Focus on Health Financing.* Policy research paper 31, MANAS Health Policy Analysis Project. Bishkek, Kyrgyzstan, 2005.

114. Buchan J. Health sector reform and the regulation and management of health professionals: a case study from Chile 2000. *Human Resources Development Journal*, 2000. 4:64–72 (http://www.who.int/hrh/hrdj/en).

115. Buchan J. What difference does ("good") HRM make? *Human Resources for Health*, 2004, 2:6 (http://www.human-resources-health.com).

116. Zaleznik A. Managers and leaders. Are they different? *Harvard Business Review*, 1977, 82:74–81.

117. Stordeur S, D'hoore W, Vandenberghe C. *Leadership, organizational stress and emotional exhaustion among nursing hospital staff. Journal of Advanced Nursing*, 2001, 35:533–542.

118. Larrabee JH, Janney MA, Ostrow CL, Withrow ML, Hobbs GR Jr, Burani CB. *Predicting registered nurse job satisfaction and intent to leave. Journal of Nursing Administration*, 2003, 33:271–283.

119. Hasselhorn H-M, Tackenberg P, Müller BH. *Working conditions and intent to leave the profession among nursing staff in Europe. NEXT – nurses early exit study, 2003.* Stockholm, National Institute for Working Life, 2004.

120. Moynihan DP, Pandey SK. Testing how management matters in an era of government by performance management. *Journal of Public Administration Research and Theory*, 2005, 15:421–439.

121. Boyne GA, Walker RM. Introducing the "determinants of performance in public organizations symposium". *Journal of Public Administration Research and Theory*, 2005, 15:483–488.

122. Boyle DK, Bott MJ, Hansen HE, Woods CQ, Taunton RL. Managers' leadership and critical care nurses' intent to stay. *American Journal of Critical Care,* 1999, 8:361–371.

123. Mathauer I, Imhoff I, *The impact of non-financial incentives and quality management tools on staff motivation. A case study from Benin and Kenya*. Eschborn, German Technical Cooperation (GTZ), 2004.

124. Blaauw D, Penn-Kekana L. Socio-Economic Inequalities and Maternal Health in South Africa. Presentation to the 22nd Conference on Priorities in Perinatal Care in Southern Africa. 2003.

125. Oulton J, International Council of Nurses, personal communication.

126. Shaw C. Managing the performance of health professionals. In: Dubois C-A, McKee M, Nolte E, eds. *Human resources for health in Europe*. Brussels, European Observatory on Health Systems and Policies, 2005: 98-115.

127. Jamtvedt G, Young JM, Kristoffersen DT, Thomson O'Brien MA, Oxman AD. *Audit and feedback: effects on professional practice and health care outcomes.* The Cochrane Database of Systematic Reviews 2003. Issue 3. Art. No.: CD000259. DOI:10.1002/14651858.CD000259.

128. Diaz-Monsalve SJ. Measuring the job performance of district health managers in Latin America. *Annals of Tropical Medicine and Parasitology*, 2003, 97:299–311.

129. De Savigny D, Kasale H, Mbuya C, Reid G. Fixing health systems. Ottawa: International Development Research centre, 2004.

130. George A. *Accountability in health services. Transforming relationships and contexts.* Cambridge, MA, Harvard Center for Population and Development Studies, 2002 (Working Paper Series, Vol 13, No. 1).

131. Averill R. Public dissemination of provider performance comparisons in the United States. *Hospital Quarterly*, 1998, 1:39–41.

132. Bhat R. Regulating the private health care sector: the case of the Indian Consumer Protection Act. *Health Policy and Planning*, 1996, 11:265–279.

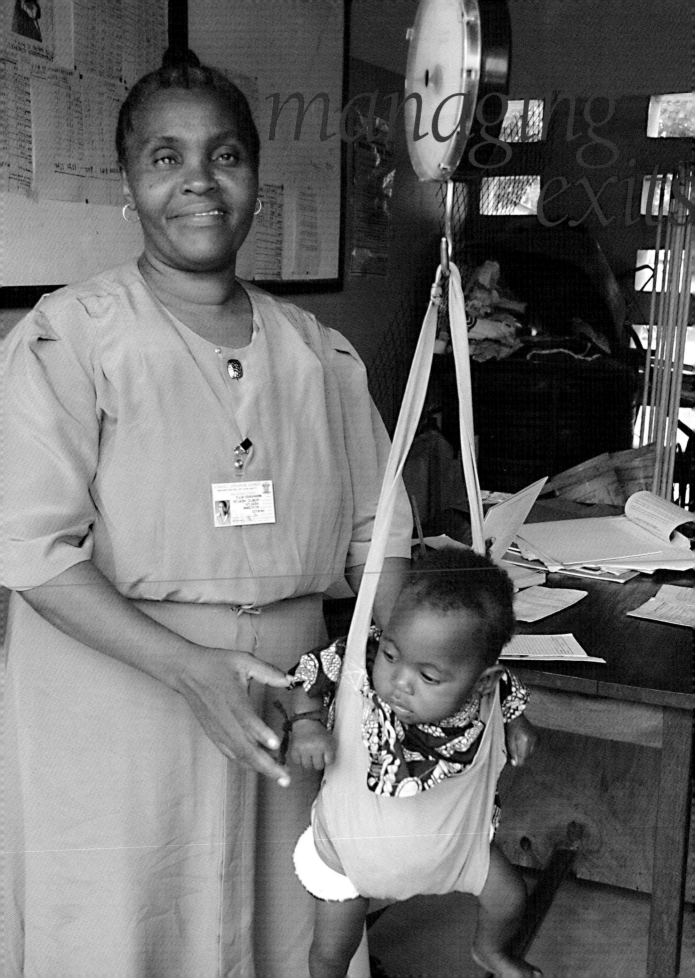

managing exits

# chapter five

# from the workforce

**Each year, substantial numbers of health workers leave the health workforce, either temporarily or permanently. These exits can provoke shortages if workers who leave are not replaced, and such shortages compromise the delivery and quality of health services *(1, 2)*. Chapter 3 discussed the routes new workers take into the workforce; this chapter examines the other end of the spectrum – the various ways in which workers depart active service. It also suggests ways of managing exits in times of worker shortage as well as in times of surplus, in order to optimize the performance of the health workforce. Finally, it reviews and analyses the factors that influence exits and proposes strategies for managing them.**

The main reasons people leave the health workforce are depicted in Figure 5.1: migration; risk of violence, illness or death; change of occupation or work status; and retirement. Some workers leave temporarily, because of illness or maternity or in order to attend advanced education courses, for example. Others are lost permanently, because of death or a change of occupation. In some cases, a health worker migrates from one country to another, thus permanently leaving one health workforce to join another. Partial exits occur when full-time health workers move to part-time employment: changes in the numbers of full-time and part-time workers can alter the health workforce equilibrium.

Over the last few decades, the working lifespan of health workers has altered because of changes in their working patterns, growing morbidity and mortality rates (in Africa, mainly attributable to HIV/AIDS and tuberculosis), increasing migration, and ageing (especially in high income countries). These factors pose serious challenges to the goal of maintaining a sufficient and effective health workforce.

High turnover rates in the health workforce may lead to higher provider costs. They are also a threat to the quality of care, because they may disrupt organizational function, reduce team efficiency, and cause a loss of institutional knowledge. Studies show that the costs associated with retention

## Figure 5.1 Exit routes from the health workforce

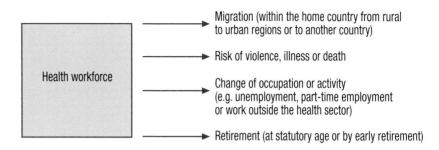

problems are often substantial (3). Turnover can have potential benefits, however, as it may provide an opportunity to match personnel skills better to workplace needs, facilitate the introduction of new ideas into well-established organizations, and increase organizational flexibility (4). In this context, it is important for policy-makers to manage exits from the health workforce to ensure the least possible disruption of services.

## EBBS AND FLOWS OF MIGRATION

Concerns about the adverse impact of the flows of skilled professionals from poorer to richer countries have thrust the migration of health workers to the forefront of the policy agenda in recent years (5). However, statistics on global flows of health workers remain far from complete (5–12). For the select number of countries that do track migration, available information is generally limited to registered doctors and nurses. Data on movements of pharmacists, occupational therapists and the many other types of health workers identified in this report are virtually non-existent.

Not knowing how many health workers are on the move, where they have come from, or where they are going makes it difficult to grasp the scale of the problem.

## Table 5.1 Doctors and nurses trained abroad working in OECD countries

| OECD country | Doctors trained abroad | | Nurses trained abroad | |
|---|---|---|---|---|
| | Number | Percentage of total | Number | Percentage of total |
| Australia | 11 122 | 21 | NA | NA |
| Canada | 13 620 | 23 | 19 061 | 6 |
| Finland | 1 003 | 9 | 140 | 0 |
| France | 11 269 | 6 | NA | NA |
| Germany | 17 318 | 6 | 26 284 | 3 |
| Ireland | NA | NA | 8 758 | 14 |
| New Zealand | 2 832 | 34 | 10 616 | 21 |
| Portugal | 1 258 | 4 | NA | NA |
| United Kingdom | 69 813 | 33 | 65 000 | 10 |
| United States | 213 331 | 27 | 99 456 | 5 |

NA, not applicable.

Data from OECD countries indicate that doctors and nurses trained abroad comprise a significant percentage of the total workforce in most of them, but especially in English-speaking countries (see Table 5.1).

It appears that doctors trained in sub-Saharan Africa and working in OECD countries represent close to one quarter (23%) of the current doctor workforce in those source countries, ranging from as low as 3% in Cameroon to as high as 37% in South Africa. Nurses and midwives trained in sub-Saharan Africa and working in OECD countries represent one twentieth (5%) of the current workforce but with an extremely wide range from as low as 0.1% in Uganda to as high as 34% in Zimbabwe (see Tables 5.2 and 5.3 overleaf).

> " *A better life and livelihood are at the root of decisions to migrate* "

### Why are health workers moving?

These OECD data on migrant flows hide the complex patterns and reasons for health workers moving. Migration takes place within countries from rural to urban areas; within regions from poorer to better-off countries and across continents. A better life and livelihood are at the root of decisions to migrate. Classically this is provoked by a (growing) discontent or dissatisfaction with existing working/living conditions – so-called push factors, as well as by awareness of the existence of (and desire to find) better jobs elsewhere – so-called pull factors. A recent study from sub-Saharan Africa points to both push and pull factors being significant *(10)*. Workers' concerns about lack of promotion prospects, poor management, heavy workload, lack of facilities, a declining health service, inadequate living conditions and high levels of violence and crime are among the push factors for migration (see Figure 5.2). Prospects for better remuneration, upgrading qualifications, gaining experience, a safer environment and family-related matters are among the pull factors

Figure 5.2  Health workers' reasons to migrate in four African countries (Cameroon, South Africa, Uganda and Zimbabwe)

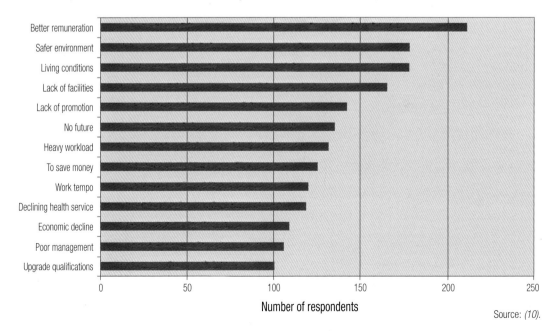

Source: *(10)*.

Table 5.2 Doctors trained in sub-Saharan Africa working in OECD countries

| Source country | Total doctors in home country | Doctors working in eight OECD recipient countries[a] | |
| | | Number | Percentage of home country workforce |
| --- | --- | --- | --- |
| Angola | 881 | 168 | 19 |
| Cameroon | 3 124 | 109 | 3 |
| Ethiopia | 1 936 | 335 | 17 |
| Ghana | 3 240 | 926 | 29 |
| Mozambique | 514 | 22 | 4 |
| Nigeria | 34 923 | 4 261 | 12 |
| South Africa | 32 973 | 12 136 | 37 |
| Uganda | 1 918 | 316 | 16 |
| United Republic of Tanzania | 822 | 46 | 6 |
| Zimbabwe | 2 086 | 237 | 11 |
| **Total** | **82 417** | **18 556** | **Average 23** |

[a] Recipient countries: Australia, Canada, Finland, France, Germany, Portugal, United Kingdom, United States of America.

Source: (11).

Table 5.3 Nurses and midwives trained in sub-Saharan Africa working in OECD countries

| Source country | Total nurses and midwives working in home country | Nurses and midwives working in seven OECD recipient countries[a] | |
| | | Number | Percentage of home country workforce |
| --- | --- | --- | --- |
| Angola | 13 627 | 105 | 0 |
| Botswana | 7 747 | 572 | 7 |
| Cameroon | 26 032 | 84 | 0 |
| Ethiopia | 20 763 | 195 | 0 |
| Ghana | 17 322 | 2 267 | 13 |
| Guinea-Bissau | 3 203 | 30 | 0 |
| Kenya | 37 113 | 1 213 | 3 |
| Lesotho | 1 123 | 200 | 18 |
| Malawi | 11 022 | 453 | 4 |
| Mauritius | 4 438 | 781 | 18 |
| Mozambique | 6 183 | 34 | 0 |
| Namibia | 6 145 | 54 | 0 |
| Nigeria | 210 306 | 5 375 | 3 |
| South Africa | 184 459 | 13 496 | 7 |
| Swaziland | 4 590 | 299 | 7 |
| Uganda | 17 472 | 21 | 0 |
| United Republic of Tanzania | 13 292 | 37 | 0 |
| Zambia | 22 010 | 1 198 | 5 |
| Zimbabwe | 9 357 | 3 183 | 34 |
| **Total** | **616 204** | **29 597** | **Average 5** |

[a] Recipient countries: Canada, Denmark, Finland, Ireland, Portugal, United Kingdom, United States of America.

Note: Data compiled by WHO from various sources.

(see Figure 5.2). In Zimbabwe, for example, a startling 77% of final university students were being encouraged to migrate by their families *(13)*.

Beyond the individual and the family, accelerated globalization of the service sector in the last two decades has helped drive migration in the health field *(14–18)*. In addition, there is a growing unmet demand for health workers in high income countries due in part to rapidly ageing populations. Two important responses in the global market are occurring. First, a growing number of middle income countries are training health workers for international export (see Box 5.1) and second, professional agencies are more actively sourcing workers internationally, raising questions about the ethics of recruitment (see Box 5.2).

> " *Losing its workforce can bring a fragile health system close to collapse* "

## Impacts of migration

The movement of health workers abroad has redeeming features. Each year, migration generates billions of dollars in remittances (the money sent back home by migrants) and has therefore been associated with a decline in poverty in low income countries *(22)*. If health workers return, they bring significant skills and expertise back to their home countries. Nonetheless, when large numbers of doctors and nurses leave, the countries that financed their education lose a return on their investment and end up unwillingly providing the wealthy countries to which their health personnel have migrated with a kind of "perverse subsidy" *(23)*. Financial loss is not the most damaging outcome, however. When a country has a fragile health system, the loss of its workforce can bring the whole system close to collapse and the consequences can be measured in lives lost. In these circumstances, the calculus of international migration shifts from brain drain or gain to "fatal flows" *(24)*.

## Strategies to manage migration

The complex combination of individual worker, workplace and market forces that generate flows of health workers defy any simple or single action related to migration. The following sections deal with managing migration in order to protect health workers and minimize inequities. Action at three levels – in source countries, in receiving countries and internationally – can diminish the negative aspects of migration.

## Box 5.1 Turning brain drain into brain gain — the Philippines

The Commission on Filipinos Overseas estimates that more than 7.3 million Filipinos – approximately 8% of the country's population – reside abroad. The government of the Philippines has encouraged temporary migration by its professionals in recent years and taken measures to turn remittances into an effective tool for national development (including health care) by encouraging migrants to send remittances via official channels. In 2004, the Central Bank of the Philippines reported total remittances of US$ 8.5 billion, representing 10% of the country's gross domestic product (GDP).

At the same time the government is taking measures to draw its migrants home after a period of service abroad.

The Philippine Overseas Employment Administration was founded in 1995 to promote the return and reintegration of migrants. Many privileges are granted to returnees, including tax-free shopping for one year, loans for business capital at preferential rates and eligibility for subsidized scholarships.

The Philippines experiment has had encouraging results and is seen by some developing countries as a role model.

Source: *(19)*.

### Source country strategies

Source countries can consider a wide range of options for managing migration, including two main strategies: providing health workers with appropriate training for their place of employment, and making it easy for them to return home after working abroad.

### Strategy 5.1 Adjust training to need and demands

Training that is focused on local conditions can help to limit workforce attrition. Lessons from longstanding efforts to improve workforce coverage in rural areas suggest that training local workers – in local languages and in skills relevant to local conditions – helps to stem exits of health workers *(25, 26)*. Such approaches to training often lead to credentials that do not have international recognition, which further limits migration. Success, however, is contingent on a wide range of on-the-job incentives and support and on the involvement of key institutions such as universities and professional associations *(25, 27)*

Even in the face of continued migration, expansion of training may help to reduce workforce shortfalls. Preserving the quality of training requires effective accreditation capacity, especially if expansion of training institutions is rapid. In low income countries with tight fiscal constraints, such an expansion would entail either significant private sector financial involvement or foreign aid. It is essential that job opportunities for graduates also grow, either through the public sector (fiscal constraints permitting) or through the private sector.

> **❝** *The Philippines has been training nurses for export for many years* **❞**

Training can also be specifically tailored to meet export requirements. The Philippines, as part of a larger policy to encourage worker migration (see Box 5.1), has been training health workers, especially nurses, for export for many years – they constitute 76% of foreign nurse graduates in the United States, for example *(28)*. Likewise, Cuba has exported thousands of health workers as part of its bilateral relations with other countries. Some countries, including China, India, Indonesia and Viet Nam, are either actively involved or contemplating export strategies *(29)*. These strategies have not been systematically evaluated, but experience indicates that they are resource intensive and require the establishment of institutional capacity for training and accreditation, and careful management of interactions with the internal or domestic health worker market.

## Box 5.2 Recruitment agencies and migration

Medical recruitment agencies are thriving, and there is widespread concern that they are stimulating the migration of health workers from low income countries. A 2004 study found that such agencies spurred the majority of recruitment from Cameroon *(10)*, and a recent analysis of nearly 400 émigré nurses in London found that as many as two thirds of them were recruited by agencies to work in Britain *(9)*. The president of the largest nursing union in Mauritius recently noted that British employers send recruitment agents to contact nurses directly and then discreetly negotiate contracts with them. Another example is in Warsaw, where dozens of agencies have sprung up in an attempt to attract Polish doctors to work in the United Kingdom.

Many people question the ethical practices of recruitment agencies. Health workers contracted by private recruitment agencies are sometimes subjected to unforeseen charges such as placement fees that put them at an immediate financial disadvantage. Studies have also shown that migrant health workers often begin jobs before their registration is completed and are paid substandard wages during the waiting period *(20–21)*.

## Strategy 5.2 Improve local conditions

As pointed out in Chapter 4, the actions related to improving employment conditions of workers help to remove the "push" factors that induce workers to migrate. Despite the absence of any systematic assessment of the effects of these interventions on migration rates, experience shows that pay, financial incentives and safety, good management and career development are all important. Efforts to improve living conditions related to transport, housing and education of family members are also used to help attract, and retain, health workers *(30)*.

In situations where the education of health workers is paid for by a prospective employer, in either the public or the private sector, contractual obligations or "bonds" are arranged whereby graduates agree to work for the employer for a specified period of time. The practice of bonding is widespread yet its effectiveness is poorly understood. Experience of bonding is mixed: it does ensure coverage, but it is strongly associated with low performance among workers and high turnover rates *(31)*.

Surveys of migrant workers indicate that in general they have a strong interest in returning to work in their home country *(32)*. As the "brain gain" strategy of the Philippines exemplifies (Box 5.1), active institutional management of migration can facilitate migrants' welfare not only abroad but also on their return home. Special migration services for health workers may also help to retain productive links with local health institutions while workers are away *(33)*.

### *Receiving country strategies*

Receiving countries should be concerned for the rights and welfare of migrant health workers and responsive to the adverse consequences in source countries associated with their absence.

## Strategy 5.3 Ensure fair treatment of migrant workers

The scant but increasing evidence on the experience of migrant health workers raises concerns related to their unmet expectations on remittances, personal security, racial and cultural isolation and unequal work conditions, with limited knowledge of their rights and the ability to exercise them *(21, 34–37)*. Migrant workers should be recruited on terms and conditions equal to those of locally recruited staff and given opportunities for cultural orientation. It is vital to have policies in place that identify and deal with racism among staff and clients *(38)*.

## Strategy 5.4 Adopt responsible recruitment policies

Receiving countries have a responsibility to ensure that recruitment of workers from countries with severe workforce shortages is sensitive to the adverse consequences. The significant investments made in training health care professionals and the immediate impact of their absence through migration must figure more prominently as considerations among prospective employers and recruitment agencies. Discussions and negotiations with ministries of health, workforce planning units and training institutions, similar to bilateral agreements, will help to avoid claims of "poaching" and other disreputable recruitment behaviour. The development of instruments for normative practices in international recruitment is discussed below.

## Strategy 5.5 Provide support to human resources in source countries

Many recipient countries are also providers of overseas development assistance for health. Through this structure, support could be more directly targeted to expanding the health workforce, not only to stem the impact of outgoing migration but also to overcome the human resources constraints to achieving the health-related Millennium Development Goals (MDGs) (see Chapter 2).

Apart from help to strengthen the health workforce in source countries, important external sources of direct human resources support are provided in humanitarian disasters and disease eradication efforts and through the proliferation of international nongovernmental organizations. Cuba's "medical brigades", for example, provide 450 health professionals to shortfall areas in South Africa and over 500 to rural areas of Haiti. The American Association of Physicians of Indian Origin, with its 35 000 practitioners, is an important pool of volunteer service (39). Direct twinning of health institutions between rich and poor countries, a popular form of development assistance (40), also involves substantial flows of health workers in both directions. With greater awareness of the human resources shortfalls in poor countries and expectations to meet the targets of the health-related MDGs, ambitious policies are being considered to increase these flows (41). More systematic efforts to understand the collective experience of these programmes could enhance the benefits for source and receiving countries in both the short and long term.

### International instruments

From an international perspective, the demand to balance the rights of migrant health workers with equity concerns related to an adequate health workforce in source countries has led to the development of ethical international recruitment policies, codes of practice and various guidelines (42). In the last five years about a dozen of these instruments have emerged from national authorities, professional associations

---

## Box 5.3 Bilateral agreement between South Africa and the United Kingdom

An agreement between South Africa and the United Kingdom was signed in 2003 aiming to create partnerships on health education and workforce issues and facilitate time-limited placements and the exchange of information, advice and expertise. Within the framework of a Memorandum of Understanding, opportunities have been provided for health professionals from one country to spend time-limited education and practice periods in the other country, to the benefit of both.

Exchange of information and expertise covers the following areas:

- professional regulation;
- public health and primary care;
- workforce planning;
- strategic planning;
- public–private partnership, including private finance initiatives;

- revitalization of hospitals, including governance;
- twinning of hospitals to share best practices and strengthen management;
- training in health care management.

The facilitation of mutual access for health professionals to universities and other training institutes for specific training or study visits is part of the agreement. It is planned that the professionals will return home after the exchange period, and for this purpose their posts will be kept open. They will use the new skills to support health system development in their own country. At the Commonwealth Ministers' meeting in May 2005, the South African Minister of Health reported on the success of the bilateral agreement in managing migration of health workers.

Source: (41).

and international bodies. Although not legally binding, they set important norms for behaviour among the key actors involved in the international recruitment of health workers. Whether these norms have sufficient influence to change behaviour remains to be seen.

Mode 4 of the General Agreement on Trade in Services (GATS) of the World Trade Organization (WTO) deals with the temporary movement of people who supply services in the territory of another WTO member. To date, this framework has not been used to assess the fairness of a trade agreement between two countries related to health service providers. As with other GATS processes, the ability of poorer countries effectively to represent and defend their interests cannot be taken for granted *(43)*.

Bilateral agreements on health service providers can provide an explicit and negotiated framework to manage migration. Cuba has had longstanding bilateral agreements regarding health workers with many countries but for many other countries this instrument is more recent (see Box 5.3). Given the complexities of migration patterns – countries may receive health workers from many countries as well as sending health workers elsewhere – there are important questions about the feasibility of managing multiple bilateral agreements for any given country. In addition, the extent to which a bilateral agreement between two governments can cover nongovernmental flows of health workers is not clear.

## OCCUPATIONAL RISKS TO HEALTH WORKERS

In many countries, health workers face the risk of violence, accidents, illness and death, and these risks may prompt them to leave their workplaces.

### Violence

Violence can strike workers in any occupation, but statistics show that health workers are at particularly high risk *(44, 45)*. In Sweden, for example, health care is the sector with the highest risk of violence, as shown in Figure 5.3 *(46)*.

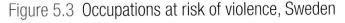

Figure 5.3  Occupations at risk of violence, Sweden

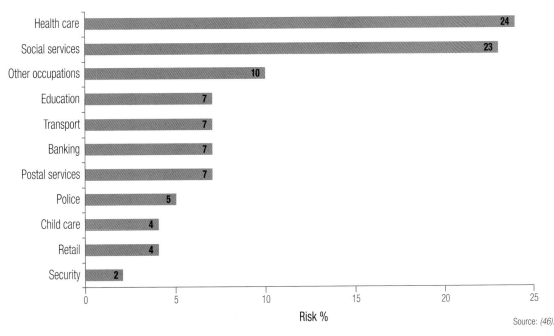

Source: *(46)*.

> **" *In many countries,*
> *health workers face*
> *the risk of violence,*
> *accidents, illness and*
> *death* "**

Violence against women health workers, in particular, has become a significant problem *(47)*. The most frequent violent acts include physical violence, assaults and bullying *(48)*. Some findings suggest a direct link between aggression and increases in sick leave, burnout and staff turnover *(49, 50)*.

## Strategy 5.6 Develop and implement tactics against violence

Through their joint programme on workplace violence in the health sector, the International Labour Organization, the International Council of Nurses, WHO and Public Services International have issued guidelines on prevention, care and support for victims, and management of workplace violence *(51)*. Measures to prevent workplace violence can require substantial investment, as illustrated by the Zero Tolerance campaign in the United Kingdom (see Box 5.4).

### Other risks

Occupational hazards and stress are also important deterrents to retention among health workers. In Canada, for example, nurses have one of the highest sick leave rates of all workers, which is mainly attributed to work-induced stress, burnout and musculoskeletal injury *(56)*. Without basic health and safety guidelines and the ability to implement them, health workers are vulnerable to accidents and exposure to infectious diseases.

One of the major risks of infection – not only to health service providers but also to health management and support workers such as cleaners and waste collectors

## Box 5.4 Strategies in action: examples of exit management

The following examples show how countries are applying some of the strategies examined in the main text to retain workers in the health sector and to minimize the effects of exits.

**Strategy 5.6 Develop and implement tactics against violence: United Kingdom**
The Zero Tolerance campaign against violence began in 1998 and was mainly advertised through a series of high-profile launches. Following its introduction, a survey of 45 NHS trusts revealed that the most common measures implemented were: closed circuit television surveillance (77%), controlled access to certain areas (73%), security guards (73%), better lighting (68%), improved signposting, (68%), improvements in space and layout (62%) and in decoration of public areas (47%), provision of smoking areas (42%) and private rooms (33%), improved cleanliness (31%), and regulation of noise (28%) and temperature (15%). Some of the changes have not been made specifically in relation to reduction of workplace violence, but as overall improvements in the institutions *(52)*.

**Strategy 5.7 Initiate and reinforce a safe work environment: Swaziland and Zambia**
The national nursing association in Swaziland has established an HIV and TB Wellness Centre of Excellence for HIV

positive health workers and their families, while in Zambia, nurses and other health care workers are the focus of a special programme to provide access to antiretroviral treatment to prevent mother-to-child transmission of HIV *(53)*.

**Strategy 5.9 Target health workers outside the health sector: Ireland**
The Irish Nurses Organisation commissioned a survey of non-practising nurses in Ireland to assess potential "returnees" and to evaluate the likely effectiveness of various strategies to encourage them to return to the health workforce. The results suggest that flexible working hours and increased pay could help bring these nurses back to work *(54)*.

**Strategy 5.11 Develop the capacity and policy tools to manage retirement: Guyana**
The government decided to recruit retired nurses to fill shortages in Guyana's HIV/AIDS Reduction and Prevention Projects (GHARP), so that nurses employed elsewhere in the health service would not be hired away from their current jobs. GHARP received 495 applications for 61 positions. When they were recruited, the "new" workers were given training to supplement and update their knowledge *(55)*.

– is injury during unsafe disposal of needles and other biomedical waste. Each year, 3 million health workers worldwide are exposed through the percutaneous route to bloodborne pathogens: 2 million are exposed to hepatitis B, 900 000 to hepatitis C and 170 000 to HIV. These injuries result in 15 000, 70 000 and 1000 infections, respectively. More than 90% of these infections occur in developing countries *(57)*.

### Strategy 5.7 Initiate and reinforce a safe work environment

Infections caused by accidental blood exposure are generally preventable if health workers use appropriate protective wear such as gloves and eye protection, spills of body fluids are cleaned up promptly, and biomedical waste is disposed of correctly. WHO also recommends routine immunization against hepatitis B and prompt management of exposure to blood and body fluids *(57)*.

### Illness and death from HIV/AIDS

In areas where rates of HIV/AIDS are high, attrition rates of health workers due to illness and death are alarming. In Zambia, deaths among female nurses in two hospitals increased from 2 per 1000 in 1980 to 26.7 per 1000 in 1991. Estimates show that Botswana lost 17% of its health workforce to AIDS between 1999 and 2005. If health workers infected with HIV are not treated, the proportion of those dying as a result of AIDS may reach 40% by 2010 *(58, 59)*. In Lesotho and Malawi, death is the largest cause of attrition *(60, 61)*. Absenteeism in the HIV/AIDS workforce can represent up to 50% of staff time in a health worker's final year of life *(62)*.

HIV/AIDS has rendered the health workplace a dangerous place in sub-Saharan Africa. Only a few African countries, notably Swaziland and Zambia, have programmes to counsel, support and treat health workers exposed to HIV (see Box 5.4). Rapid expansion of such programmes is imperative *(63)*.

In 2005 WHO, the International Labour Organization and a panel of experts *(64)* established guidelines on HIV/AIDS and health services that provide specific recommendations on prevention, training, screening, treatment and confidentiality (see Box 5.5).

## CHANGE OF OCCUPATION OR WORK STATUS

Health workers who leave the health labour market or limit the time they spend working can leave gaps in the workforce.

### Choosing a reduced work week

There is an emerging trend in OECD countries for people to seek a more comfortable balance between work, leisure and family time; and health workers are no exception.

Evidence suggests that many doctors – especially young doctors, who tend to place greater emphasis on personal time – are working fewer hours *(65, 66)*. In addition workers, especially women, are increasingly seeking part-time work *(67–71)*.

### Strategy 5.8 Accommodate workers' needs and expectations

Offering part-time jobs and facilitating the return of workers who have taken maternity leave can prevent departures from the workforce and encourage the return

> " *Each year, 3 million health workers worldwide are exposed to bloodborne HIV and hepatitis viruses* "

of workers who have left. Incentives such as affordable child care, financial support for children, and provision of leave adapted to family needs can encourage entry into the workforce, especially nursing *(72, 73)*.

## Health workers not employed in their field

There is little reliable information on how many workers below retirement age have left the health sector, but it is certain that their reasons vary. Some workers may find available jobs unacceptable or in the wrong location; others may lack job opportunities. The example of nursing is illustrative. In the United States, of the approximately 500 000 registered nurses who are not in the nursing labour market, 36 000 are seeking employment in nursing and 136 000 are working in non-nursing occupations, despite the fact that the estimated number of vacancies exceeds 100 000 *(74)*. In contrast, some 5000 nurses in Kenya are not currently working in their field due in part to ceilings or caps placed on public sector recruitment of health workers *(75)*. South Africa has about 35 000 registered nurses who are inactive or unemployed, despite 32 000 vacancies *(76)*.

## Strategy 5.9 Target health workers outside the health sector

Evidence is scarce on the effectiveness of policies to recruit workers from outside the health sector, but there are some indications that they could make a difference. Research could reveal the sort of conditions that would encourage health workers to return to the jobs for which they were trained (see Box 5.4 for an example from Ireland).

## Absentees and ghost workers

Although anecdotal evidence of absenteeism among health workers abounds (especially in South-East Asia), researchers have begun only recently to measure the problem systematically. A recent study involving unannounced visits to primary health facilities in six countries – Bangladesh, Ecuador, India, Indonesia, Peru and Uganda – found medical personnel absenteeism rates from 23% to 40%, with generally higher numbers in lower income countries and in lower income regions within countries *(77)*.

One study in Bangladesh revealed, unsurprisingly, that remoteness and difficulty of access were major correlates of absenteeism. Personnel in facilities in villages or towns that had roads and electricity were far less likely to be absent. Absentee rates

## Box 5.5 Measures for a safe work environment: HIV/AIDS

Key principles of the joint ILO/WHO guidelines on health services and HIV/AIDS:
- Prevention and containment of transmission risks: measures should be taken for hazard identification, risk assessment and risk control and provisions made for post-exposure management.
- Ongoing national dialogue, including all types of negotiation, consultation and information-sharing among governments, employers and workers, should be a key mechanism for the introduction of HIV/AIDS policies and programmes that build a safer and healthier working environment.
- Information, education and training should be offered to sensitize the health care workplace to issues related to HIV/AIDS and the rights and needs of patients as well as workers. Mandatory HIV screening, for the purpose of exclusion from employment, should not be required, and employment of workers living with HIV/AIDS should continue while they are medically fit.
- Gender focus: as the health services sector is a major employer of women, special emphasis should be placed on the particular challenges faced by them in the health care working environment. Programmes, education, and training initiatives should ensure that both men and women understand their rights within the workplace and outside it.

Source: *(64)*.

among doctors tended to correlate positively with conditions such as poor latrine facilities, lack of access to piped and potable water, and the absence of visual privacy at the health centre *(78)*.

Ghost workers are individuals who are listed on the payroll but who do not exist, or who work only part time *(78)*. Eliminating ghost workers is a complex task and can be costly. Moreover, in some cases authorities may condone dual employment as a coping strategy that allows health workers to earn a satisfactory income and as a means to attract health workers to otherwise unattractive locations. This complacency about ghost work may explain why legislation forbidding dual employment has failed in many countries. Another drain on health workforce financing in some countries is the continued presence on the books of workers who have left the health sector or died. For example, in Ghana, of the 131 000 civil servants on the payroll at the end of August 1987, 1500 had actually left the service *(79)*.

### Strategy 5.10 Keep track of the workforce

Regular audits, physical head counts, questionnaires, and reconciliation of different data sources could help to identify ghost workers and reduce the number of unauthorized absences. Such information should be made available to the public, and affected institutions should be empowered to take corrective actions.

## RETIREMENT

The average statutory pensionable age varies by as much as 8.2 years across WHO regions. Europe and the Americas have the highest retirement ages, while South-East Asia has the lowest (see Table 5.4) The statutory pensionable age is younger for women than for men across all regions.

The statutory pensionable age often differs from the actual age of retirement *(82)*. Evidence suggests that some independent health workers continue working after they have reached pensionable age *(83, 89)*. At the same time, workers in many countries are choosing to retire before they reach the statutory pensionable age *(85)*. The trend towards earlier retirement seems to be taking hold among health workers as well *(84)* and is likely to be reinforced by the increasing presence of women, who retire earlier than their male counterparts *(86–88)*.

> " *In the United Kingdom, about 10 000 nurses retire every year* "

### Retirement rates and the risk of shortages

Information about the retirement rate of health workers is very scarce. An expected working life of 30 years for doctors and 23 for nurses *(89)*, as well as a uniform age distribution, would result in a retirement rate of 3% for doctors and 4% for nurses. However, these figures do not account for other attrition factors such as death, different working patterns such as part-time employment, and the actual age distribution. As a result, the retirement rate in reality is lower. In the United Kingdom, estimates show that about 10 000 nurses (2% of the nursing workforce) retire each year *(87)*. In countries with the greatest needs-based shortages, little information is available about exits from the health workforce. In sub-Saharan Africa, the number of health service providers who retire annually is estimated to be between 8780 and 13 070 *(90)*, representing 0.6–1% of the health workforce. Although these retirement figures for Africa might seem low, they become significant when other attrition factors are taken into account and when they are compared with the figures related to the inflow of health workers.

## Table 5.4 Statutory pensionable age

| WHO region | Number of Member States | | Pensionable age (years) | |
|---|---|---|---|---|
| | In region | Reporting | Average for men (range) | Average for women (range) |
| Africa | 46 | 37 | 58 (50– 65) | 57 (50–65) |
| Americas | 35 | 34 | 62 (55–65) | 61 (55–65) |
| South-East Asia | 11 | 6 | 55 (55–57) | 55 (50–57) |
| Europe | 52 | 49 | 64 (60–67) | 61 (55–67) |
| Eastern Mediterranean | 21 | 15 | 60 (50–65) | 57 (50–64) |
| Western Pacific | 27 | 20 | 58 (50–65) | 58 (50–65) |

Sources: *(80, 81)*.

## Health workforce ageing

In many countries, a trend towards earlier retirement dovetails with a rise in the average age of health workers, and these dual shifts could lead to mass exits from the health workforce *(88, 91, 92)*. Middle-aged nurses, who are part of the "baby boom" generation born after the Second World War, dominate the workforce in many countries and will reach retirement age within the next 10 to 15 years. In the United States, for example, progressive ageing of the registered nurse population since

## Figure 5.4 Ageing nurses in the United States of America

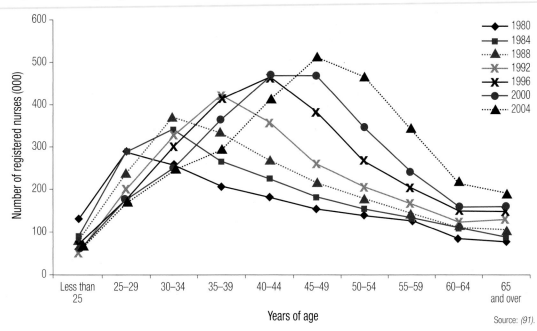

Source: *(91)*.

1980 indicates that there will be accelerated attrition of experienced nurses from the workforce at a time of growing demand *(93, 94)*, as shown in Figure 5.4.

The ageing trend is not systematic across countries, however. Some developing countries, like Lesotho, have a younger physician workforce, for example, than industrialized countries such as Switzerland (see Figure 5.5).

Unlike illness and migration, retirement is relatively predictable. Proactive retirement policies could prevent any shortages connected to early retirement and an ageing workforce.

## Strategy 5.11 Develop the capacity and policy tools to manage retirement

Information systems can capture details of age patterns, yearly outflows caused by retirement and patterns of retirement, which lay the groundwork for effective management policies that reduce or increase retirement outflows. Once those policies are in place, employers may provide incentives to workers to retire earlier or later, and governments may offer subsidies or taxes to change the costs of employing older people or consider making changes to the statutory pensionable age. Retirees represent a pool of health workers who could be recruited back into the health workforce to provide a much needed increase in numbers and experience in resource-constrained environments around the world. Box 5.4 describes one such scheme in Guyana.

### The need for knowledge transfer

Retirement removes from the health care delivery system not just workers themselves, but also their hands-on experience and institutional knowledge. Failure to transfer the experience and knowledge of exiting workers to those who remain, through succession planning, can deprive the workforce of key competencies and skills. Poor succession planning has been identified as a key challenge associated with nursing in rural and remote areas *(96)*.

### Strategy 5.12 Develop succession planning

Succession planning – which entails such strategies as having prospective retirees mentor younger staff and participate in knowledge sharing mechanisms such as communities of practice – can transmit knowledge from experienced health workers to their successors and minimize the impact of retirement on the workforce.

## Figure 5.5 Age distribution of doctors

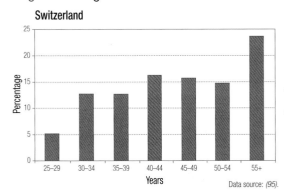
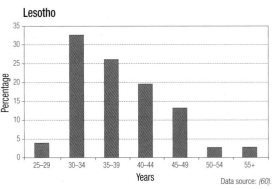

Data source: *(95)*.

Data source: *(60)*.

## CONCLUSION

Although this chapter is not an exhaustive treatment of the factors leading to temporary or permanent exit from the workforce, it has nonetheless dealt with four major dimensions: migration; risk of violence, illness and death; occupational change; and retirement. Each requires careful analysis in its own right with its respective responses, yet when examined as a group, the bigger picture of workforce exits or attrition emerges. This picture reveals the rate of worker outflow, and along with information on inflows, permits an assessment of the relative balance in terms of entry and exits. In a steady state, or workforce equilibrium, the flows into the workforce – primarily from training and recruitment – should equal the outflows. However, if at the baseline there is a major shortfall of workers, as in the case of the 57 countries with critical shortages identified in Chapter 1, then inflows should greatly exceed outflows.

The case of sub-Saharan Africa is instructive in this regard. This chapter has revealed major exits of health professionals from the workforce due to migration, ill-health and absenteeism and to a much lesser degree from retirement. Redressing the critical shortages in Africa requires not only expanding inflows through training more workers but significantly diminishing the rate of outflow through better retention, improved worker health, and reducing the wastage that is inherent in absenteeism and ghost workers.

The set of factors linked to taking workers out of the workforce draws attention to the importance of looking forward and being aware of trends. The age distribution of the workforce in many richer countries discloses a "greying" trend that will result in accelerated attrition through retirement in the medium term. Likewise, the sex distribution reveals patterns of "feminization", especially in the medical profession, with patterns of work and retirement among women that differ significantly from those of men. Such trends cannot afford to be ignored. Rather, they call for forward planning to avoid significant imbalances. In the case of women, greater efforts must be made to retain health work as a career of choice by providing greater protection at the workplace from abuse and insecurity, more flexibility in work patterns that accommodate family considerations, and promotion ladders that allow them to advance to senior management and leadership positions in the health sector.

Finally, as exemplified by the case of international migration, the health workforce is strongly linked to global labour markets. Shortages in richer countries send strong market signals to poorer countries with an inevitable response through increased flows of migrant workers. In articulating their plans for the workforce, countries must recognize this and other linkages beyond their borders. The next two chapters focus on the challenges of formulating national strategies in the current global context.

# REFERENCES

1. Zurn P, Dal Poz MR, Stilwell B, Adams O. Imbalance in the health workforce. *Human Resources for Health*, 2004, 2:13 (http://www.human-resources-health.com/content/2/1/13, accessed 2 February 2006).

2. Egger D, Lipson D, Adams O. *Achieving the right balance: the role of policy-making processes in managing human resources for health problems.* Geneva, World Health Organization, 2000 (Issues in health services delivery. Discussion paper 2; WHO/EIP/OSD/00.2; http://www.who.int/hrh/documents/en/right_balance.pdf, accessed 23 January 2006).

3. Zurn P, Dolea C, Stilwell B. *Nurse retention and recruitment: developing a motivated workforce.* Geneva, International Council of Nurses, 2005 (Issue Paper 4; http://www.icn.ch/global/Issue4Retention.pdf, accessed 2 February 2006).

4. Buchan J, Thompson M, O'May F. *Health workforce incentive and remuneration strategies: a research review.* Geneva, World Health Organization, 2000 (Issues in health services delivery, Discussion paper 4. Incentive and remuneration strategies; WHO/EIP/OSD/00.14; http://www.who.int/health-services-delivery/disc_papers/Incentives_remuneration.pdf, accessed 23 January 2006).

5. Stilwell B, Diallo K, Zurn P, Dal Poz MR, Adams O, Buchan J. Developing evidence-based ethical policies on the migration of health workers: conceptual and practical challenges. *Human Resources for Health*, 2003, 1:8.

6. Aiken LH, Buchan J, Sochalski J, Nichols B, Powell M. Trends in international nurse migration. *Health Affairs,* 2004, 23:69–77.

7. Buchan J, Calman L. *The global shortage of registered nurses: an overview of issues and actions.* Geneva, International Council of Nurses, 2004 (http://www.icn.ch/global/shortage.pdf, accessed 2 February 2006).

8. Buchan J, Parkin T, Sochalski J. *International nurse mobility: trends and policy implications.* Geneva, World Health Organization, 2003.

9. Buchan J, Jobanputra R, Gough P, Hutt R. *Internationally recruited nurses in London: profile and implications for policy.* London, King's Fund, 2005 (http://www.kingsfund.org.uk/resources/publications/internationally.html, accessed 2 February 2006).

10. Awases M, Gbary A, Nyoni J, Chatora R. *Migration of health professionals in six countries.* Brazzaville, World Health Organization Regional Office for Africa, 2004.

11. *Trends in international migration.* Paris, Organisation for Economic Co-operation and Development, 2005.

12. Hagopian A, Thompson M, Fordyce M, Johnson K, Hart LG. The migration of physicians from sub-Saharan Africa to the United States of America: measures of the African brain drain. *Human Resources for Health*, 2004, 2:17.

13. Tevera D. *Early departures: the emigration potential of Zimbabwean students.* Cape Town, Southern African Migration Project, 2005 (Migration Policy Series no. 39; http://www.queensu.ca/samp/sampresources/samppublications/policyseries/policy39.htm, accessed 2 February 2006).

14. Iredale R. The migration of professionals: theories and typologies. *International Migration*, 2001, 39:7–26.

15. Findlay A, Stewart E. S*killed labour migration from developing countries.* Geneva, International Labour Organization, 2002 (ILO International Migration Papers, No. 55).

16. Lowell BL, Findlay A. *Skilled Labour Migration from developing countries.* Geneva, International Labour Organization, 2002 (ILO International Migration Papers, No. 56).

17. Mejía A, Pizurki H, Royston E. *Physician migration and nurse migration: analysis and policy implications.* Geneva, World Health Organization, 1979.

18. Stilwell B, Diallo K, Zurn P, Vujicic M, Adams O, Dal Poz MR. Migration of health workers from developing countries: strategic approaches to its management. *Bulletin of the World Health Organization,* 2004, 82:595–600.

19. *Unlocking the human potential for public sector performance.* New York, United Nations Department of Economic and Social Affairs, 2005 (World Public Sector Report, ST/ESA/PAD/SER.E/63).

20. Anderson B, Rogaly B. *Forced labour and migration to the UK.* Oxford, Centre for Migration Policy and Society, 2005.

21. Van Eyck K. *Who cares? Women health workers in the global labour market*. Ferney-Voltaire, Public Services International, 2005.
22. *Global economic prospects: economic implications of remittances and migration*. Washington, DC, The World Bank, 2005.
23. Mensah K, Mackintosh M, Henry L. The "skills drain" of health professionals from the developing world: a framework for policy formulation. London, Medact, 2005 (http://www.medact.org/article_health.php?articleID=337, accessed 2 February 2006).
24. Chen LC, Boufford JI. Fatal flows – doctors on the move. *New England Journal of Medicine*, 2005, 353:1850–1852.
25. Wibulpolprasert S. Economic uncertainties: future challenges to world health. Lessons learned from Thailand. In: *Health by the people: a celebration of the life of Ken Newell*. Liverpool, Liverpool School of Tropical Medicine, 2001.
26. *The migration of skilled health personnel in the Pacific Region*. Manila, World Health Organization Regional Office for the Western Pacific, 2004.
27. *Health Priorities in the World Bank's Pacific Member Countries*. Washington, DC, The World Bank, 1994.
28. Choy CC. *Empire of care: nursing and migration in Filipino American history*. Durham, NC, Duke University Press, 2003.
29. Commander S. *Brains: what can they do for export?* Sussex Development Lecture 2004 (http://www.london.edu/assets/documents/PDF/brains_lecture.pdf, accessed 2 February 2006).
30. Denham L, Shaddock A. Recruitment and retention of rural allied health professionals in developmental disability services in New South Wales. *Australian Journal of Rural Health*, 2004, 12:28–29.
31. Reid S. Community service for health professionals: coercion, change and challenge. In: *South African Health Review, 2002*. Durban, Health Systems Trust, 2002 (http://www.hst.org.za, accessed 2 February 2006).
32. Turrittin J, Hagey R, Guruge S, Collins E, Mitchell M. The experiences of professional nurses who have migrated to Canada: cosmopolitan citizenship or democratic racism? *International Journal of Nursing Studies*, 2002, 39:655–667.
33. Connell J, Brown R. *Remittances in the Pacific: an overview*. Manila, Asian Development Bank, 2005 (http://www.adb.org, accessed 2 February 2006).
34. Van Eyck K. *Women and international migration in the health sector*. Ferney-Voltaire, Public Services International, 2004.
35. Hagey R, Choudhry U, Guruge S, Turrittin J, Collins E, Lee R. Immigrant nurses' experience of racism. *Journal of Nursing Scholarship*, 2001, 33:389–394.
36. Turrittin J, Hagey R, Guruge S, Collins E, Mitchell M. The experiences of professional nurses who have migrated to Canada: cosmopolitan citizenship or democratic racism? *International Journal of Nursing Studies*, 2002, 39:655–667.
37. Rokoduru A. *The contemporary migration of skilled labour from Fiji to Pacific Island countries*. Canberra, Asia Pacific Migration Research Network, 2002 (Working Paper No. 12:43–48).
38. Allen H, Aggergaard LJ. *"We need respect" – experiences of internationally recruited nurses in the UK*. London, Royal College of Nursing, 2003 (http://www.rcn.org.uk/downloads/international/irn-report-we-need-respect.pdf, accessed 2 February 2006).
39. Barré R, Hernandez V, Meyer J-P, Vinck D. *Diasporas scientifiques*. Paris, Institut de recherche pour le développement (IRD), 2003.
40. *Building bridges: a report to the Massachusetts–South Africa Health Care Task Force* Boston, MA, South Africa Partners, 2000 (http://www.sapartners.org/documents/Doc4.pdf, accessed 2 February 2006).
41. Mafubelu D. *Using bilateral arrangements to manage migration of health care professionals: the case of South Africa and the United Kingdom*. Paper presented at: IOM/WHO/CDC Seminar on Health and Migration, Geneva, June 2004 (http://www.iom.int/documents/officialtxt/en/pp%5Fbilateral%5Fsafrica.pdf, accessed 2 February 2006).
42. *Management of international health worker migration. Instruments on ethical recruitment and other policy options*. Geneva, World Health Organization, 2004 (unpublished report).
43. *World migration report – Costs and benefits of international migration*. Geneva, International Organization for Migration, 2005.

44. Cooper C, Swanson N, eds. *Workplace violence in the health sector. State of the art.* Geneva, ILO/ICN/WHO/PSI Joint Programme on Workplace Violence in the Health Sector, 2002 (Working paper; http://www.who.int/violence_injury_prevention/injury/en/WVstateart.pdf, accessed 2 February 2006).

45. Di Martino V. *Workplace violence in the health sector. Country case studies: Brazil, Bulgaria, Lebanon, Portugal, South Africa, Thailand and an additional Australian study, Synthesis report.* Geneva, ILO/ICN/WHO/PSI Joint Programme on Workplace Violence in the Health Sector, 2002 (Working paper; http://www.who.int/violence_injury_prevention/injury/en/WVsynthesisreport.pdf, accessed 2 February 2006).

46. Chappell D, Di Martino V. Violence at work. *Asian-Pacific Newsletter on Occupational Health and Safety,* 1999, 6(1) (http://www.ilo.org/public/english/protection/safework/violence/violwk/violwk.pdf, accessed 2 February 2006).

47. Dalphond D, Gessner M, Giblin E, Hijazzi K, Love C. Violence against emergency nurses. *Journal of Emergency Nursing*, 2000, 26:105.

48. Jackson D, Clare J, Mannix J. Who would want to be a nurse? Violence in the workplace – a factor in recruitment and retention. *Journal of Nursing Management*, 2002, 10:13–20.

49. Farrell GA. Aggression in clinical settings: nurses' views – a follow-up study. *Journal of Advanced Nursing*, 1999, 29:532–541.

50. O'Connell B, Young J, Brooks J, Hutchings J, Lofthouse J. Nurses' perceptions of the nature and frequency of aggression in general ward settings and high dependency areas. *Journal of Clinical Nursing*, 2000, 9:602–610.

51. International Labour Organization (ILO), International Council of Nurses (ICN), World Health Organization (WHO) and Public Services International (PSI). *Framework guidelines for addressing workplace violence in the health sector.* Geneva, ILO/ICN/WHO/PSI Joint Programme on Workplace Violence in the Health Sector, 2002 (http://www.who.int/violence_injury_prevention/violence/interpersonal/en/WVguidelinesEN.pdf, accessed 2 February 2006).

52. Wiskow C. *Guidelines on workplace violence in the health sector – Comparison of major known national guidelines and strategies: United Kingdom, Australia, Sweden, USA.* Geneva, ILO/ICN/WHO/PSI Joint Programme on Workplace Violence in the Health Sector (forthcoming working paper).

53. *Healthy and valued health workers are essential to save health systems in sub-Saharan Africa.* Geneva, International Council of Nurses, 2005 (Press release ICN/PR05, No. 21; http://www.icn.ch/PR21_05.htm, accessed 25 February 2006).

54. Egan M, Moynihan M. *An examination of non practising qualified nurses and midwives in the Republic of Ireland and an assessment of their intentions and willingness to return to practice.* Dublin, Irish Nurses Organisation/Michael Smurfit Business School, 2003.

55. Morgan R. *Addressing health worker shortages: recruiting retired nurses to reduce mother-to-child transmission in Guyana. Snapshots from the field.* Arlington, VA, Family Health International, 2005.

56. Shamian J, O'Brien-Pallas L, Thomson D, Alksnis C, Kerr MS. Nurse absenteeism, stress and workplace injury: what are the contributing factors and what can/should be done about it? *International Journal of Sociology and Social Policy*, 2003, 23:81–103.

57. *Aide-mémoire for a strategy to protect health workers from infection with bloodborne viruses.* Geneva, World Health Organization, 2003 (http://www.who.int/injection_safety/toolbox/docs/en/AM_HCW_Safety.pdf, accessed 1 February 2006).

58. Cohen D. *Human capital and the HIV epidemic in sub-Saharan Africa.* Geneva, International Labour Organization, 2002 (Working Paper 2).

59. Buve A, Foaster SD, Mbwili C, Mungo E, Tollenare N, Zeko M. Mortality among female nurses in the face of the AIDS epidemic: a pilot study in Zambia. *AIDS,* 1994, 8:396.

60. Schwabe C, McGrath E, Lerotholi K. *Lesotho human resources consultancy: health sector human resources needs assessment.* Silver Spring, MD, Medical Care Development International, 2004.

61. *Challenges facing the Malawian health workforce in the era of HIV/AIDS. Final draft.* Washington, DC, Commonwealth Regional Health Community Secretariat (CRHCS), United States Agency for International Development, Bureau for Africa (USAID/AFR), and Support for Analysis and Research in Africa (SARA) Project, 2004.

62. Kober K, Van Damme W. Scaling up access to antiretroviral treatment in southern Africa: who will do the job? *Lancet,* 2004, 364:103–107.

63. Tawfik L, Kinoti S. *The impact of HIV/AIDS on the health workforce in developing countries.* Arlington, VA, Management Sciences for Health and Bethesda, MD, University Research Co., LLC, 2005.

64. *Joint ILO/WHO guidelines on health services and HIV/AIDS.* Geneva, International Labour Organization and World Health Organization, 2005.

65. Schroeder SA. How many hours is enough? An old profession meets a new generation. *Annals of Internal Medicine*, 2004, 140:838–839 (http://www.annals.org/cgi/content/full/140/10/838, accessed 2 February 2006).

66. Buske L. Younger physicians providing less direct patient care. *Canadian Medical Association Journal*, 2004, 170:1217.

67. Knaul F, Frenk J, Aguilar A. The gender composition of the medical profession in Mexico: implications for employment patterns and physician labor supply. *Journal of American Medical Women's Association*, 1999, 55:32–35.

68. Higginbotham E. Celebrating women in ophthalmology. *Archives of Ophthalmology*, 1998, 116:1227–1228.

69. Reamy J, Pong R. *Physician workforce composition by gender: the implications for managing physician supply.* Paper presented at: 4th FICOSSER General Conference, Cuernavaca, Mexico, 1998.

70. Hojat M, Gonnella J, Xu G. Gender comparisons of young physicians' perceptions of their medical education, professional life, and practice: a follow-up study of Jefferson Medical College graduates. *Academic Medicine*, 1995, 70:305–312.

71. Woodward C, Hurley J. Comparison of activity level and service intensity of male and female in five fields of medicine in Ontario. *Canadian Medical Association Journal*, 1995, 153:1097–1106.

72. *Babies and bosses: reconciling work and family life, Canada, Finland, Sweden and the United Kingdom. Vol. 4.* Paris, Organisation for Economic Co-operation and Development, 2005.

73. Phillips VL. Nurses' labor supply: participation, hours of work, and discontinuities in the supply function. *Journal of Health Economics*, 1995, 14:567–582.

74. Lafer G, Moss H, Kirtner R, Rees V. *Solving the nursing shortage.* Eugene, OR, University of Oregon, 2003.

75. *Health workforce challenges: lessons from country experiences.* Background paper for the High-Level Forum on the Health MDGs, Abuja, 2004 (http://www.hlfhealthmdgs.org/Documents/HealthWorkforceChallenges-Final.pdf, accessed 2 February 2006)

76. The international mobility of health professionals: an evaluation and analysis based on the case of South Africa. In: *Trends in international migration, Part III.* Paris, Organisation for Economic Co-operation and Development, 2004.

77. Chaudhury N, Hammer J, Kremer M, Muralidharan K, Rogers FH. Provider absence in schools and health clinics. *Journal of Economic Perspectives* (forthcoming; http://post.economics.harvard.edu/faculty/kremer/webpapers/MissinginAction.pdf, accessed 2 February 2006).

78. Chaudhury N, Hammer J. *Ghost doctors: absenteeism in Bangladeshi health facilities.* Washington, DC, The World Bank, 2003 (Policy Research Working Paper No. 3065).

79. Dovlo D. 2005: Wastage in the health workforce: some perspectives from African countries. *Human Resources for Health*, 2005, 3:6 (http://www.human-resources-health.com/content/3/1/6, accessed 2 February 2006).

80. McCallum N, Tyler V. *International experience with civil service censuses and civil service databases*. London, International Records Management Trust, 2001 (http://www.irmt. org/download/DOCUME~1/DEVELO~1/RESEAR~1/Census.pdf, accessed 2 February 2006).
81. *Social security programs throughout the world*. Washington, DC, Social Security Administration and International Social Security Association, 2003–2005 (http://www. ssa.gov/policy/docs/progdesc/ssptw, accessed 23 January 2006).
82. Keese M, Hirsch D. *Live longer, work longer*. Paris, Organisation for Economic Co-operation and Development (forthcoming).
83. Starkiene L, Smigelskas K, Padaiga Z, Reamy J. The future prospects of Lithuanian family physicians: a 10-year forecasting study. *BMC Family Practice*, 2005, 6:41.
84. Greene J. Physicians enticed into early retirement. *American Medical News*, 2000, 43:1–2.
85. Auer P, Fortuny M. *Ageing of the labour force in OECD countries: economic and social consequences*. Geneva, International Labour Organization, 2000 (http://www.ilo. org/public/english/employment/strat/download/ep2.pdf, accessed 23 January 2006).
86. Canadian Labour and Business Centre, for Task Force Two: A Physician Human Resource Strategy for Canada. *Physician workforce in Canada: literature review and gap analysis. Final report*. Ottawa, Government of Canada, 2003 (http://www.physicianhr.ca/reports/ literatureReviewGapAnalysis-e.pdf, accessed 23 January 2006).
87. Watson R, Manthorpe J, Andrews J. *Nurses over 50: options, decisions and outcomes*. Bristol, Policy Press in association with the Joseph Rowntree Foundation, 2003.
88. Schofield DJ, Beard JR. Baby boomer doctors and nurses: demographic change and transitions to retirement. *Medical Journal of Australia*, 2005, 183:80–83.
89. Netten A, Knight J. Annuitizing the human capital investment costs of health service professionals. *Health Economics*, 1999, 8:245–255.
90. Kinfu Y, Mercer H, Dal Poz MR, Evans DB. *Estimating inflows and outflows of health service providers in sub-Saharan Africa*. Geneva, World Health Organization, 2006 (background paper for The world health report 2006. available at: http://www.who. int/hrh/documents/enl).
91. Buerhaus P, Staiger D, Auerbach D. Implications of an ageing registered nurse workforce. *JAMA*, 2000, 283:2948–2954.
92. Buchan J. The "greying"of the United Kingdom nursing workforce: implications for employment policy and practice. *Journal of Advanced Nursing*, 1999, 30:818–826.
93. *The registered nurse population: national sample survey of registered nurses, March 2004. Preliminary findings*. Washington, DC, United States Department of Health and Human Services, 2005 (ftp.hrsa.gov/bhpr/nursing/rnpopulation/ theregisterednursepopulation.pdf, accessed 23 January 2006).
94. Janiszewski Goodin H. The nursing shortage in the United States of America: an integrative review of the literature. *Journal of Advanced Nursing*, 2003, 43:335–343.
95. Swiss Medical Association, 2004 (http://www.fmh.ch/shared/data/pdf/import_fmh/ict/ statistik/2004/sts2004-14.pdf, accessed 2 February 2006).
96. National Rural Health Alliance. *Nursing in rural and remote areas*. Deakin, Association for Australian Rural Nurses Inc., 2002 (Position paper; http://www.aarn.asn.au/pdf/papers/ position_paper.pdf, accessed 2 February 2006).

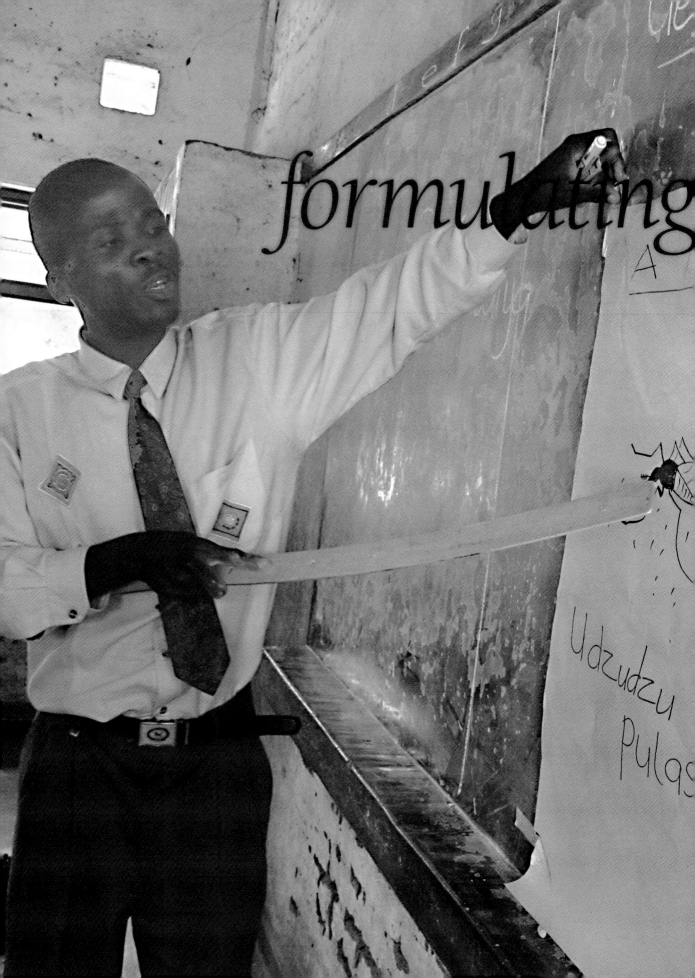

formulating

Udzudzu
Pulas

## chapter six
# national health workforce strategies

**The ultimate goal of health workforce strategies is a delivery system that can guarantee universal access to health care and social protection to all citizens in every country. There is no global blueprint that describes how to get there – each nation must devise its own plan. Effective workforce strategies must be matched to a country's unique situation and based on a social consensus.**

The workforce presents a set of interrelated problems that cannot be quickly tidied up or solved by a "magic bullet". Workforce problems are deeply embedded in changing contexts, fraught with uncertainty and exacerbated by a lack of information. Most significantly, the problems can be emotionally charged because of status issues and politically sensitive because of divergent interests. That is why workforce solutions require all stakeholders to be engaged together, both in diagnosing problems and in solving them.

The key is to mobilize political commitment to tackle workforce challenges. But this is difficult because achieving a health impact from an investment in the workforce takes time, extending well beyond election cycles. Disgruntled workers can paralyse a health system, stall health-sector reform, occasionally even bring down a government. Yet, successful strategies have been demonstrated that can energize the workforce and win public support. The political challenge is to apply known solutions, to craft new approaches, to monitor progress, and to make mid-course corrections.

Previous chapters have focused on dealing with workforce problems through the management of entry, workforce and exit. These aspects determine the performance of a health system and its ability to meet present and future challenges.

However, such problems cannot only be discussed in managerial and technical terms. The perspective of people who use the health care system must also be considered. Their expectations are not about the efficient delivery of cost-effective interventions to target populations; they are about getting help and care when faced with a health problem that they cannot cope with by themselves. In the relationship between individual health workers and individual clients, trust is of paramount importance, and it requires fair governing and effective regulations to build and sustain – which in turn involves leadership, strategic intelligence and capacity building in institutions, tools and training. These essential elements of national workforce strategies are the focus of this chapter.

## BUILDING TRUST AND MANAGING EXPECTATIONS

To the general public, the term "health workers" evokes doctors and nurses. While this does not do justice to the multitude of people who make a health care system work, it does reflect the public's expectations: encounters with knowledgeable, skilled – and trustworthy – doctors and nurses who will help them to get better and who will act in their best interests.

Trust is not automatic: it has to be actively produced and negotiated. It is "slowly gained but easily lost in the face of confounded expectations" (1). In many countries the medical establishment has lost its aura of infallibility, even-handedness and dedication to the patient's interests. Fuelled by press reports of dysfunctional health care provision, public trust in health workers is eroding in the industrialized world (2) as well as in many developing countries (3–5). Poor people in particular may be sceptical or cynical when talking about their doctors, nurses or midwives: "We would rather treat ourselves than go to the hospital where an angry nurse might inject us with the wrong drug" (6). Trust is jeopardized each time patients do not get the care they need, or get care they do not need, or pay too much for the care they do receive. When patients experience violence, abuse or racketeering in health facilities their fragile trust is shattered.

The consequences of loss of trust go beyond the individual relationship between user and provider. A society that mistrusts its health workers discourages them from pursuing this career. The erosion of trust in health workers also affects those who manage and steer the health system (7). The administrations in charge of the health care system – governments, health-insurance institutions and professional organizations – have to make difficult trade-offs. They have to decide between competing demands: each citizen's entitlement of access to health care goods and services; the need to govern the cost of the uptake of these goods and services; and the needs of the professionals and other human resources who deliver these goods and services. The characteristics of the health sector with its large number of actors, asymmetry of information and conflicting interests make it particularly vulnerable to the abuse of entrusted power for private gain (8). The public no longer takes for granted that these trade-offs are always made fairly and effectively, nor do the front-line health workers.

### Strategy 6.1 Design and implement a workforce strategy that fosters trust

The design of a strategy for a national health workforce might include measures actively to produce and negotiate trust in providers and managers of the health system (9, 10). This requires explicit measures that:

- address personal behaviour in the interaction between care providers and patients, between employers and employees, and between managers and institutions (this requires training as well as political leadership, and civil society organizations play a key role);
- set up managerial and organizational practices that give space for responsiveness, caring, interpersonal interaction and dialogue, and support the building of trust;
- take visible steps to eliminate exclusion and protect patients against mismanagement and financial exploitation;
- establish decision-making processes that are seen as fair and inclusive.

# FAIR AND COOPERATIVE GOVERNING

Building and sustaining trust and protecting the public from harm require good governance and effective oversight, as well as fair regulation of the operations of health care facilities and the behaviour of health workers. The problem is that, in many countries, the regulatory environment is opaque and dysfunctional. All too often, weak professional and civil society organizations with few resources or little political clout exist alongside an equally weak state bureaucracy that lacks the structures, the people and the political will for the effective regulation of the health care sector.

## Self-regulation

In many countries, professional organizations decide who can provide care and how providers should behave. Self-regulation can indeed be effective and positive: professional associations can promote professional ethics and positive role models, sanction inappropriate behaviour, and maintain the technical competence of their members. The way health workers balance their own interests and those of their patients depends to a large extent on what is considered "good professional behaviour" by their teachers and peers. Professional associations can play an active role in shaping that image (see Box 6.1).

Self-regulation by professional associations is not always effective, for a number of reasons. First, unlike doctors and nurses, some categories of health workers are not organized in this way. Second, each professional category tends to have its own organization, which results in energy being wasted in battles over boundaries and in defence of professional privileges. Third, in contrast to Europe and the Americas, where the majority of professional organizations are well established and date back at least 100 years, four out of 10 associations in low income countries are less than 25 years old *(11)*. These younger organizations tend to be under-resourced and less well connected politically, and, crucially, to have less authority over their members.

The professional self-regulation model is also showing signs of strain because employers increasingly override it. This has long been the case where the state is the traditional employer of health workers, but in countries where large numbers of health workers were self-employed and autonomous, most of them now work in an employer–employee relationship. As a result of this "proletarianization" of health workers *(12)*, it is employers and not professional organizations who exert the most influence on professional behaviour. This is the case whether the employer is the state, a not-for-profit nongovernmental organization, a financial corporation or an international organization. This shift to employer-power is so pronounced that, in some countries, health professionals have started to form unions in reaction to employer challenges to their autonomy and income *(13)*. As a result, professional associations by themselves can no longer claim to provide coherent governance, in the public interest, of the health workforce as a whole.

## "Muddling through" and command-and-control

Driven by political pressure for universal access and financial protection, governments have taken an increasingly prominent role in financing and regulating the collective consumption of health care (14). This has overriden the autonomous governance of professional organizations, and self-regulation has been gradually replaced by a more elaborate institutional control by public administration (15).

The way this control operated varied from place to place. In much of Europe and the Americas, where a large part of the workforce was self-employed or employed by private institutions, much of the state's regulatory efforts focused on payment mechanisms and on training and accreditation mechanisms to define the territory of the various health professions. Given the resistance of professional associations to state encroachment on their autonomy, the process of governing health workers was very much a process of "muddling through" a low-intensity conflict (16, 17). There is a tradition, however, of negotiated regulation that has effectively built up the regulatory capacities of state and social security organizations.

In many socialist and developing countries, where a large proportion of health workers are in the employ of government, a more elaborate kind of institutional control has effectively replaced self-regulation. In these countries the public administration tends to rely on a command-and-control approach: the use of hierarchy and administrative rules to govern the health workforce. It is true that a well-functioning command-and-control structure is advantageous in controlling epidemics and responding to environmental catastrophes. As a strategy to regulate and orient the health care market, however, the approach has its limitations.

At worst, when a health system is structurally underfunded or near collapse or the legitimacy of the state is questioned, the command-and-control approach simply does not work. At best, it is ill-adapted to what is expected of health systems today. First of all, administrative rules are a rather blunt instrument to steer the interaction between individual patients and caregivers – particularly when the expectations of the former are rising. Second, such an approach to policy-making and regulation generally focuses on government employees, leaving health workers and institutions

## Box 6.1 Self-regulation opportunities

In 2001, a group of national nursing associations, government nurses and regulators from east, central and southern Africa developed and published a prototype regulatory framework and guidance on the accreditation of nursing and midwifery education programmes. As a result, those countries in the region that already had registers have begun moving away from lifetime registrations to ones that require periodic licensure.

In Uganda, the registrar of the Nurses and Midwives Council recently closed down a number of health training schools that did not meet the required standards. These measures were taken despite the fact that some of the schools that were closed, and some of the students who were affected, had powerful connections in political and senior civil service circles.

In Angola, the national nurses associations and the Order of Nurses of Portugal are equipping districts with nursing textbooks.

In Thailand, the Rural Doctors Association has played an important role in ensuring the commitment – and the presence – of doctors in rural and underserved areas.

The "evidence-based medicine" movement is another way of self-regulating the behaviour of health-care providers in a manner that serves the public interest.

outside the public sector to take care of themselves. The regulations that do exist (e.g. prohibiting moonlighting in private practice) are not or cannot be enforced. The failure of the traditional command-and-control approach to stem the unregulated commercialization of the health sector *(18)* has contributed greatly to the erosion of trust in health care providers and in health systems.

## Watchdogs and advocates

Civil society organizations that act on behalf of citizens (consumer groups, HIV/AIDS activists, etc.) have gained a large amount of influence in the health sector. These organizations have often had an important role for a long time in resource mobilization and improving health care delivery. In more recent years they have also found many ways to put pressure on providers, professional associations and health care bureaucracies and institutions *(3)*. Some provide citizens with information that puts them in a stronger position when they have to deal with a health care provider. In France, for example, the lay press publishes a ranking of hospitals in the performance of different procedures

Other civil society groups function as watchdog organizations to sound the alarm when citizens are denied their health entitlements or are discriminated against. In Sierra Leone, for example, women's groups demonstrated in the streets of Freetown demanding that the military government guarantee emergency care for all pregnant women, following newspaper reports that women had died after being denied treatment they could not afford. In many countries, civil society groups contribute to priority setting by participating in the planning process, as in Bangladesh *(19)*, or by providing checks and balances on government budgeting, as in Mexico *(20)*.

Consumer defence movements are gaining strength because they can push for mechanisms to be put in place to protect people against exclusion, poor-quality care, over-medicalization and catastrophic expenditures. They can also ensure that procedures are adopted that give people the possibility to redress harm. It is clear that a great many people currently lack such protection. For example, in contrast to industrialized countries, regulation of fees charged by private institutions or self-employed care providers is almost non-existent in most developing countries. Even where regulations exist, governments may have major problems enforcing them *(21)*. There are three results: first, each year approximately 44 million households worldwide are faced with catastrophic health expenditures *(22)*; second, many more people are excluded from access to care; and third, this situation favours supply-induced over-medicalization *(23)*. One example is the high incidence of caesarean sections around the world *(24)*. Within a single country, mothers with the financial means may be subject to an unnecessary and potentially dangerous intervention, while the same procedure is denied to another who needs it to save her life or that of her baby but who cannot mobilize the funds.

## A model for effective governance

None of the models described above – self-regulating professional associations, the command-and-control approach of institutional regulators, and the advocacy of civil society – is sufficient on its own to regulate the behaviour of health workers and institutions. Rather than relying on one single regulatory monopoly, national health workforce strategies should insist on cooperative governing. Regulations resulting from the participation of all three bodies, as well as health care institutions and the workforce, are more likely to generate trust and cooperation.

### Strategy 6.2 Ensure cooperative governance of national workforce policies

In order to ensure public safety and good governance of health care providers, capacity building requires investment in the overall regulatory architecture outlined in Figure 6.1. Simultaneous efforts are needed to reinforce the potential contributions of the state and social insurance institutions, as well as those of professional and civil society organizations. This means that, along with the creation of the specific technical bodies for licensing, accreditation and so on, forums must be established that allow for interaction among these various groups, which in turn implies the recognition and support, including financial, of their contributions *(19)*. Ministries of health may be reluctant to strengthen the very institutions that act as checks and balances on their own work, but in the long run it is in their own interest to have a strong system of dialogue and cooperation.

Figure 6.1  Organizations influencing the behaviour of health workers and the health institutions

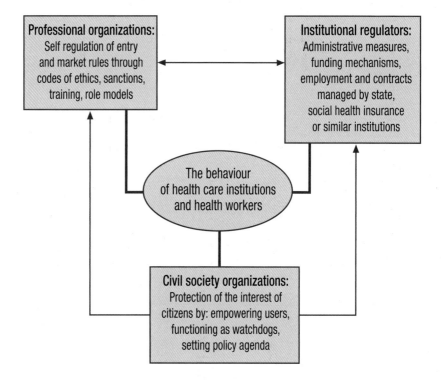

# STRONG LEADERSHIP

Because the health workforce is a domain of many conflicting interests, policy-making cannot be exclusively consensual and sometimes there has to be the possibility of arbitrage. Without strong leadership, national policies tend to flounder in a combination of ad hoc solutions, many of which focus on defending the interests of particular professional categories and create problems of their own. National leadership is necessary to initiate the process, push for breakthroughs, engage key stakeholders (workers, government and civil society), promote the synergistic roles of each, and encourage them to adopt a partnership approach.

The responsibility for that leadership lies with public authorities: the policy-makers and managers of the public and parapublic sectors. In recent years, however, little or no investment has been made in leadership in the public sector. In an environment of widespread scepticism about public sector and state involvement, stewardship functions have suffered from the stranglehold of macroeconomic constraints on public sector development, along with, if not more than, other public health functions.

The need for administrative and stewardship capacities is perhaps most obvious in extreme situations, such as post-conflict reconstruction in Afghanistan or the Democratic Republic of the Congo. It is also evident in many stable countries, where sector-wide approaches or poverty reduction strategies fail to perform as expected for want of leadership capacity, or where the unregulated commercialization of the health sector is undermining both workforce and health system performance.

Leadership is also crucial to deal with competing vested interests and to obtain high-level political endorsement of health workforce strategies. The work of the "change team" that brought about the health reforms in Colombia in the early 1990s exemplifies some of the tactical capacities that are crucial to successful reform *(25)*. At an early stage the team strictly controlled access to the decision-making process, and drew attention away from the health reforms by including proposals in a wider social security reform, the main spotlight of which was on pensions. Nevertheless, the team understood the need to allow certain voices, such as those of senators, to be heard. In working with groups that championed change, they focused their attention on the development of new institutions, such as new insurance agencies, that would take part in the new system. The reform of the old institutions, which would clearly be difficult, was tackled in a later phase.

Developing leadership skills depends on leadership structures and tactical capacities. The lack of both is recognized. The problem is that most people are inclined to believe that political know-how is an innate quality and therefore ill-suited to capacity building. Those who have attempted to develop training courses for leadership have often come to the disenchanting conclusion that they did not make a great deal of headway. There is little empirical evidence on what, if anything, can be done. Interviews with policy-makers, however, show that individual tactical capacities are built through coaching and mentoring, particularly within structured projects, whereas the strongest influence on the creation of the leadership structures comes from the organized sharing of knowledge and experiences with other countries. Coaching, mentoring and intercountry exchange are less straightforward capacity-building tools than training, but they can be organized. If this could be done effectively and on a large scale, it would help remove one of the key constraints to health worker development – the lack of people and structures to provide policy leadership, even in resource-poor or fragile countries.

# STRENGTHENING STRATEGIC INTELLIGENCE

In all too many cases, the health workforce information that is available to national decision-makers is extremely poor. Many, if not most, ministries of health, for example, do not know how many health professionals there are in the country, let alone how they are distributed. That major stakeholders have such poor knowledge of their own situation underscores the lack of connection between the acuteness of human resources problems and a coherent policy response.

## Strategy 6.3 Obtain better intelligence on the health workforce in national situations

For a thorough understanding of health workforce problems, systematic work is required in four areas: the extent and nature of the problem in the specific national context; what is being done and what can be done; the national politics around the issue; and the potential reactions of health workers and the institutions that employ them.

## Extent and nature of the national workforce problem

In most countries, this information is patchy at best. Among others, Malawi has recently demonstrated that a proper understanding of the nature of local health worker problems can help it to make a quantum leap in the formulation of more coherent policies and strategies (26). Accurate information on medical demography, shortages and oversupply is essential, but there is also a need to cover the range of problems that relate to entry, workforce and exit as well as to performance and trust; there is a need to cover the entire range of health workers, not merely doctors and nurses, and not merely the public sector; and there is a need to look at what there is in the field as well as at the expectations of the staff and the public, in the light of the present crisis and the future challenges.

## Action taken and further options

This is an area where even less is being done than in documenting the magnitude and determinants of health workforce problems. Much can be learnt from innovation and problem-solving which takes place at the grass-roots level and escapes the notice of policy-makers. Making assessments of actions and options requires specific skills as well as a systematic and institutional approach that involves inventory keeping, monitoring, evaluation, documentation and exchange. Much can also be learnt from experiences in other countries; that assessment, too, has to be carried out in a systematic way, with methodical evaluation, sharing and exchange.

## National politics around the health workforce

To build a workable strategy by changing a dysfunctional situation, it is often useful to understand the forces that have created such a situation in the first place: otherwise there is a real risk of making a bad situation worse. Much of the rigidity that characterizes the public sector workforce, for example, comes from attempts to protect the workforce from political interference: ill-thought-out policies to create more flexibility may then introduce opportunities for discrimination and favouritism, which would add to the malfunction. To take another example, if the reason for excessively centralized human resource management is insufficient management expertise or a lack of accountability mechanisms at more decentralized levels, then rapid administrative decentralization may not be a wise choice.

## Reactions of health workers and their employers

The good intentions of policy-makers when designing health system structures, processes and reform programmes are often undermined by a failure to consider how health workers are likely to respond. It is of particular importance to understand the reasons for their resistance to change. For example, one would expect staff in a centralized system to welcome the increased autonomy that comes with decentralization. In Uganda and Zimbabwe, however, decentralization was perceived as a threat to job security and raised concerns that the politics of ethnicity would govern both recruitment and personnel *(27, 28)*. Where public services are downsized or shifted to the private sector, health workers can experience the triple stress of fear of job loss, fear of failure to secure alternative employment, and growing workload *(29)*. In other situations, health workers may resist change because they are uncomfortable with the increased responsibility associated with reform proposals. It is possible to prevent many of these problems through a better understanding of the reactions of the different stakeholders. Informal dialogue goes a long way towards achieving such understanding, but it is also possible to organize more systematic exercises in order to appreciate potential reactions *(30)*.

## INVESTING IN WORKFORCE INSTITUTIONS

When governments have little capacity for policy design, regulatory measures are easily appropriated by interest groups. Policy-making then becomes ineffective at best and counter-productive at worst. Some countries have done well: Malawi's human resource plan is one example (see Box 2.2). In recent years, however, most countries have not made adequate investments in developing policy-making and regulatory capacities. Indeed, during the 1990s a considerable number of health departments in ministries of health around the world fell victim to public sector downsizing and rationalization.

Building or rebuilding country capacities for policy-making in health care delivery requires much more than just tools and training: there is a hierarchy of tools, people and structures *(31)*. Without the policy-makers and managers who can interpret and contextualize the output of costing and budgeting tools, making such tools available and training staff to implement them will be of little benefit. At the same time, without the institutions, structures and committees that have the authority to make decisions, managers and policy-makers have no way of transforming intellectual exercises into political facts.

National-level health workforce institutions are needed to build public trust, facilitate fair and cooperative governing, produce strong leaders, and gather strategic intelligence. These reasons alone should be enough to justify their financing, but in reality it is not easy for policy-makers to sell the idea that such institutions need to be built and strengthened – if only because of the long time perspective and the lack of visibility of issues such as return on investment.

Since investment in training or tools is more readily accepted and since significant amounts of funding are now being directed towards training, the way forward is probably to link these directly to institution building. The key is to identify specific areas where insufficiencies are greatest and where distinct institutional efforts can yield concrete results.

Some of these efforts have already been discussed in previous sections of this chapter: building capacity for regulation; leadership structures and tactical capacities; and strategic information on core indicators. Two other areas that warrant highlighting are learning from microlevel innovations and scenario building and planning. Both are explored below; they can best be organized through the creation of national health workforce observatories (see Box 6.2) or by linking ministry of health departments, academic institutions and nongovernmental organizations in learning networks and communities of practice.

## Learning from microinnovations

Perhaps nowhere has there been as much creative problem-solving and innovation at the microlevel as in the health workforce. Many examples have been mentioned throughout this report. The idea is to learn from these innovations, encouraging what works and discouraging what does not. Making these assessments requires specific skills as well as a systematic and institutional approach that involves inventory keeping, monitoring, evaluation, documentation and exchange.

An accurate assessment is necessary in order to decide which actions merit inclusion in a national health worker strategy: they must be cost-effective, provide quick results, correct present distortions and prevent further deterioration of health care services (34). One such innovation was a stop-gap solution for a lack of doctors in one area of Mozambique, where *tecnicos de cirurjia*, or assistant medical officers, were trained in surgical skills. Their excellent results led policy-makers to generalize the experiment and today *tecnicos de cirurjia* are a characteristic feature of district hospitals across the country (35).

## Box 6.2 Human resources for health observatories in Latin America

National observatories for human resources for health were set up in 22 countries in 1998 as part of an initiative by the Pan American Health Organization (PAHO), WHO's Regional Office for the Americas, to counteract the neglect of health workforce issues in Latin America during the 1980s and early 1990s. PAHO established an Observatory of Human Resources in Health to link these national observatories, which have helped raise the profile of the health workforce agenda, improve the information base, and strengthen health sector stewardship (32). The observatories provide continuity in settings where there may be a significant turnover of decision-makers and policies. Their common characteristic is multiple stakeholder participation involving universities, ministries of health, professional associations, corporate providers, unions and user representatives.

The institutional arrangements, however, are specific to each country. The Brazilian Observatory (33) provides a number of important lessons about state–non-state interactive capacity building. It consists of a network of university institutes, research centres and one federal office dealing with human resources for health. There are 13 network "nodes" or "workstations" coordinated by a secretariat staffed by the Ministry of Health and the Brasilia office of PAHO. The Observatory's remit since 1999 has been to contribute to, and inform the development, regulation and management of, human resources in the health sector and related policy areas.

The Observatory has produced much valuable information and analytical work and its capacities have developed considerably. It has built on existing informal networks where managers and academics were motivated by professional interest in investigating the relevance of planning, management and training in human resources for the health sector. Much of the network's success and resilience can be attributed to the initial focus on content as well as to its working style. The focus on content allowed network members to build their technical and professional capabilities in a spirit of intellectual independence and autonomy that continues to characterize interactions today. The style of working is characterized by flexibility, creativity, pragmatism, inventiveness and entrepreneurial spirit . The combination of pursuing technical excellence and informal collaboration resulted in group learning, and consolidated shared ideas.

On this basis the networks were formalized and institutionalized in the late 1990s. This move further enhanced productivity, largely by intensifying exchanges nationally and internationally with the help of a number of personalities in Brazil and in other countries.

The Brazilian Observatory shows that informal networking can develop into more formal structures that produce concrete outputs and outcomes. Within the network there are demands for an intensification of exchanges in terms of content and policy relevance, and for the introduction of monitoring and evaluation mechanisms to ensure quality and relevance of the network's outputs.

## Scenario building and planning

Scenario building and planning, which are essential to determine long-term orientations, also require specific capacities that lend themselves to an institutional approach. National strategists have to make fundamental choices that define what the future workforce will look like and how it will relate to the value systems of the society in which it operates. The demands on health workers are changing fast, and one can only guess what they will be in the future, but the time of omniscient professionals working on their own is definitely past. The provision of health care in the future lies in teamwork, with overlapping and complementary skills that constantly adapt to rapid changes in society and technology. At the same time, the health care team will be asked to be much closer to their clients, with a family doctor type of contact point who acts as the hub for the team and as the interface between clients and the health system. The model of separate and independent health care professions will soon be overtaken.

More than a planning problem, preparing for these changes is a matter of organizing a broad discussion around entitlements and scenarios for the future. Such discussions may emerge from the civil society movement as in Thailand *(36)*, from local authorities as in Oregon, United States *(37)*, or from the public health establishment as in New Zealand or the Netherlands *(38, 39)*. Debates on scenarios for the future have to take into account the spectrum of drivers shaping the workforce, including changing health needs, demographic trends such as ageing, consumer expectations, growth in private health services, and the global labour market for health workers (see Figure 2 in the Overview to this report). In terms of content, future scenarios are likely to focus on the tensions between commercialization on the one hand and universal access and social protection on the other, and between a technocratic disease orientation and social demands for a more patient-centred approach.

It is the process that is of prime importance. Just as fair governance requires cooperation, so too does planning for the future. Experience from priority-setting debates shows that the legitimacy of the choices that are made is less a function of what is actually decided than the perception of procedural fairness *(40)*. If the way decisions are made is inclusive and transparent, societal support follows. There is a clear association between the intensity of dialogue with multiple stakeholders and the strength and sustainability of the policy choices *(30, 41)*. A failure to be inclusive means that opportunities are missed and resistance and resentment build up.

## CONCLUSION

National health workforce strategies must move beyond salary and training in the public sector to strategies for the entire work cycle of entry–workforce–exit in both the public and private sectors. Workforce development is both a technical and political exercise, requiring the building of trust among stakeholders and linking people's expectations with health worker performance.

Whether in fragile states focusing on short-term and medium-term perspectives, or in more stable countries that focus on longer-term strategies that command more resources, the quality and the success of policy-making and regulation depend firstly on the inclusion of key stakeholders. Also crucial are the availability of people and resources to carry out the policy formulation work, and the capacity to base the policy on a proper understanding of the nature of the problems.

All country strategies should prioritize the following actions.

- Build national strategies out of concrete action points that cover management of entry, workforce and exit as well as: building or rebuilding trust; multi-stakeholder management of the regulatory environment; and leadership capacities.
- Pay attention to the process. The choices to be made may be difficult and controversial: it is essential to ensure procedural fairness by being inclusive and transparent, but with the courage to arbitrate when vested interests are taking over.
- Strengthen strategic intelligence, focusing on: (i) understanding the extent and nature of health workforce problems; (ii) evaluating what is being done and determining what can be done; (iii) identifying the political drivers that led to the current situation; and (iv) understanding workers' viewpoints and anticipating their possible reactions to change.
- Build the country's health workforce institutional capacity, with a focus on regulation, leadership and strategic information, including: (i) analysis and evaluation of microinnovations; and (ii) scenario building and planning for the future.

# REFERENCES

1. Davies H. Falling public trust in health services: implications for accountability. *Journal of Health Services Research and Policy*, 1999, 4:193–194.
2. Mechanic D. Changing medical organization and the erosion of trust. In: Conrad P, ed. *The sociology of health and illness*, 6th ed. New York, NY, Worth Publishers, 2001:198–204.
3. Van Lerberghe W, Ferrinho P. *Civil society organizations and the poor: the unfulfilled expectations.* Washington, DC, The World Bank, 2003 (background paper 28028 for *World Development Report 2004*).
4. Gilson L. Trust and the development of health care as a social institution. *Social Science and Medicine,* 2003, 56:1453–1468.
5. Jaffré Y, Olivier de Sardan JP. *Une médecine inhospitalière: les difficiles relations entre soignants et soignés dans cinq capitales d'Afrique de l'Ouest [Inhospitable medicine: difficult relations between carers and cared for in five West African capital cities].* Paris, Karlhala, 2003.
6. Narajan D. *Voices of the poor: can anyone hear us?* New York, NY, Oxford University Press, 2000:97.
7. Robinson R. Rationing health care: a national framework and local discretion. *Journal of Health Services Research and Policy*, 1997, 2:67–70.
8. Transparency International. *Corruption and health. Global corruption report 2006.* London, Pluto Press, 2006.
9. Benington J. Risk and reciprocity: local governance rooted within civil society. In: Coulson A, ed. *Trust and contracts: relationships in local government, health and public services.* Bristol, The Polity Press, 1998.
10. Taylor-Gooby P. Markets and motives: Trust and egoism in welfare markets. *Journal of Social Policy*, 1999, 28:97–114.
11. Mercer H, Ineson S, McCarty P. *National regulation of medical profession capacities.* Geneva, World Health Organization, 2006 (background paper for *The world health report 2006*; available at: http://www.who.int/hrh/documents/en/).
12. McKinlay JB, Stoeckle JD. Corporatization and the social transformation of doctoring. In: Conrad P, ed. *The sociology of health and illness,* 6th ed. New York, NY, Worth Publishers, 1999:175–185.
13. Krause EA. *Death of the guilds. Professions, states and the advance of capitalism, 1930 to the present.* New Haven and London, Yale University Press, 1996.
14. Frenk J, Donabedian A. State intervention in medical care: types, trends and variables. *Health Policy and Planning*, 1987, 2:17–31.
15. Moran M. *Governing the health care state. A comparative study of the United Kingdom, the United States and Germany.* Manchester and New York, Manchester University Press, 1999.
16. Lindblom CE. The science of "muddling through". *Public Administration Review*, 1959, 19:79–88.
17. Bennet AE, Holland WW. Rational planning or muddling through? Research allocation in the NHS. *Lancet*, 1977, 8009:464–466.
18. Bloom G, Standing H. *Pluralism and marketisation in the health sector: meeting health needs in context of social change in low and middle-income countries.* Brighton, Institute of Development Studies, 2001 (IDS Working Paper 136).
19. Jahan R, Germain A. Mobilizing support to sustain political will is the key to progress in reproductive health. *Lancet*, 2004, 364:742–744.
20. *Dignity counts: a guide to using budget analysis to advance human rights.* Mexico, Fundar, 2004 (International Budget Project, International Human Rights Internship Program).
21. Van Lerberghe W, el Rashidi AR, Sales A, Mechbal A. Reform follows failure: unregulated private care in Lebanon. *Health Policy and Planning,* 1997, 12:296–311.
22. Xu K, Evans D, Carrin G, Aguilar-Rivera AM. *Designing health financing systems to reduce catastrophic health expenditure.* Geneva, World Health Organization, 2005 (Department of Health System Financing, Technical Brief for Policy-Makers, No. 2).
23. Pongsupap Y, Van Lerberghe W. Choosing between public and private or between hospital and primary care? Responsiveness, patient-centredness and prescribing patterns in outpatient consultations in Bangkok. *Tropical Medicine and International Health*, 2006, 11:81–89.

24. *The world health report 2005 – Make every mother and child count*. Geneva, World Health Organization, 2005.

25. Gonzalez-Rossetti A. *Enhancing the political feasibility of health reform: the Colombia case*. Data for Decision-making Project, 2000 (Health Sector Reform Initiative, Paper No. 39; http://www.hsph.harvard.edu/ihsg/publications/pdf/lac/Colombiafinal-pp2.PDF, accessed 22 February 2006).

26. Palmer D. *Human resources for health case study: Malawi's emergency human resources programme*. DFID–Malawi, December 2004.

27. Pangu KA. Health workers motivation in decentralized settings: waiting for better times? In: Ferrinho P, Van Lerberghe W, eds. *Providing health care under adverse conditions: health personnel performance and individual coping strategies*. Antwerp, ITG Press, 2000 (Studies in Health Services Organization and Policy, 16):19–29.

28. Mutizwa-Mangiza D. *The impact of health sector reform on public sector health worker motivation in Zimbabwe*. Bethesda, MD, Abt Associates, 1998 (Partnerships for Health Reform, Major Applied Research 5, Working Paper No. 4).

29. Wiscow C. *The effects of reforms on the health workforce*. Geneva, World Health Organization, 2005 (background paper for *The world health report 2006,* available at: http://www.who.int/hrh/documents/en/).

30. Ammar W. *Health system and reform in Lebanon*. Beirut, Entreprise universitaire d'Etudes et de Publications, 2003.

31. Potter C, Brough R. Systemic capacity building: a hierarchy of needs. *Health Policy and Planning*, 2004, 19:336–345.

32. Rigoli F, Arteaga O. *The experience of the Latin America and Caribbean Observatory of Human Resources in Health* http://www.lachsr.org/en/observatorio.cfm, accessed 22 February 2006).

33. Campos FE, Hauck V. *Networking collaboratively: The Brazilian Observatório on Human Resources in Health. A case study prepared for the project 'Capacity, Change and Performance'*. Maastricht, European Centre for Development Policy Management, 2005 (Discussion Paper, 57L); http://www.ecdpm.org/Web_ECDPM/Web/Content/Navigation.nsf/index2?ReadForm, accessed 22 February 2006).

34. *Rehabilitating the workforce: the key to scaling up MNCH* (*The world health report 2005*, Policy Brief 2). Geneva, World Health Organization, 2005.

35. Vaz F, Bergstrom S, Vaz Mda L, Langa J, Bugalho A. Training medical assistants for surgery. *Bulletin of the World Health Organization,* 1999, 77:688–691.

36. Tangcharoensathien V, Jongudomsuk P. *From policy to implementation: historical events during 2001-2004 of universal coverage in Thailand*. Bangkok, National Health Security Office, 2004.

37. Kitzhaber JA. Prioritizing health services in an era of limits: the Oregon experience. In: R Smith, ed. *Rationing in action*. London, BMJ Publishing Group, 1993.

38. *Core services 1993/4*. Wellington, National Advisory Committee, 1992.

39. *Choices in health care: a report by the Government Committee on Choices in Health Care*. Rijswijk, Ministry of Health, Welfare and Cultural Affairs, 1992.

40. McKee M, Figueras J. Setting priorities: can Britain learn from Sweden? *BMJ,* 1996, 312:691–694.

41. Stewart J, Kringas P. *Change management – strategy and values: six case studies from the Australian public sector*. University of Canberra, Centre for Research in Public Sector Management, 2003 (http://www.dmt.canberra.edu.au/crpsm/research/pdf/stewartkringas.pdf, accessed 21 February 2006).

# working together

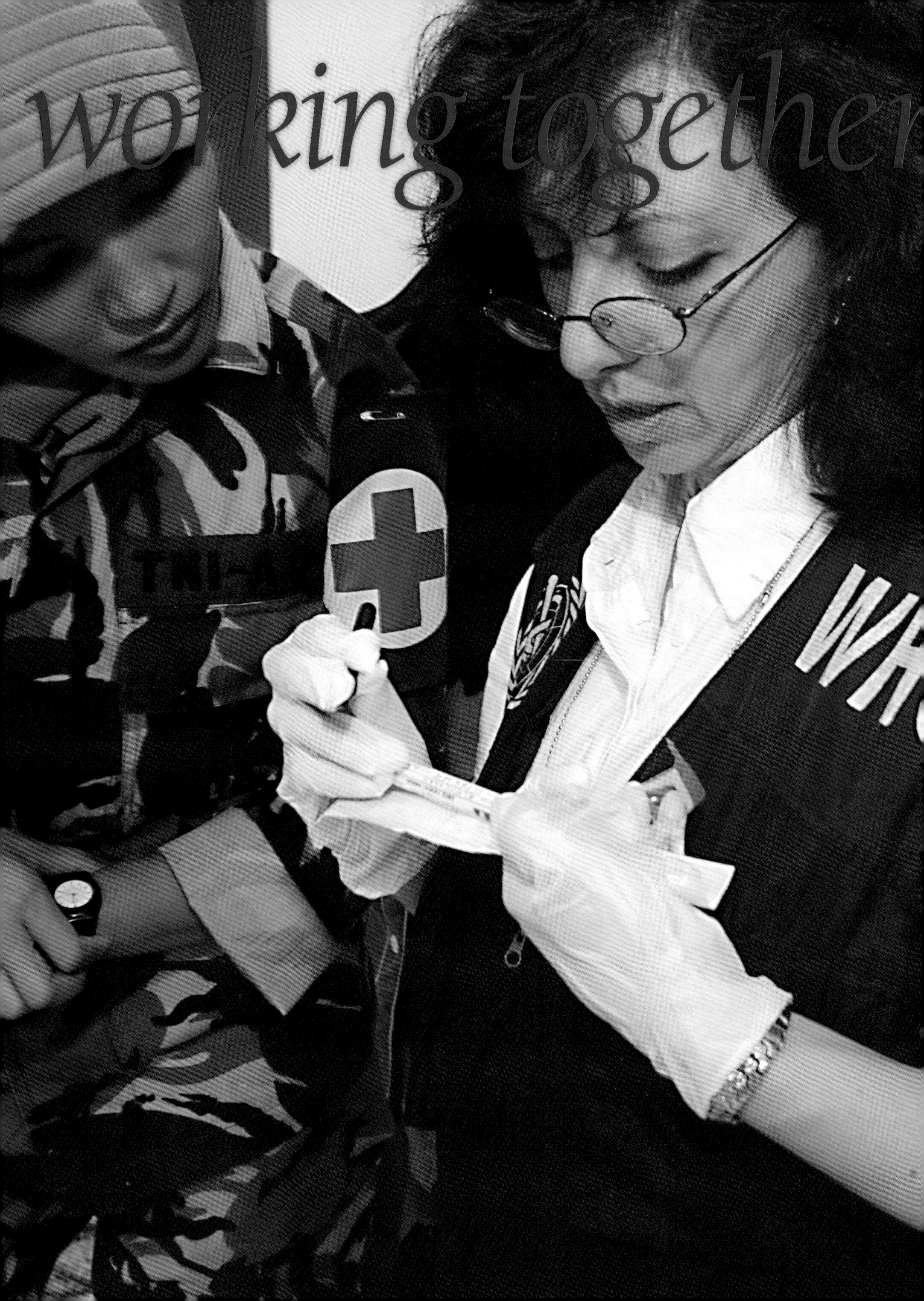

# chapter seven
# within and across countries

**There are five broad areas of concern that impel countries to look beyond their borders and work together with others in order to address issues of human resources for health more effectively:**

- The profound lack of information, tools and measures, the limited amount of evidence on what works, and the absence of shared standards, technical frameworks and research methodologies are all imperatives for regional and international collaboration.
- The scarcity of technical expertise available to develop better metrics, monitor performance, set standards, identify research priorities, and validate methodologies means that a collective global effort is the only way to accelerate progress in these areas.
- The changes in demographics, demand for care, and technological advances cut across borders and are manifested in increasingly global labour markets. Cooperative arrangements and agreements between countries are essential to manage these flows and minimize adverse effects.
- The reality that a violent conflict, an outbreak of an infectious disease, or an unexpected catastrophic event can lay waste even to the most well-prepared national health system demonstrates that no country will ever have the human resource capacity to be able always to mount an effective response entirely on its own.
- The enormous workforce crisis that constrains health development so profoundly in the world's poorest countries requires an international response.

This chapter focuses on the rationale for working together and concludes with a plan of action that is based on national leadership and global solidarity.

## CATALYSING KNOWLEDGE AND LEARNING

As has been pointed out in this report, basic information on the workforce that is required in order to inform, plan and evaluate resources is in very short supply in virtually all countries. The scant information that does exist is difficult to aggregate and compare over time and across sources and countries (1–4). This limitation is reflected not only in the challenges inherent in coordinating information flows across sectors – education, health, labour/employment – but more fundamentally in the absence of agreed frameworks and standards for health workforce assessment. Investment should be made in developing these frameworks and standards so that better tools to understand and respond to health workforce challenges can be made widely available more quickly and at lower cost.

## A firm foundation for information

An important first step towards strengthening the foundations of information about health workers is to develop a clear conceptual framework that describes the boundaries and make-up of the workforce. Encouragingly, there is a global effort under way to develop a common technical framework (see Box 7.1). Even with such a framework, however, there remain a number of fundamental challenges related to health workforce information that must be taken up.

One problem area is the classification of the health workforce. Until 2006, WHO reported only on health professionals – doctors, nurses, midwives, pharmacists and dentists – thus rendering invisible other important service providers as well as all health management and support workers (who account for around one third of the workforce). This oversight reflects the shortcomings of using instruments whose primary purpose is not the collection of information on the health workforce. It underlines the need to develop special health workforce classification tools that can be more effectively integrated into existing census, survey and occupational reporting instruments.

Another important information need is for metrics to assess performance. Policy-makers and donors are increasingly demanding evidence showing that their decisions and investments are indeed strengthening the health workforce. In the area of health information systems, a performance assessment instrument has been developed that permits cross-country comparisons (see Figure 7.1). A similar instrument for human resources could lead to more and wiser investments in the health workforce. Among the indicators that can be used in the development of health workforce performance metrics are sufficient numbers, equitable distribution, good competencies, appropriate sociocultural and linguistic background, responsiveness to clients, and productivity.

Human resource information is also needed to understand global labour markets, migratory flows of health workers, and the activities of multinational companies that

## Figure 7.1 Health information system (HIS) performance

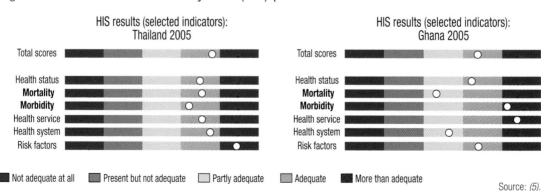

Source: *(5).*

## Box 7.1  Seeking a common technical framework for human resources for health: a public good useful to all countries?

Could a common technical framework help governments and national planners understand the myriad and complex problems of human resources for health – and find feasible solutions? Could such a framework address all sides of the issue in a comprehensive manner, be collaboratively developed, and be universally used – a public good of benefit to all countries?

A common framework would have several benefits. First, it would define the key dimensions of technical competence needed to develop and implement a strategy for human resources. This is particularly important given the limited pool of expertise available globally. Second, it would help inform the growing number of groups interested in this area of the complexities of the health workforce and prevent the spread of simplistic and limited views on what is involved (e.g. that developing human resources for health is simply about training and increasing salaries). Third, it would be a common reference point for all health workforce stakeholders and save policy-makers, implementers, donors, academics and others the effort of "re-inventing the wheel".

An attempt to develop a common technical framework began in December 2005, when WHO and USAID invited 35 representatives from multilateral and bilateral agencies, donor countries, nongovernmental organizations and the academic community to meet at the Pan American Health Organization in Washington, DC. They drew on 11 technical frameworks that had been developed over the years by researchers and human resources professionals in various parts of the world. Some of these applied to very specific contexts; others offered broad conceptual roadmaps for

thinking through the issues. Many focused on just one aspect of the health workforce, for example human resources planning.

The participants agreed that the desired common framework needed to be scientifically-based, operationally useful (field-tested), and useful in a multisectoral and multi-stakeholder context. It had to capture the content and processes involved in developing and implementing a national strategy for human resources for health, be simple but comprehensive, and show the interdependencies among the various players, institutions and labour markets involved in the health workforce.

The figure below shows the framework that was produced at the meeting. All seven interlinking thematic areas – human resource management systems, policy, finance, education, partnership and leadership – must be taken into account in dealing with health workforce development, and this calls for multisector involvement. However, the diagram shows only the upper layer of a conceptual orientation that also has underlying secondary and tertiary levels.

Work continues to develop and complete the framework. The goal is to produce an interactive CD-ROM that will convey the detailed content and processes underlying each thematic area. In the meantime, more information on the elements in each thematic area, on action that can be taken, and on the overall process for using the framework to develop a national strategy can be found in the WHO publication *Tools for planning and developing human resources for HIV/AIDS and other health services* (available at: http://www.who.int/hrh/tools/en/).

### Human resources for health technical framework: achieving a sustainable health workforce

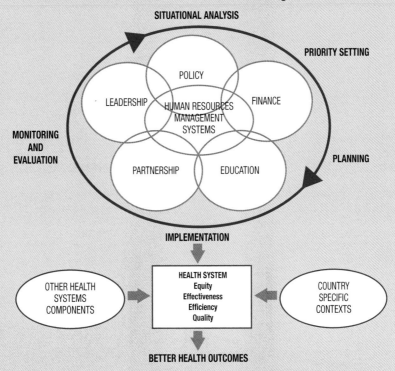

Table 7.1 Short description of results of three Cochrane systematic reviews on human resources for health

| Title of Cochrane systematic review | Research question | Number of studies (initial/final) | Total number of subjects | Results |
|---|---|---|---|---|
| **Substitution of doctors by nurses in primary care** | To investigate the impact of nurses working as substitutes for primary care doctors on:<br><br>health outcomes<br><br><br>process of care<br><br><br><br><br>resource use<br><br>costs | 4253 articles initially<br><br><br><br><br><br>25 articles, relating to 16 studies, met inclusion criteria | Not applicable | No difference in quality of care and health outcomes between appropriately trained nurses and doctors<br><br>Nurses tend to provide more health advice and achieve higher levels of patient satisfaction, compared with doctors<br><br>Even though using nurses may save salary costs, nurses may order more tests and use other services, which may decrease the cost savings of using nurses instead of doctors |
| **Lay health workers (LHWs) in primary and community health care** | To assess the effects of LHWs' interventions in primary and community health care on health care behaviours, patients' health and well-being, and patients' satisfaction with care | 8637 abstracts initially<br><br><br><br><br><br><br>400 potentially eligible<br><br><br>43 eventually included | 210 110 consumers | LHWs show promising benefits in promoting immunization uptake and improving outcomes for acute respiratory infections and malaria, when compared to usual care.<br>For other health issues, evidence is insufficient to justify recommendations for policy and practice.<br>There is also insufficient evidence to assess which LHW training or intervention strategies are likely to be most effective. |
| **Audit and feedback: effects on professional practice and health care outcomes** | Are audit and feedback effective in improving professional practice and health care outcomes? | 85 randomized controlled trials<br><br>Only 10 of the 85 included studies to be of high methodological quality | > 3500 health professionals | Audit and feedback can improve professional practice, but the effects are variable.<br>When it is effective, the effects are generally small to moderate.<br><br>The results of this review do not provide support for mandatory or unevaluated use of audit and feedback. |

Source: (10).

employ significant numbers of health workers. In addition to good country data, an accurate, consistent and coherent view of the big picture also requires effective regional and global aggregation and analytical capacities. Reaching agreement on what information will be collected, how data will be aggregated and the necessary institutional arrangements is an important priority for concerned international partners.

## Generation and management of knowledge

Strongly linked to building a foundation for health workforce information are challenges related to both the generation and management of knowledge. Given that close to half of health expenditure is spent on the health workforce, it seems incredible that there is so little research investment or solid evidence in this area. The evidence base within and across countries related to the health workforce is perilously weak, especially when compared with the strength of evidence in other domains of the health sector *(6)*. The absence of a formal designation of the health workforce as a research priority has resulted in a patchy knowledge base. There is considerable research on curricula and teaching methods (see Box 3.8), rural retention schemes and various aspects of health worker management, but large subject areas related to health training institutions, recruitment, management of incentives and attrition lack a critical research mass. Moreover, the existing knowledge base is largely skewed towards high income countries, medical doctors, and descriptive reports as opposed to intervention studies or best practice assessments *(7–9)*. The paucity of research in general is reflected in the fact that there are only 12 systematic reviews on human resource issues available through the Cochrane Collaboration *(10)*. Table 7.1 presents details of three of the most recent systematic reviews on human resources for health.

## Figure 7.2 Immunization coverage and density of health workers

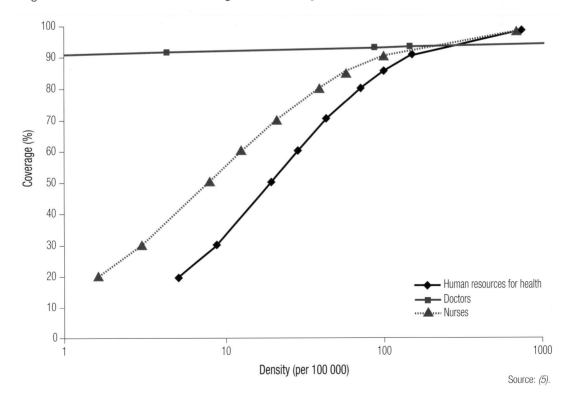

Source: *(5)*.

Although the knowledge generation agenda is most important at the country level and in specific workplaces, the return from well-designed and rigorous research cross-nationally should not be discounted. For example, simply assessing the relationship of the health workforce to key health outcomes across countries has helped to identify very important relationships such as that between nurse density and immunization coverage *(11)*. Figure 7.2 shows that to achieve wider immunization coverage, the density of nurses and other health workforce staff is more important than the density of doctors – simply because in many countries it is nurses, and not doctors, who administer vaccinations. Scaling up and effectively deploying community health workers as a common response to critical shortages in the health workforce would benefit from insights into a number of important questions (see Box 7.2).

In an attempt to draw attention to this neglected area of investigation, the Mexico Summit on Health Research, in 2004, identified health systems research into subjects such as the health workforce as one of three priorities for global action *(12)*, echoing the recommendations emerging from an international gathering in Cape Town *(13)* and the work of a WHO-convened task force *(14)*.

In general, preference for research activities should be given to the following:

■ a better balance between primarily descriptive studies and more conceptual or fundamental policy and operations research;

■ more international comparative research, drawing on multiple contexts such as the African migration study *(15)* and the European nursing exit study *(16)*;

■ the integration of research into specific health workforce interventions and more general health sector reforms, so as to document experiences across countries more systematically.

This last point underlines the importance of developing more systematic mechanisms to disseminate and share knowledge once it is generated. As stressed in Chapters 2 and 6, in the context of tackling urgent health needs or pursuing ambitious national programmes, there is significant "micro-innovation" that, if critically assessed, could help to accelerate the identification of more effective strategies for human resources. Regional and national observatories are potential mechanisms for harvesting and disseminating new knowledge, provided they effectively engage the full range of stakeholders and their institutions (see Box 6.2).

## Box 7.2 Research priorities related to community health workers

- Recruitment and retention – what factors and policies enhance recruitment of community health workers and reduce attrition?
- Roles – if community health workers do better with specific roles, how many roles can they undertake with a given level of training and support? How can these be integrated with other community level work and with other levels in the health system?
- Improving performance, incentive systems and remuneration – what level and method of remuneration and types of non-financial incentives maximize cost–effectiveness but are sustainable? What are the other effective approaches to improving performance?

- Referral linkages – how can referral linkages be operationalized, especially if communications and transport systems are weak?
- Communications – can mobile technologies be used to improve communications with community health workers and to help improve health outcomes in isolated communities?
- Routine supplies – how can basic supplies be made regularly available, and what is the best mix of social marketing, community-based distribution and strengthened health system logistics to ensure equitable access?

## Pooling of expertise

Effective technical cooperation relies on being able to draw on appropriate expertise and on having a set of tools that corresponds to the diverse challenges of the health workforce. Global collaboration can improve access to quality tools and expertise. There is a general lack of awareness of the range of tools available as well as un-certainty about which ones work best in specific situations. Consequently, a working group of international specialists is developing a compendium of tools to facilitate their greater and more appropriate use (see Box 7.3).

Much can also be done to improve the way expertise is managed and used. Countries rely on technical cooperation for three distinct purposes, depending on their particular needs. First, there are quite a number of countries that can benefit from outside opinion to refine their diagnostic overview, ranking and determina-tion of the nature of the country's human resources for health problems, with their entry, workforce and exit dimensions. Second, countries may have a need for expert collaboration in developing and planning the implementation of human resource policies, especially where the task of scaling up health systems is substantial. There may be a need, for example, to design and monitor financial solutions to increase coverage, as well as to build scenarios based on production and retention projec-tions. Third, there may be specific sub-areas where highly specialized technical skills are needed (see Box 7.4).

## Box 7.3 Tools for health workforce assessment and development

Reliable tools have been developed to strengthen techni-cal inputs in the planning, management and development of human resources in health. However, a Joint Learning Initiative report *(7)* pointed out that many practitioners are unaware of the large number of such aids available, or have difficulty in choosing those appropriate to their need. A working group of international human resources specialists was therefore established in June 2005 to put together a compendium of tools consisting of guidelines, models and analytical methodologies.

Known as "THE Connection", the group identifies new tools which are then reviewed by at least two people using a simple protocol developed by the group. If accepted for inclusion in the compendium, a short review is written up in standard format for each tool, with a section called "Will it work?" (information on testing and users' experiences). Reviews are organized in a colour-coded system around two general topics: tools for a comprehensive analysis of the human resources situation, and those that are specific to particular workforce functions.

By December 2005, 15 reviews had been completed and at least a further 10 are expected to be available by mid-2006. The compendium is constantly evolving as new tools are developed, new reviews added and existing reviews up-dated. To facilitate this process, the compendium is available as a CD-ROM and also on the Internet (available at: http://

www.who.int/hrh/tools/en/), where users can see the range of tools with a brief description; a detailed review is also available, with a link to access the tool (mostly as documents in pdf format). All those reviewed so far are free, and all but one are available on the Internet.

In preparing the compendium, researchers have found some areas with several tools to choose from, but no tools in other areas such as recruitment/retention and employee relations/change management. If indeed none exist THE Connection will request funding bodies to sup-port the development of new ones to fill these gaps. The group is well aware that many management tools never get used or even distributed to the appropriate users, and is trying to establish what works in the process of developing and disseminating tools. It will pass on this information to developers.

One of the key aims of THE Connection has been to establish a network of human resources practitioners. The interaction between members of the working group – some of whom have never met personally – and the inclusion of other individuals in the process has already expanded that network. Including a feedback mechanism on the reviews, the tools themselves and the identifica-tion of important gaps should stimulate an even wider dialogue among practitioners, facilitating greater techni-cal cooperation in this challenging area of work.

Whatever the specific needs that technical cooperation is responding to, it has to be organized in such a way that it becomes an instrument for institutional and individual capacity building: this implies that technical cooperation has to shift from assistance and gap-filling to exchange and joint learning. Countries can adopt a number of measures to facilitate this shift. The first relates to how expertise and technical cooperation are sourced: for example, pooling funds with transparent sourcing rules; avoiding sourcing from tied funds; sourcing through technical partners that can act as honest brokers; and going through global mechanisms and networks that help to identify quality expertise. Second, countries can keep track of expertise that is provided and set up mechanisms to evaluate systematically its cost and effectiveness, including capacity building. Third, they can accelerate the shift from passive use of expertise towards exchange of experience on a regional and subregional basis, engaging their own experts and institutions in technical networks. As an illustration, in a Memorandum of Understanding between Uganda and its development partners in 2005, the Government of Uganda said it would request technical assistance on a demand-driven basis according to the needs and priorities of the Government in consultation with development partners. Use of Ugandan regional consultants would be encouraged where expertise is available *(17)*. Lastly, countries can rationalize the way they negotiate technical cooperation, for example by establishing codes of conduct.

In countries with severely constrained capacities of their own, the most promising avenue for a structural improvement is to federate and expand regional and national observatories and networks of resources (see Box 6.2). Open collaborative structures will make it possible to pool existing knowledge and skills, to set standards and to assess effectiveness in collaboration with countries: a virtuous circle of improved access to possibilities for collaboration, exchange and joint learning that will also lead to an expansion of the global expertise base.

## Box 7.4 Technical skills for human resource policy-making

The development of policy for human resources for health in national health workforce planning requires a diversity of expertise in the following areas:

- **Policy and planning**: policy development and/or analysis, workforce planning, medical demographics and modelling, public health priorities, policy implementation, scenario building.
- **Institutional and management development**: change management; change processes analysis and monitoring; partnership and consensus building; leadership and team building; sociology of organization and professions.
- **Legal frameworks and policies**: laws/regulation/conditions of work, strategy development, regulation of professions.

- **Health workforce economics**: labour economics, labour market analysis, workforce financing.
- **Education**: scope of education: public health, medical, nursing, pharmacy, dentistry, community; educational process: curricula, pedagogy, technology; educational stages: pre-service/prior to work, continuous/in-service; governance: accreditation, financing, administration.
- **Workforce management systems and tools**: data collection and analysis; information systems design; monitoring and evaluation of workforce development; guidelines development; operational research; technology development; performance of workforce; costing tool development.
- **Professionally focused workforce development**: medicine, nursing, midwifery, pharmacy, dentistry.

## STRIKING COOPERATIVE AGREEMENTS

In planning their health workforce strategies, countries cannot overlook the dynamics of the global labour markets affecting health workers. Pushed by population trends towards ageing, changes in consumer expectations and technological innovations, the health sector globally continues to defy expectations in terms of its rate of growth. Demand for service providers will escalate markedly in all countries – rich and poor *(18, 19)*. The workforce shortfalls identified in this report would pale in comparison with *total shortages* if all health workforce demands for all countries were projected into the future *(20)*. Demographic changes in Europe and Japan are such that, were the health workforce to remain at its present share of the total workforce, the ratio of health workers to citizens over 65 years of age would drop by 38–40% by 2030. In contrast, were the health workforce to continue to grow at its present rate, its share of the total workforce would more than double *(21)*.

"*Demand for service providers will escalate markedly in all countries – rich and poor*"

These trends are likely to accelerate the international flow of health workers, thus raising the importance of global cooperative mechanisms to minimize the adverse affects of migration. As discussed in Chapter 5, managing migration entails rules that protect the rights and safety of individual workers as well as multilateral principles and bilateral agreements related to recruitment. The emergence of an export and import industry in health workers, the growth of medical tourism, and the volume of workers moving back and forth between countries will increase the need for international arrangements related to accreditation, quality assurance and social security. As in other areas related to the health workforce, the capacity of interested institutions and the ability of processes to be sufficiently inclusive of key stakeholders will be important determinants of the ability to reach cooperative agreements.

Beyond the increasing demands emerging from the market, human conflicts, epidemics and natural disasters (such as avian influenza, SARS and the tsunami of December 2004) raise further demands for effective health workforce cooperation across countries (see Chapter 2). Global training centres for specific categories of workers, standardized curricula and codes of practice for volunteers are among the types of agreement that will facilitate more effective international responses.

## RESPONDING TO THE HEALTH WORKFORCE CRISIS

The severity of the health workforce crisis in some of the world's poorest countries is illustrated by WHO estimates that 57 of them (36 of which are in Africa) have a deficit of 2.4 million doctors, nurses and midwives. The exodus of skilled professionals from rural areas to urban centres or other nations is one of the factors that have led to severe shortages, inappropriate skill mix and gaps in service coverage in poorer countries. Other factors include the HIV/AIDS epidemic and the policies of resource-poor governments that have capped public sector employment and limited investment in education. Paradoxically, insufficiencies in workforce requirements often coexist with large numbers of unemployed health professionals. Poverty, flawed private labour markets, lack of public funds, bureaucratic red tape and political interference are partly responsible for the underutilization of skilled workers.

Given the projections for high attrition rates attributable to illness, death and accelerated migration, it seems likely that the crisis of health care providers in many poorer countries will worsen before it gets better. In the WHO African Region, where

> *" The crisis requires nothing short of an outstanding global response "*

the shortage of health workers stands at about 1.5 million, there are many countries where the annual outflows caused by worker deaths, migration and retirement exceed the inflows of newly trained doctors and nurses *(22)*.

## An extraordinary global response is needed

The dire situation provoked by the global health workforce crisis requires nothing short of an outstanding global response. International action necessitates: coalitions around emergency national plans for health care providers; health worker-friendly practices among global partners; and sufficient and sustained financing of the health workforce.

### Coalitions around emergency plans

The first imperative – emergency national plans for the health workforce – must combine credible technical input across the spectrum of human resource issues with intrepid and innovative strategies to make significant changes in the short term as well as in the medium and longer terms. As explained in Chapter 6, engaging diverse stakeholders across sectors in a clear process at the outset of strategy development will help to forge shared ownership of the coalition. The conditions for developing these strategies in the crisis countries are suboptimal because of the scarcity of expertise, inadequate public sector capacity to lead a complex process, and the difficulties of convening stakeholders in the midst of multiple competing priorities. High-level political support both nationally and internationally is necessary to ensure priority attention to the development of these plans. Malawi's Emergency Human Resources Plan benefited from close involvement of the ministers of health and finance as well as from visits from heads of international bilateral and multilateral agencies *(23)*.

### Towards more worker-friendly practices

There is no longer any question that the massive international efforts under way to treat people living with HIV/AIDS and to achieve the Millennium Development Goals (MDGs) must start dealing with workforce constraints more directly. If not, the billions of dollars that are being poured into these programmes are at risk of being wasted. For their part, countries have identified human resources as the area of the health system most in need of investment *(5)* (see Figure 7.3).

Current practices among international stakeholders for supporting the health workforce tend to be antiquated in terms of content, ad hoc with respect to process and unintentionally adverse as regards impact. All multilateral, bilateral and civil society actors involved in health development in countries with a health workforce crisis could benefit enormously from a thorough review and impact assessment of their activities in this direction. They should ensure that their practices embrace the working lifespan approach of entry, workforce and exit, in order to decrease the risk of focusing too narrowly on single issues such as on-the-job training. Any direct investments by partners in workforce-related issues should be based on a clear rationale of comparative advantage relative to pooling support to national emergency plans for health care providers.

Directing support to countries in crisis defies a single approach, and no such process should be seen as exempt from incorporating a dimension to strengthen the health workforce. This includes – but is not limited to – sector-wide approaches, poverty reduction strategies, medium-term expenditure frameworks, and instruments

such as the country coordinating mechanisms of the Global Fund to Fight AIDS, Tuberculosis and Malaria and the national control programmes for HIV/AIDS. All of these processes should be brought into line with national emergency plans for human resources, and mechanisms should be identified to put the cooperation into place. The decision by the Global Alliance for Vaccines and Immunization (GAVI) to support a health systems strengthening strategy inclusive of the health workforce is now being translated through country applications with principles, requirements and minimal criteria summarized in clear guidelines. Importantly, the strategy seeks to ensure that GAVI's prospective assistance to the health workforce (and other elements of health systems) in a country is aligned with existing strategies for strengthening the workforce. As the experience of sector-wide approaches and poverty reduction strategies has shown, the promise of more effectively integrating policies for the health workforce is constrained by insufficient numbers of adequately supported national staff *(24)*. This underlines the need to develop national capacities for strategic intelligence (see Chapter 6) and to facilitate access to technical cooperation.

### *The imperative of sufficient, sustained financing*

Overcoming the workforce shortage will require substantial financial commitments to train and pay the additional health workers. The cost of very rapid scaling up of training aimed at eliminating the shortfall by 2015 – the target date for achieving the goals of the Millennium Declaration – was shown in Chapter 1 to be about US$ 136 million per year for the average country. The additional cost of paying health workers once the shortage has been met is just over US$ 311 million per country at current salary levels *(25)*.

Assuming that scaling up takes place over a 20-year period – which many observers might argue is more realistic – the required annual investment in training is US$ 88 million per country. Additional salary costs when the workforce is fully

## Figure 7.3 Country priorities for health systems strengthening

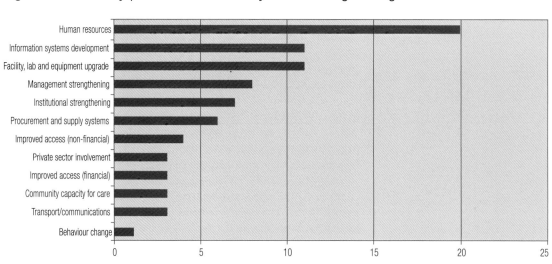

Number of proposals to the Global Fund for Tuberculosis, HIV/AIDS and Malaria, round 5

Source: *(5)*.

staffed would be higher under this scenario (because the population will increase substantially between 2015 and 2025 and so will the need for health workers), reaching in excess of US$ 400 million per country.

Translating the figures into per capita expenditure in health for the average country gives further perspective on the costs of scaling up the health workforce. To meet the investment costs for training over a 20-year period, the average country would need to increase its overall level of health expenditure per capita by about US$ 1.60 each year. By 2025, a minimum increase of US$ 8.30 per capita would be required to pay the salaries of the appropriate workforce.

While such costing models are indicative rather than precise, they do reveal important issues. Firstly, scaling up the health workforce on either a 10-year or 20-year trajectory will require very significant dedicated funding. Next, these estimates of the training and salary costs of scaling up are based on doctors, nurses and midwives. Although there are no data, strategies that depend on lower paid cadres with less formal training may be more affordable and therefore merit serious consideration. Finally, the results are sensitive to the age of retirement of health workers, their mortality rates, and the extent to which they remain in the country and choose to be employed in the health sector after training. Policies to improve workers' health, extend retirement age and increase retention may reduce the numbers that need to be trained and may result in cost savings.

It is clear from the above that a major expansion of the health workforce has both immediate and long-term cost implications. Understandably, governments with few financial resources may be reluctant to commit to such long-term costs without clear signals of support from the international donor community. As the nature and magnitude of the health worker crisis comes into greater focus and national strategies to scale up the workforce emerge, now is the time to clarify the role of international financial assistance.

## A global guideline for financing

The financing challenge has two distinct aspects: generating sufficient volume to cope realistically with the crisis, and sustaining adequate levels of funding over time. Mobilizing the sizeable funds required for the financing of the health workforce must be carried out through a combination of improved government budgets and international development assistance. There are some promising signs. For example, the recent dedication of funds for strengthening health systems amounting to US$ 500 million, budgeted by GAVI over five years, indicates how the health workforce is becoming one of the priority areas for systems support. Similarly, the Emergency Health Workforce Plan in Malawi has dedicated US$ 278 million over six years through a coalition of country and global partners.

While bottom-up budgeting around emergency plans is the optimal way to proceed, there is nonetheless a need for a financing guideline that can ensure that the response is commensurate with need and around which the international community can mobilize. With respect to the total flows of international development assistance for health, approximately US$ 12 billion per annum in 2004 *(26)*, this report recommends a 50:50 principle – that 50% of this financing be directed to health systems strengthening, of which at least half is dedicated to supporting emergency health workforce plans. The rationale for this proportional investment relates to the reliance of health workers on functioning health systems and the need for dedicated financing of workforce strategies above and beyond the human resources activities that may be inherent in specific priority programmes of global health organizations.

In so far as the proposed expansion is publicly financed – through taxes, social health insurance or international solidarity – it is subject to the rules of public financing. In an effort to preserve macroeconomic stability and fiscal sustainability, international finance institutions and ministers of finance use criteria such as the public expenditure:GDP ratio to set ceilings. The most visible consequences for the health sector are the ceilings on recruitment and the stagnant salaries of health workers in public employment. Hiring moratoriums are limiting the expansion of health services and creating unemployment of health workers, particularly in sub-Saharan Africa. Poverty reduction strategies, for example, often refer explicitly to such restrictions. Authorities in Kenya, Mozambique, Zambia and many other countries are thus refraining from hiring health workers because they cannot find a way around these stipulations (27).

Greater attention to this issue has produced a menu of options to manage better within current public sector financing rules. Examples include effective outsourcing as a means of lowering costs and eliminating ghost workers (28, 29). Although such efficiency measures would be helpful, they are unlikely to be sufficient on their own. Recognition of the need to expand fiscal space (i.e. make more budget room for health) calls for a status of exception to be accorded to public financing of health and its workforce. Negotiating fiscal space safeguards for the health workforce will require the health development world to engage productively with ministries of finance, international finance institutions and major international stakeholders. Strengthened evidence on the health and economic returns on investment in the health workforce may assist in these negotiations. At the same time, the moral and political rationales related to placing the people's health first and pursuing universal access can help to achieve a health workforce exception.

Part of the concern in public financing of workforce expansion relates to the ability of governments to pay for staff throughout the length of their careers. Because countries are reluctant to expose themselves to a potentially unsustainable public debt, they need predictability of donor back-up over the long term (30). Donor funds, however, are expressions of current government priorities, and mechanisms for long-term reassurance or guarantees of support are generally not forthcoming. The challenges of funding the scaling up of the health workforce in the longer term, therefore, cannot be separated from the broader dilemma of resource mobilization for health. Bold commitments and new mechanisms may help to provide greater predictability of global aid flows (31). These must be complemented by national strategies that build towards sustainable financing of the health sector.

## MOVING FORWARD TOGETHER

Over the last decade much has been done to raise the awareness that, unless problems of the health workforce are dealt with squarely, health systems are going to founder. There are still huge gaps in knowledge about the extent of the fundamental drivers that shape the human resources predicament, and the range of solutions that can be suggested. There is, however, a way out of the crisis.

By working together through inclusive stakeholder alliances – global as well as national – problems that cross sectors, interest groups and national boundaries can be tackled: limited expertise can be pooled, and opportunities for mutual learning, sharing and problem-solving can be seized. Global solidarity will make it possible to exploit synergies between the specific inputs of bodies such as WHO, international finance institutions, academia and professional associations. It is particularly

important to monitor carefully the effects of these inputs so as to build up gradually a critical mass of evidence – and to share this knowledge with all who might benefit from it.

There is not a country in the world that is not facing major health workforce challenges – challenges that affect its health system, its economy and its obligations towards its citizens. All countries need to build or strengthen their institutional capacities to deal with their own predicaments and problems of human resources for health. Some countries need a significant amount of external assistance to succeed in doing so; if such support is not forthcoming, they will fall even further behind because the global forces that drive health workforce development will accelerate distortions. From a global perspective, this would mean an exacerbation of inequalities as health workers move to countries where policy-makers are more responsive to their concerns. From a national perspective, it would mean rising political tensions as citizens' rightful expectations fail to materialize.

Momentum for action has grown steadily over recent years. Member States of WHO, spearheaded by health leaders from Africa, adopted two resolutions at recent World Health Assemblies calling for global action to build a workforce for national health systems, including stemming the flow of unplanned professional emigration. Europe and Latin America have promoted regional observatories in human resources for health, and the WHO South-East Asia and Eastern Mediterranean Regional Offices have launched new public health training initiatives. One hundred global health leaders in the Joint Learning Initiative recommended urgent action to overcome the crisis of human resources for health. Calls for action have come from a series of High-Level Forums for the health-related MDGs in Geneva, Abuja and Paris, and two Oslo Consultations have nurtured a participatory stakeholder process to chart a way forward. A clear mandate has emerged for a global plan of action bringing forth national leadership backed by global solidarity.

## National leadership

Strong country strategies require both solid technical content and a credible political process. This involves embracing the breadth of issues inherent in the entry–workforce–exit framework while cultivating trust and brokering agreements through effective engagement of stakeholders in planning and implementation. In addition, national strategies are likely to be more successful if they adopt three priorities: acting now, anticipating the future and acquiring critical capabilities.

- Acting now for workforce productivity by cutting waste (such as eliminating ghost workers and absenteeism) and improving performance through compensation adjustments, work incentives, safer working conditions, and worker mobilization efforts. Better intelligence gathering is crucial, in order to understand national situations and monitor progress or setbacks.
- Anticipating the future by engaging stakeholders to craft national strategic plans through evidence-based information and scenarios on likely future trends. Significant growth of private education and services should be anticipated, necessitating the targeting of public funds for health equity, promotion and prevention. Public action in information, regulation and delegation are key functions for mixed public and private systems.
- Acquiring critical capacities by strengthening core institutions for sound workforce development. Leadership and management development in health and other related sectors such as education and finance are essential for strategic

planning and implementation of workforce policies. Standard setting, accrediting and licensing must be effectively established to improve the work of worker unions, educational institutions, professional associations and civil society.

## Global solidarity

National strategies on their own, however well conceived, are insufficient to deal with the realities of health workforce challenges today and in the future. Strategies across countries are similarly constrained by patchy evidence, limited planning tools and a scarcity of technical expertise. Outbreaks of disease and labour market inflections transcend national boundaries, and the depth of the workforce crisis in a significant group of countries requires international assistance. National leadership must therefore be complemented by global solidarity on at least three fronts: knowledge and learning; cooperative agreements; and responsiveness to health workforce crises.

> "*National leadership and global solidarity can result in significant improvements in all countries*"

- Catalysing knowledge and learning. Low-cost but significant investments in the development of better metrics for the workforce, agreement on common technical frameworks, and the identification of and support for priority research will accelerate progress in all countries. Effective pooling of the diverse technical expertise and breadth of experiences can assist countries in accessing the best talent and practices.

- Striking cooperative agreements. The growing international nature of the health workforce related to the flows of migrants, relief workers and volunteers calls for cooperative agreements to protect the rights and safety of workers and to enhance the adoption of ethical recruitment practices. The current global situation regarding avian influenza is indicative of a more fundamental need for effective international capacity to marshal the requisite human resources for acute health and humanitarian emergencies.

- Responding to health workforce crises. The magnitude of the crisis in the world's poorest countries cannot be overstated and requires an urgent, sustained and coordinated response from the international community. Donors must facilitate the immediate and longer-term financing of human resources as a health systems investment. The costs of scaling up the workforce over a 20-year period corresponds to an annual increase of about US$ 1.60 in per capita expenditure on health. A 50:50 guideline is recommended, whereby 50% of all priority initiative funds are devoted to health systems, with half of this funding devoted to national health workforce strengthening strategies. Development financing policies must find ways to ensure that hiring ceilings are not the primary constraint to workforce expansion. All partners should critically evaluate their modalities for supporting the workforce with a view to shedding inefficient practices and aligning more effectively with national leadership.

National leadership and global solidarity can result in significant structural improvements of the workforce in all countries, especially those with the most severe crises. Such advances would be characterized by universal access to a motivated, competent and supported health workforce, greater worker, employer and public satisfaction, and more effective stewardship of the workforce by the state, civil society and professional associations.

## Plan of action

National leadership must urgently jump-start country-based actions and sustain them for at least a decade. Table 7.2 summarizes targets in the plan of action over the decade 2006–2015.

■ Immediate actions over the next few years should consist of lead countries pioneering national plans for scaling up effective strategies, increasing investments, cutting waste, and strengthening educational institutions. Global support should accelerate progress in countries, with immediate policy attention given to intelligence, technical cooperation, policy alignment of fiscal space and migration, and harmonization of priority initiatives and donor assistance.

■ At the decade's mid-point, over half of all countries should have sound national plans with expanded execution of good policies and management practices concerned with workforce incentives, regulation and institutions. Global advances will include shared norms and frameworks, strong technical support, and improved knowledge management. Responsible recruitment and alignment of priority programmes and development instruments to support the health workforce should be in place.

■ The decade goal in all countries is to build high-performing workforces for national health systems to respond to current and emerging challenges. This means that every country should have implemented national strategic plans and should be planning for the future, drawing on robust national capacity. Globally, a full range of evidence-based guidelines should inform good practice for health workers. Effective cooperative agreements will minimize adverse consequences despite increased international flows of workers. Sustained international financing should be in place to support recipient countries for the next 10 years as they scale up their workforce.

## Table 7.2 Ten-year plan of action

| | | 2006<br>Immediate | 2010<br>Mid-point | 2015<br>Decade |
|---|---|---|---|---|
| **Country leadership** | **Management** | Cut waste, improve incentives | Use effective managerial practices | Sustain high performing workforce |
| | **Education** | Revitalize education strategies | Strengthen accreditation and licensing | Prepare workforce for the future |
| | **Planning** | Design national workforce strategies | Overcome barriers to implementation | Evaluate and redesign strategies, based on robust national capacity |
| **Global solidarity** | **Knowledge and learning** | Develop common technical frameworks | Assess performance with comparable metrics | Share evidence-based good practices |
| | | Pool expertise | Fund priority research | |
| | **Enabling policies** | Advocate ethical recruitment and migrant workers' rights | Adhere to responsible recruitment guidelines | Manage increased migratory flows for equity and fairness |
| | | Pursue fiscal space exceptionality | Expand fiscal space for health | Support fiscal sustainability |
| | **Crisis response** | Finance national plans for 25% of crisis countries | Expand financing to half of crisis countries | Sustain financing of national plans for all countries in crisis |
| | | Agree on best donor practices for human resources for health | Adopt 50:50 investment guideline for priority programmes | |

## Figure 7.4 Global stakeholder alliance

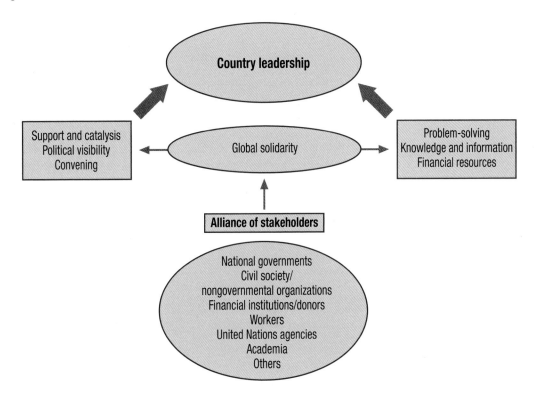

## JOINT STEPS TO THE FUTURE

Moving forward on the plan of action necessitates that stakeholders work together through inclusive alliances and networks – local, national and global – across health problems, professions, disciplines, ministries, sectors and countries. Cooperative structures can pool limited talent and fiscal resources and promote mutual learning. Figure 7.4 proposes how a global workforce alliance can be launched to bring relevant stakeholders to accelerate core country programmes.

A premier challenge is advocacy that promotes workforce issues to a high place on the political agenda and keeps them there. The moment is ripe for political support as problem awareness is expanding, effective solutions are emerging, and various countries are already pioneering interventions. Workforce development is a continuous process that is always open for improvement. However, immediate acceleration of performance can be attained in virtually all countries if well-documented solutions are applied. Some of the work should be implemented immediately; other aspects will take time. There are no short cuts and there is no time to lose. Now is the time for action, to invest in the future, and to advance health – rapidly and equitably.

# REFERENCES

1. Dubois C-A, McKee M. Cross-national comparisons of human resources for health. What can we learn? *Health Economics, Policy and Law*, 2006, 1:59–78.

2. Moore J, Karnaukhova J, McGinnis S, Ricketts T, Skillman S, Paul E et al. *Human resources for health: options for analysis and monitoring* (unpublished document, 2005).

3. Diallo K, Zurn P, Gupta N, Dal Poz MR. Monitoring and evaluation of human resources for health: an international perspective. *Human Resources for Health*, 2003, 1:3.

4. *Human resources of European health systems: final report*. Paris, Organisation for Economic Co-operation and Development, 2001.

5. *Opportunities for global health initiatives in the health systems action agenda*. Geneva, World Health Organization, 2005 (Making health systems work, Working Paper No.4).

6. *Report on WHO Workshop on Formulating a Global Research Agenda for Human Resources for Health, Cape Town, 6–8 September 2004*. Geneva, World Health Organization, 2004.

7. *Human resources for health: overcoming the crisis*. Cambridge, MA, Joint Learning Initiative, 2004.

8. Hongoro C, McPake B. How to bridge the gap in human resources for health. *Lancet*, 2004, 364:1451–1456.

9. Black N. Health care workforce: how research can help. *Journal of Health Services Research and Policy*, 2004, 9(Suppl. 1):1–2.

10. Cochrane Database of Systematic Reviews (available at: http://www.mrw.interscience.wiley.com/cochrane/cochrane_clsysrev_articles_fs.html, accessed 12 February 2006).

11. Anand S, Bärnighausen T. *Human resources for health and vaccination coverage in developing countries* (unpublished document, Oxford University, 2005).

12. *Report from the Ministerial Summit on Health Research: identify challenges, inform actions, correct inequities*. Geneva, World Health Organization, 2005.

13. *Cape Town recommendations for scaling up research on human resources for health*. World Health Organization Workshop on Formulating a Global Research Agenda on Human Resources for Health, 6 to 8 September 2004, Cape Town, South Africa. (http://www.who.int/reproductive-health/tcc/meeting_documents/cape_town_recommendations.pdf, accessed 26 February 2006).

14. *Report of the Task Force on Health Systems Research*. Geneva, World Health Organization, 2005 (http://www.who.int/rpc/summit/Task_Force_on_HSR_2.pdf, accessed 12 February 2006).

15. Awases M, Nyoni J, Gbary A, Chatora R. *Migration of health professionals in six countries: a synthesis report*. Brazzaville, World Health Organization Regional Office for Africa, 2004.

16. Hasselhorn H-M, Tackenberg P, Müller BH. *Working conditions and intent to leave the profession among nursing staff in Europe: NEXT – nurses early exit study, 2003*. Stockholm, National Institute for Working Life, 2004.

17. Ministry of Health, the Government of Uganda (http://www.health.go.ug/, accessed 26 February 2006).

18. *Towards a society for all ages. Employment, health, pensions and intergenerational solidarity*. Brussels, European Commission, 1999 (Conference Paper, European Symposium; available at: http://europa.eu.int/comm/employment_social/soc-prot/ageing/vienna/vienna_en.pdf, accessed 26 February 2006).

19. *Jobs of the future.* Accenture/The Lisbon Council, 2005 (available at: http://www.accenture.com/Global/Research_and_Insights/Policy_And_Corporate_Affairs/JobsFuture.htm, accessed 26 February 2006).

20. Cooper RA, Getzen TE, McKee HJ, Laud P. Economic and demographic trends signal an impending physician shortage. *Health Affairs*, 2002, 21:140–154.

21. Matthews Z, Van Lerberghe W. *Notes on workforce implications of demographic change* (background paper for *The world health report 2006*; available at: http://www.who.int/hrh/documents/en/).

22. Kinfu Y, Mercer H, Dal Poz MR, Evans DB. *Estimating inflows and outflows of health service providers in sub-Saharan Africa.* Geneva, World Health Organization, 2005 (background paper prepared for *The world health report 2006*; available at: http://www.who.int/hrh/documents/en/).

23. Palmer D, United Kingdom Department for International Development–Malawi, personal communication.

24. *PRSPs: their significance for health – second synthesis report.* Geneva, World Health Organization, 2004 (document WHO/HDP/PRSP/04.1).

25. Verboom P, Tan-Torres Edejer T, Evans DB. *The cost of eliminating critical shortages in human resources for health.* Geneva, World Health Organization, 2005 (background paper prepared for *The world health report 2006;* available at: http://www.who.int/hrh/en).

26. Michaud C. Development assistance for health (DAH): recent trends and resource allocation. Paper prepared for the Second Consultation Commission on Macroeconomics and Health, World Health Organization, Geneva, 29–30 October, 2003 (http://www.who.int/macrohealth/events/health_for_poor/en/dah_trends_nov10.pdf, accessed 26 February 2006) .

27. *Human resources for health strategic plan 2006–2010.* Lusaka, Ministry of Health Zambia, 2005.

28. Heller PS. *Finding sustainable "fiscal space" for the health sector.* Paper presented at: High Level Forum on the Health MDGs, Paris, November 2005 (http://www.hlfhealthmdgs.org/November2005Mtg.asp, accessed 12 February 2006).

29. Vujicic M. *Macroeconomic and fiscal issues in scaling up human resources for health in low-income countries.* Washington, DC, The World Bank, Human Development Network, 2005 (background paper for *The world health report 2006;* available at: http://www.who.int/hrh/documents/en/).

30. Williams G, Hay R. *Fiscal space and sustainability from the perspective of the health sector.* Background paper for the High Level Forum on the Health MDGs, Paris, November 2005 (http://www.hlfhealthmdgs.org/November2005Mtg.asp; accessed 12 February 2006).

31. Foster M. *Fiscal space and sustainability – towards a solution for the health sector.* Background paper for the High Level Forum on the Health MDGs, Paris, November 2005 (http://www.hlfhealthmdgs.org/Documents/FiscalSpaceTowardsSolution.pdf, accessed 26 February 2006).

# statistical annex
# *explanatory*
# *notes*

## ANNEX TABLE 1

All estimates of population size and structure for 2004 are based on the demographic assessments prepared by the United Nations Population Division *(1)*. These estimates refer to the de facto population, and not the de jure population in each Member State.

The annual growth rate, the dependency ratio, the percentage of population aged 60 years and more, and the total fertility rate are obtained from the same United Nations Population Division database.

To assess overall levels of health achievement, it is crucial to develop the best possible assessment of the life table for each country. Life tables have been developed for all 192 Member States for 2004 starting with a systematic review of all available evidence on levels and trends in under-five and adult mortality rates. It is worth noting the efforts of WHO regional offices in collecting vital registration data from Member States *(2)*. International agencies such as the United Nations Children's Fund (UNICEF) also maintain historical databases on under-five mortality rates, which have been generously shared and incorporated in these analyses. Other sources of information include data from national censuses or household surveys such as the Demographic and Health Survey (DHS) undertaken by ORC Macro, the World Bank Living Standards Measurement Study, and the Multiple Indicator Cluster Survey (MICS) conducted by UNICEF. Finally, national statistical documents such as statistical yearbooks, reports from specialized agencies and periodical paper findings were also incorporated into the database.

This review of data sources benefited greatly from a collaborative assessment of under-five mortality levels for 2004 by UNICEF, WHO, the World Bank and the United Nations Population Division responsible for monitoring child mortality trends.

The four agencies have established the Child Mortality Coordination Group including an independent group of academics which aims to conduct a critical review of current procedures used in each institution for compiling data and arriving at point estimates *(3)*.

WHO uses a standard method to estimate and project life tables for all Member States using comparable data. This may lead to minor differences compared with official life tables prepared by Member States.

Life expectancy at birth, the probability of dying before five years of age (under-five mortality rate) and the probability of dying between 15 and 60 years of age (adult mortality rate) derive from life tables that WHO has estimated for each Member State.

Procedures used to estimate the 2004 life table differed for Member States depending on the data available to assess child and adult mortality. Because of increasing heterogeneity of patterns of adult and child mortality, WHO has developed a model life table system of two-parameter logit life tables, and with additional age-specific parameters to correct for systematic biases in the application of a two-parameter system *(4)*. This system of model life tables has been used extensively in the development of life tables for those Member States without adequate vital registration and in projecting life tables to 2004 when the most recent data available are from earlier years. Estimates for 2004 have been revised to take into account new data received since publication of *The world health report 2005* for many Member States and may not be entirely comparable with those published in previous reports. The methods used to construct life tables are summarized below and a full detailed overview has been published *(4, 5)*.

For Member States with vital registration and sample vital registration systems, demographic techniques (Preston–Coale method, Brass Growth–Balance method, Generalized Growth–Balance method and Bennett–Horiuchi method) were first applied to assess the level of completeness of recorded mortality data in the population above five years of age and then those mortality rates were adjusted accordingly *(6)*. Where vital registration data for 2004 were available, these were used directly to construct the life table. For other countries where the system provided a time series of annual life tables, the parameters ($l_5$, $l_{60}$) were projected using a weighted regression model giving more weight to recent years (using an exponential weighting scheme such that the weight for each year *t* was 25% less than that for year *t+1*). For countries with a total population of less than 750 000 or where the root mean square error from the regression was greater than or equal to 0.011, a shorter-term trend was estimated by applying a weighting factor with 50% annual exponential decay. Projected values of the two life table parameters were then applied to a modified logit life table model, using the most recent national data as the standard, which allows the capture of the most recent age pattern, to predict the full life table for 2004.

For all Member States, other data available for child mortality, such as surveys and censuses, were assessed and adjusted to estimate the probable trend over the past few decades in order to predict the child mortality in 2004. A standard approach to predicting child mortality was employed to obtain the estimates for 2004 *(7)*.

Those estimates are, on the one hand, used to replace the under-five mortality rate in life tables of the countries that have a vital registration or sample vital registration system, but with incomplete registration of numbers of deaths under the age of five years; on the other hand, for countries without exploitable vital registration systems, which are mainly those with high mortality, the predicted under-five mortality rates are used as one of the inputs to the modified logit system. Adult mortality rates were derived from either surveys or censuses where available; otherwise the most likely corresponding level of adult mortality was estimated based on regression models of child versus adult mortality as observed in the set of approximately 1800 life tables. These estimated child and adult mortality rates were then applied to a global standard, defined as the average of all the life tables, using the modified logit model to derive the estimates for 2004.

It should be noted that the logit model life table system using the global standard does not capture high HIV/AIDS epidemic patterns, because the observed underlying life tables do not come from countries with the epidemic. Similarly, war deaths are not captured because vital registration systems often break down in periods of war *(8)*. For these reasons, for affected countries, mortality without deaths attributable to HIV/AIDS and war was estimated and separate estimates of deaths caused by HIV/AIDS and war in 2004 were added.

The main results in Annex Table 1 are reported with uncertainty intervals in order to communicate to the user the plausible range of estimates for each country on each measure. For the countries with vital registration data projected using time series regression models on the parameters of the logit life table system, uncertainty around the regression coefficients has been accounted for by taking 1000 draws of the parameters using the regression estimates and variance covariance matrix of the estimators. For each of the draws, a new life table was calculated. In cases where additional sources of information provided plausible ranges around under-five and adult mortality rates the 1000 draws were constrained such that each life table produced estimates within these specified ranges. The range of 1000 life tables produced by these multiple draws reflects some of the uncertainty around the projected trends in mortality, notably the imprecise quantification of systematic changes in the logit parameters over the time period captured in available vital registration data.

For Member States where complete death registrations were available for the year 2004 and projections were not used, the life table uncertainty reflects the event count uncertainty, approximated by the Poisson distribution, in the estimated age-specific death rates arising from the observation of a finite number of deaths in a fixed time interval of one year.

For countries that did not have time series data on mortality by age and sex, the following steps were taken. First, point estimates and ranges around under-five and adult mortality rates for males and females were developed on a country-by-country basis *(5)*. In the modified logit life table system described *(4)*, values on these two parameters may be used to identify a range of different life tables in relation to a global standard life table. Using the Monte Carlo simulation methods, 1000 random life tables were generated by drawing samples from normal distributions around these inputs with variances defined according to ranges of uncertainty. In countries where uncertainty around under-five and adult mortality rates was considerable because of a paucity of survey or surveillance information, wide distributions were sampled but the results were constrained based on estimates of the maximum and minimum plausible values for the point estimates.

For 55 countries, mainly in sub-Saharan Africa, estimates of life tables were made by constructing counterfactual life tables excluding the mortality impact of the HIV/AIDS epidemic and then combining these life tables with exogenous estimates of the excess mortality rates attributable to HIV/AIDS. The estimates were based on back-calculation models developed as part of collaborative efforts between WHO and the Joint United Nations Programme on HIV/AIDS (UNAIDS) to derive country-level epidemiological estimates for HIV/AIDS. In countries with substantial numbers of war deaths, estimates of their uncertainty range were also incorporated into the life table uncertainty analysis.

## ANNEX TABLE 2

Annex Table 2 (Annex Table 5 in last year's report) provides a set of policy-relevant indicators on major health expenditure aggregates. The indicators include the total expenditure on health, broken down into public/general government expenditure on health and private health expenditure. Selected components are presented of public health expenditures (social security expenditure on health) and private health expenditures (health insurance and prepaid schemes and out-of-pocket expenditure). General government expenditure on health is also presented as a ratio to total general government expenditure (GGE). Data on external resources, which are flows earmarked for health originating outside the country and treated as a financing source, are also available. External resources represent all outside funds that finance the above-mentioned general government health expenditure and private health expenditure.

The data include the best figures that were accessible to WHO until the end of 2005 for its 192 Member States. Subsequent updates, additional years and detailed information are available on the WHO National Health Accounts (NHA) web site at http://www.who.int/nha/en/.

During the past half decade, an increasing number of countries have been releasing more comprehensive data on health spending: about 100 countries produced full national health accounts (for one year or more) or report expenditure on health to the Organisation for Economic Co-operation and Development (OECD), released as *OECD health data*. WHO publishes data collated from national and international sources and reports. Data are consolidated, triangulated and harmonized in the NHA framework, using international classifications and standard national accounts procedures. Standard accounting estimation and extrapolation techniques have been used to provide time series. As in previous years, a draft template of the estimates was sent to ministers of health seeking their comments and assistance in obtaining additional information. Their responses and those of other government agencies, such as statistical offices, provided valuable feedback that has improved the estimates for the health expenditure indicators reported here. WHO staff at headquarters and in regional and country offices facilitate this process. Years of regular consultation and discussion have established extensive communication channels with ministries of health and other agencies, domestic and international experts and networks and have also helped in developing national capacity.

### Measurement of expenditure on health

Health accounting (HA) is a synthesis of the financing and spending flows recorded in the operation of a health system. It offers the potential to monitor all transactions from funding sources to the distribution of benefits according to geographical, demographic, socioeconomic and epidemiological characteristics. NHA are further related to the macroeconomic and macrosocial accounts whose methodological approach they borrow.

An important methodological contribution to the construction of HA is the *Guide to producing national health accounts with special applications for low-income and middle-income countries (9)*, itself grounded on the OECD *System of health accounts (10)* principles. This methodology rests on the foundations of the United Nations *System of national accounts* (commonly referred to as SNA93) *(11)*.

WHO has been publishing a moving five-year series on NHA indicators since 2002, and updates the figures every year with the best estimates accessible. Each five-year series exhibits internal consistency among the included years. Because HA is a discipline in development – not only regarding methods but also regarding implementation by countries – several Member States have modified previous estimates in order to improve measurement. Some of the reasons for improved estimates can be categorized into five groups: 1) new NHA reports, where countries make their first ever NHA report; 2) improved NHA reports, where an additional report offers improved estimates over preliminary NHA work; 3) new data sources, where there is access to new data such as social security data or new households expenditure survey results released; 4) improved data sources, where governments provide better data or instances of double counting were identified; and 5) macro data updated. Caution is required when comparing newly published estimates with previously published series or when trying to construct a series longer than the currently available multiyear series (please refer to the web site for longer reconciled series).

## Definitions

Total health expenditure (THE) has been defined as the sum of general government expenditure on health (commonly called public expenditure on health), and private expenditure on health. General government health expenditure (GGHE) is estimated as the sum of outlays by government entities to purchase health care services and goods: notably by ministries of health and social security agencies. Private health expenditure (PvtHE) includes total outlays on health by private entities: notably commercial insurance, non-profit institutions, households acting as complementary funders to the previously cited institutions or disbursing unilaterally on health commodities. The revenue base of these entities may comprise multiple sources, including external funds. This necessitates taking into account essential attributes of health accounting such as comprehensiveness, consistency, standardization and timeliness when building estimates. Figures are originally estimated in million national currency units (million NCU) and in current prices.

GGHE comprises the outlays earmarked for health maintenance, restoration or enhancement of the health status of the population, paid for in cash or in kind by the following financing agents:

- central/federal (ministry of health or other ministries), state/provincial/regional, and local/municipal authorities;
- extrabudgetary agencies, principally social security schemes;
- direct expenditure on health care by parastatals and public firms (which operate as though they were private sector firms but are controlled by the government).

All three can be financed through domestic funds or through external resources (mainly as grants passing through the government or loans channelled through the national budget).

GGHE includes both recurrent and investment expenditures (including capital transfers) made during the year. The classification of the functions of government (COFOG) promoted by the United Nations, the International Monetary Fund (IMF), OECD and other institutions sets the boundaries for public outlays. In many instances, the data contained in the publications accessed are limited to those supplied by ministries of health. Expenditure on health, however, should include all expenditure when the primary intent is to improve health, regardless of the implementing entity. An effort has been made to obtain data on health expenditure by other ministries, the armed forces, prisons, schools, universities and others, to ensure that all resources accounting for health expenditures are included. Furthermore, all expenditures on health include final consumption, subsidies to producers, and transfers to households (chiefly reimbursements for medical and pharmaceutical bills).

The figures for social security expenditure on health include purchases of health goods and services by schemes that are mandatory and controlled by government. A major hurdle faced by accountants is the need to avoid double counting and exclude cash benefits for periods of sickness or loss of employment, which are classified as income maintenance expenditure. Government-controlled and mandatory social security schemes that apply only to a selected group of the population, such as public sector employees only, are also included here.

PvtHE has been defined as the sum of expenditures by the following entities:

■ Prepaid plans and risk-pooling arrangements: the outlays of private insurance schemes and private social insurance schemes (with no government control over payment rates and participating providers but with broad guidelines from government), commercial and non-profit (mutual) insurance schemes, health maintenance organizations, and other agents managing prepaid medical and paramedical benefits (including the operating costs of these schemes).

■ Firms' expenditure on health: the outlays by private enterprises for medical care and health-enhancing benefits other than payment to social security or other pre-paid schemes.

■ Non-profit institutions serving mainly households: the resources used to purchase health goods and services by entities whose status does not permit them to be a source of income, profit or other financial gain for the units that establish, control or finance them. This includes funding from internal and external sources.

■ Household out-of-pocket spending: the direct outlays of households, including gratuities and in-kind payments made to health practitioners and to suppliers of pharmaceuticals, therapeutic appliances and other goods and services, whose primary intent is to contribute to the restoration or the enhancement of the health status of individuals or population groups. This includes household payments to public services, non-profit institutions or nongovernmental organizations and non-reimbursable cost sharing, deductibles, copayments and fees for services. It excludes payments made by enterprises which deliver medical and paramedical benefits, mandated by law or not, to their employees and payments for overseas treatment. It also excludes transport and food costs (except those paid officially to the providers) and contributions to pre-paid pooling schemes.

The external resources appearing in Annex Table 2 are those entering the system as a financing source, i.e. all external resources (grants and loans) whether passing through governments or private entities are included. The other institutions and entities reported are public or private expenditures on health acting as financing agents. Financing agents are entities that pool health resources collected from different financing sources (such as households, government, external agencies, firms and nongovernmental organizations) and pay directly for or purchase health care.

Gross domestic product (GDP) is the value of all goods and services provided in a country by residents and non-residents without regard to their allocation among domestic and foreign claims. This (with small adjustments) corresponds to the total sum of expenditure (consumption and investment) of the private and government agents of the economy during the reference year.

General government expenditure (GGE) includes consolidated direct outlays and indirect outlays (for example, subsidies to producers, transfers to households), including capital, of all levels of government (central/federal, provincial/regional/state/district, and local/municipal authorities), social security institutions, autonomous bodies, and other extrabudgetary funds.

## Data sources

Annex Table 2 provides both updated and revised figures for 1999–2003. Estimates for additional years along with sources and methodology are available at http://www.who.int/nha. National sources include: national health accounts reports, public expenditure reports, statistical yearbooks and other periodicals, budgetary documents, national accounts reports, central bank reports, nongovernmental organization reports, academic studies, and reports and data provided by central statistical offices, ministries of health, ministries of finance and economic development, planning offices, and professional and trade associations, statistical data on official web sites, and household surveys.

Specific health accounts or comprehensive health financing documents and studies (including both private and public sectors) are available in the following countries presented by WHO regional groupings:

- African Region: Algeria, Burkina Faso, Cameroon, Ethiopia, Guinea, Kenya, Malawi, Mauritius, Mozambique, Namibia, Niger, Nigeria, Rwanda, Senegal, South Africa, Togo, Uganda, United Republic of Tanzania, Zambia, Zimbabwe.
- Region of the Americas: Argentina, Bahamas, Bolivia, Brazil, Canada, Chile, Colombia, Costa Rica, Ecuador, El Salvador, Guatemala, Honduras, Mexico, Nicaragua, Panama, Paraguay, Peru, Suriname, Trinidad and Tobago, United States of America, Uruguay.
- South-East Asia Region: Bangladesh, India, Indonesia, Sri Lanka, Thailand.
- European Region: Albania, Austria, Belgium, Bulgaria, Czech Republic, Denmark, Estonia, Cyprus, Finland, France, Georgia, Germany, Greece, Hungary, Iceland, Ireland, Israel, Italy, Kyrgyzstan, Latvia, Lithuania, Luxembourg, Netherlands, Norway, Poland, Portugal, Romania, Russian Federation, Slovakia, Slovenia, Spain, Sweden, Tajikistan, Turkey, United Kingdom.
- Eastern Mediterranean Region: Bahrain, Djibouti, Egypt, the Islamic Republic of Iran, Jordan, Lebanon, Morocco, Oman, Tunisia, Yemen.
- Western Pacific Region: Australia, China, Japan, Malaysia, Mongolia, New Zealand, Papua New Guinea, Philippines, Republic of Korea, Samoa, Tonga, Viet Nam.

*OECD health data series* supply GGHE and PvtHE entries for OECD's 30 Member countries. For GGHE, a larger number of reports on expenditure on health from non-OECD countries has been made available in the recent years. This has allowed a more complete estimation than in previous World Health Reports. The IMF *Government finance statistics* now reports central government expenditure on health for over 120 countries, as well as regional and local government outlays on health for a third of these countries. Government finance data, together with statistical yearbooks, public finance reports, reports from social security agencies, and status reports on the implementation of health policies, facilitate the estimation of GGHE for Member States which do not yet release this information.

Most data on private expenditure on health come from NHA reports, statistical yearbooks and other periodicals, statistical data on official web sites, reports of nongovernmental organizations, household expenditure surveys, academic studies, and relevant reports and data provided by central statistical offices, ministries of health, insurance agencies, professional and trade associations and planning councils. Standard extrapolation and estimation techniques are used to obtain the figures for missing years.

Information on external resources is taken from the Development Action Committee of the OECD (DAC/OECD). Where some Member States explicitly monitor the external resources entering their health system, that information has been used to validate or amend the order of magnitude derived from the DAC entries. DAC entries used by WHO relate to disbursements (which reports only bilateral flows from certain countries), wherever available, otherwise commitments are presented.

For macro variables, several international references facilitate the compilation of needed estimates, including the latest estimates from IMF *Government finance statistics yearbook (12)*, *International financial statistics yearbook (13)* and *International financial statistics (14)*; the Asian Development Bank *Key indicators (15)*; *OECD health data (16)*; *International development statistics (17)*; the United Nations *National accounts statistics: main aggregates and detailed tables (18)*; United Nations Statistics Division, the Economic Commission for Europe of the United Nations, and United Nations Economic and Social Commission for Western Asia; The World Bank's *World development indicators*, unpublished data from the IMF research department, the Caribbean Community Secretariat (CARICOM); and national series from ministries of finance or central banks.

The main sources of GDP are latest current year estimates from *OECD national accounts* and *OECD health data* for the OECD countries; for non OECD countries, the United Nations *National accounts statistics* and data from other United Nations agencies are used. When United Nations data are unavailable, other sources as mentioned above are used.

## Methodological notes

Variations in the boundaries used in the original sources have been adjusted as far as possible to allow standardized definition. For example, in some countries, GGHE and hence THE may include expenditure on environmental health, education of health personnel and health research activities, whereas other countries treat these expenses as a memorandum item. In the tables reported here, the principles outlined in the *Guide to producing national health accounts with special applications for low-income and middle-income countries (9)* have been followed, which consider these expenditures as health-related and hence have not been included in THE. Inability to exclude these has sometimes led to publication of overestimated ratios of THE to GDP. Availability of new information and subsequent adjustment have then produced lower figures than previously reported.

External resources in these Annex Tables are treated differently from the Rest of the World (ROW) resources under the OECD System of Health Accounts. Under OECD, ROW funds are classified under sources of financing (same as financing agents under

NHA categories) and include only grants passing through the countries. These tables also report expenditure on health by parastatal institutions as public, while others include it as private.

In some cases, expenditures reported under the government finance classification are limited to those of the ministry of health rather than all expenditures on health regardless of source. In such cases, wherever possible, other series have been estimated to supplement that source. GGHE and, therefore, the figures for THE, may sometimes be an underestimate in the cases when it has not been possible to obtain data for local government, nongovernmental organizations, other ministries and insurance expenditures.

The IMF *International financial statistics* provides central government disbursement (CGD) which approximates GGE in many developing countries without autonomous local taxing power. The CGD figures have been complemented whenever possible by data for local/municipal governments as well as some social security payments for health. Several public finance audits, executed budgets, budget plans, statistical yearbooks, web sites, World Bank and Regional Development Bank reports, and academic studies have been consulted to verify GGE.

The entries are not always a continuous time series for all countries, leading to a more thorough search for the relevant national publications to triangulate and complete the information. Also, previous time series have been updated when benchmarking revisions or changes in methodology to estimate particular items, especially out-of-pocket expenditures, for an extensive HA reconstruction are undertaken. Changes in ratios will occur when estimates of GDP are made using the current *System of national accounts* SNA93 instead of the 1968 version (SNA68).

Several quality checks have been used to assess the validity of the data. The data are triangulated with information from different sources and with the macro data available from the country to obtain the best estimates. For example, the aggregate government health expenditure data are compared with total GGE, or out-of-pocket expenditure is compared with total or household private consumption expenditure. Furthermore, estimated expenditure on health is compared against inpatient care expenditure, pharmaceutical expenditure data and other records (including programme administration) to ensure that the outlays for which details have been compiled constitute the bulk of the government and private expenditure on health. The estimates obtained are thus plausible in terms of a system's description.

## ANNEX TABLE 3

Annex Table 3 (Annex Table 6 in last year's report) presents total expenditure on health and general government expenditure on health in per capita terms. The methodology and sources to derive THE and GGHE are those discussed in the notes to Annex Table 2. Ratios are represented in per capita terms by dividing the expenditure figures by population figures. The per capita figures are expressed in US dollars at an average exchange rate (the observed annual average or year end number of units at which a currency is traded in the banking system). The per capita values in local currency units are also presented in international dollar estimates, derived by dividing these by an estimate of their purchasing power parity (PPP) compared with US dollars, i.e. a rate or measure that minimizes the consequences of differences in price levels existing between countries.

*OECD health data* is the major source for population estimates for the 30 OECD Member countries, just as it is for other health expenditure and macroeconomic variables. All estimates of population size and structure, other than for OECD countries, are based on demographic assessments prepared by the United Nations Population Division *(1)*. The estimates are of de facto population, and not the de jure population, in each Member State.

The exchange rates have mainly been obtained from the IMF *International financial statistics*. For remaining countries, United Nations, World Bank, and Asian Development Bank reports have been used. While official rates are mostly used, market exchange rates sometimes have also been used. Further, complete change in currency in a particular year have at times led to a revision of the full series.

For OECD Member countries, the OECD PPP has been used to calculate international dollars. For European and central Asian countries that are part of the UNECE but are not members of OECD, the UNECE PPPs are used. For non-European and non-OECD countries, international dollars have been estimated by WHO using methods similar to those used by the World Bank.

## ANNEX TABLE 4

Human resources for health are defined as "the stock of all individuals engaged in the promotion, protection or improvement of population health" *(19)*. However, for the purpose of the report, we focus only on paid activities, and divide the health workforce into two main groups: "health service providers" and "health management and support workers" (see Chapter 1).

The indicators needed to describe the characteristics of the health workforce and monitor its development over time are often generated from a multitude of sources and cover many areas (such as profession, training level and industry of employment). The data used in Annex Table 4 were compiled from four major sources: establishment surveys, household and labour force surveys, population and housing censuses and records from professional and administrative sources. The diversity of sources meant that harmonization had to be undertaken to arrive at comparable estimates of the health workforce for each Member State. The harmonization process was based on internationally standardized classification systems, mainly the International Standard Classification of Occupations (ISCO), but also the International Standard Classification of Education (ISCED) and the International Standard Industrial Classification of all Economic Activities (ISIC).

Some difficulties in harmonizing data based on a variety of definitions and classification systems could not be solved through the application of the ISCO. For example, in order to include country-specific types of workers, many ministries of health apply their own national classification system. Community health workers and traditional birth attendants are not captured through the standard ISCO system, but sometimes account for up to a third of the health workforce and form an important part of the infrastructure for service delivery. Therefore, for the purposes of this report, we have kept community health workers and traditional birth attendants as a separate group, whereas most of the country specific cadres were mapped with the common ISCO classification.

The following occupational categories are used in Annex Table 4:

■ Physicians – includes generalists and specialists.

■ Nurses – includes professional nurses (and midwives), auxiliary nurses and enrolled nurses, and other nurses such as dental nurses or primary care nurses.

■ Midwives – includes auxiliary midwives and enrolled midwives. Does not include traditional birth attendants, who are counted as community health workers. While much effort has been made, caution needs to be exercised in using the data for nurses and midwives; for some countries the available information does not clearly distinguish between the two groups.

- Dentists – includes dentists, dental assistants and dental technicians.
- Pharmacists – includes pharmacists, pharmaceutical assistants and pharmaceutical technicians.
- Lab workers – includes laboratory scientists, laboratory assistants, laboratory technicians and radiographers.
- Environment and public health professionals – includes environmental and public health officers, sanitarians, hygienists, environmental and public health technicians, district health officers, malaria technicians, meat inspectors, public health supervisors and similar professions.
- Community health workers – includes traditional medicine practitioners, faith healers, assistant/community health education workers, community health officers, family health workers, lady health visitors, health extension package workers, community midwives, and traditional birth attendants.
- Other health workers – includes a large number of occupations, such as clinical officers, dieticians and nutritionists, medical assistants, occupational therapists, operators of medical and dentistry equipment, optometrists and opticians, physiotherapists, podiatrists, prosthetic/orthetic engineers, psychologists, respiratory therapists, respiratory therapy technicians, speech pathologists, trainees and interns.
- Health management and support workers – includes general managers, statisticians, teaching professionals, lawyers, accountants, medical secretaries, gardeners, computer technicians, ambulance staff, cleaning staff, building and engineering staff, skilled administrative staff and general support staff.

Apart from questions concerning the harmonization of health workforce categories, an additional challenge was the triangulation of various data from different sources. Generally, when data were available from more than one source, we opted for the census as a first choice as it provides information on both "health service providers" and "health management and support workers". However, not many recent censuses with sufficiently detailed ISCO coding were both available and accessible. In the present data set, a total of 12 countries fall into this category: Australia, Bolivia, Brazil, Costa Rica, Honduras, Mexico, Mongolia, New Zealand, Panama, Paraguay, Thailand and Turkmenistan. For a further three, namely Estonia, the United Kingdom and the United States, the data presented in Annex Table 4 were from representative labour force or household surveys: collected in the Luxemburg Income (or Employment) Study (http://www.lisproject.org/). These surveys were as detailed as census data in terms of the occupation categories they provide and at the same time were based on ISCO classification system (in the case of Estonia) or we mapped them to corresponding ISCO codes (in the cases of the UK and US surveys).

For all countries in the African Region as well as for a large number of countries in South-East Asia and the Eastern Mediterranean Region, the data presented in Annex Table 4 were obtained through a special survey developed by WHO and executed through its regional and country offices. As much as possible, the survey attempted to obtain information on both "health service providers" and "health management and support workers" and used the ISCO system, while maintaining some country-specific classifications for selected types of occupations (23). The following is a list of countries in which the survey was implemented:

Algeria, Bahrain, Bangladesh, Benin, Bhutan, Botswana, Burkina Faso, Burundi, Cameroon, Cape Verde, Central African Republic, Chad, Comoros, Congo, Côte d'Ivoire, Democratic People's Republic of Korea, Democratic Republic of the Congo, Djibouti, Egypt, Equatorial Guinea, Eritrea, Ethiopia, Gabon, Gambia, Ghana, Guinea, Guinea-Bissau, India, Indonesia, Iraq, the Islamic Republic of Iran, Jordan, Kenya, Lebanon, Lesotho, Liberia, Madagascar, Malawi, Maldives, Mali, Mauritania, Mauritius, Morocco, Mozambique, Myanmar, Namibia, Nepal, Niger, Nigeria, Oman, Pakistan, Rwanda, Sao Tome and Principe, Saudi Arabia, Senegal, Seychelles, Sierra Leone, South Africa, Sri Lanka, Sudan, Swaziland, Timor-Leste, Togo, Tunisia, Uganda, United Republic of Tanzania, Yemen, Zambia, Zimbabwe.

For the following countries, data were obtained from miscellaneous sources, namely records of the departments of health, lists maintained by public service commissions or other administrative sources:

Argentina, Belize, Brunei, Cambodia, Chile, China, Colombia, Cook Islands, Cuba, Dominican Republic, Ecuador, El Salvador, Fiji, Finland, Jamaica, Malaysia, Nicaragua, Uruguay, Venezuela, Papua New Guinea, Philippines, Tonga, Tuvalu, Viet Nam.

For the remaining countries, the required data were compiled from the *OECD health data*, the *European health for all database* (http://data.euro.who.int/hfadb/index.php) or the previous version of WHO's *Global database on the health workforce*. These data were the least detailed of all, containing information on only four to five occupations and almost always containing no information on health management and support workers.

The countries for which data was obtained from these sources are the following:

Afghanistan, Albania, Andorra, Angola, Antigua and Barbuda, Armenia, Austria, Azerbaijan, Bahamas, Barbados, Belarus, Belgium, Bosnia and Herzegovina, Canada, Croatia, Cyprus, Czech Republic, Denmark, Dominica, France, Georgia, Germany, Greece, Grenada, Guatemala, Guyana, Haiti, Hungary, Iceland, Ireland, Israel, Italy, Japan, Kazakhstan, Kiribati, Kuwait, Kyrgyzstan, Lao People's Democratic Republic, Latvia, Libya, Lithuania, Luxembourg, Malta, Marshall Islands, Micronesia (Federated States of), Moldova, Monaco, Nauru, Netherlands, Niue, Norway, Palau, Peru, Poland, Portugal, Qatar, Republic of Korea, Romania, Russian Federation, Samoa, San Marino, Serbia and Montenegro, Slovak Republic, Slovenia, Solomon Islands, Somalia, Spain, Saint Kitts and Nevis, Saint Lucia, Saint Vincent and the Grenadines, Suriname, Sweden, Switzerland, Syrian Arab Republic, Tajikistan, The Former Yugoslav Republic of Macedonia, Trinidad and Tobago, Turkey, Ukraine, United Arab Emirates, Uzbekistan, Vanuatu.

The table provides the best figures that were available to WHO up to January 2006 for each of the 192 Member States. Any subsequent updates will be made available on the WHO *Global atlas for the health workforce* web site (www.who.int/globalatlas/autologin/hrh_login.asp).

# REFERENCES

1. United Nations Population Division. *World population prospects – the 2004 revision*. New York, NY, United Nations, 2005.
2. *WHO mortality database*. Geneva, World Health Organization, 2006.
3. Child Mortality Coordination Group. Tracking progress in the Millennium Development Goals: towards a consensus about child mortality levels and trend. *Bulletin of the World Health Organization*, 2006, 84:225–232.
4. Murray CJL, Ferguson BD, Lopez AD, Guillot M, Salomon JA, Ahmad O. Modified logit life table system: principles, empirical validation and application. *Population Studies*, 2003. 57:1–18.
5. Lopez AD, Ahmad O, Guillot M, Ferguson B, Salomon J, Murray CJL et al. *World mortality in 2000: life tables for 191 countries*. Geneva, World Health Organization, 2002.
6. Mathers CD, Ma Fat D, Inoue M, Rao C, Lopez AD. Counting the dead and what they died of: an assessment of the global status of cause-of-death data. *Bulletin of the World Health Organization*, 2005, 83:171–177.
7. Hill K, Pande R, Mahy M, Jones G. *Trends in child mortality in the developing world: 1990 to 1996*. New York, NY, United Nations Children's Fund, 1998.
8. Mathers CD, Bernard C, Iburg KM, Inoue M, Ma Fat D, Shibuya K. *Global burden of disease in 2002: data sources, methods and results*. Geneva, World Health Organization, 2003 (GPE Discussion Paper No. 54).
9. WHO/World Bank/United States Agency for International Development. *Guide to producing national health accounts with special applications for low-income and middle-income countries*. Geneva, World Health Organization, 2003 (http://whqlibdoc.who.int/publications/2003/9241546077.pdf, accessed 20 February 2006).
10. *A system of health accounts*. Paris, Organisation for Economic Co-operation and Development, 2000 (http://www.oecd.org/dataoecd/41/4/1841456.pdf, accessed 20 February 2006).
11. Organisation for Economic Co-operation and Development/International Monetary Fund/World Bank/United Nations/Eurostat. *System of national accounts 1993*. New York, NY, United Nations, 1994.
12. *Government finance statistics yearbook, 2004*. Washington, DC, International Monetary Fund, 2004.
13. *International financial statistics yearbook, 2005*. Washington, DC, International Monetary Fund, 2005.
14. *International Financial Statistics*, 2005, November.
15. *ADB Key indicators 2003*. Manila, Asian Development Bank, 2004.
16. *OECD health data 2004*. Paris, Organisation for Economic Co-operation and Development 2004.
17. *International development statistics 2004*. Organisation for Economic Co-operation and Development, Development Assistance Committee, 2004.
18. *National accounts statistics: main aggregates and detailed tables, 2001*. New York, NY, United Nations, 2004.
19. *The world health report 2000 – Health systems: improving performance*. Geneva, World Health Organization, 2000.
20. Diallo K, Zurn P, Gupta N, Dal Poz M. Monitoring and evaluation of human resources for health: an international perspective. *Human Resources for Health*, 2003, 1:3.
21. Gupta N, Zurn P, Diallo K, Dal Poz MR. Uses of population census data for monitoring geographical imbalance in the health workforce: snapshots from three developing countries. *International Journal for Equity in Health*, 2003, 2:11.
22. Hoffmann E, Dal Poz MR, Diallo K, Zurn P, Wiskow C. *Defining the scope of human resources in health, as basis for requesting national statistics*. Geneva, International Labour Organization, World Health Organization, 2003 (Unpublished technical note; available at: http://www.who.int/hrh/documents/en/).
23. Dal Poz MR, Kinfu Y, Dräger S, Kunjumen T, Diallo K. *Counting health workers: definitions, data, methods and global results*. Geneva, World Health Organization, 2006 (background paper for *The world health report 2006*; available at: http://www.who.int/hrh/documents/en/).

## Annex Table 1 Basic indicators for all Member States

Figures computed by WHO to ensure comparability;[a] they are not necessarily the official statistics of Member States, which may use alternative rigorous methods.

| | Member State | POPULATION ESTIMATES | | | | | | | | | LIFE EXPECTANCY AT BIRTH (YEARS) | | | PROBABILITY OF DYING (PER 1000) | | |
| | | Total population (000) | Annual growth rate (%) | Dependency ratio (per 100) | | Percentage of population aged 60+ years | | Total fertility rate | | Both sexes | | | Under age 5 years (under-5 mortality rate[b]) Both sexes | | |
| | | 2004 | 1994–2004 | 1994 | 2004 | 1994 | 2004 | 1994 | 2004 | 2004 | Uncertainty | | 2004 | Uncertainty | |
|---|---|---|---|---|---|---|---|---|---|---|---|---|---|---|---|---|
| 1 | Afghanistan | 28 574 | 3.9 | 96 | 97 | 4.6 | 4.4 | 8.0 | 7.4 | 42 | 30 – | 53 | 257 | 179 – | 333 |
| 2 | Albania | 3 112 | −0.2 | 61 | 56 | 8.9 | 11.8 | 2.7 | 2.2 | 72 | 71 – | 72 | 19 | 15 – | 22 |
| 3 | Algeria | 32 358 | 1.6 | 79 | 54 | 5.7 | 6.4 | 3.7 | 2.5 | 71 | 69 – | 72 | 40 | 33 – | 47 |
| 4 | Andorra | 67 | 0.7 | 46 | 44 | 20.5 | 21.3 | 1.3 | 1.3 | 80 | 78 – | 83 | 7 | 4 – | 9 |
| 5 | Angola | 15 490 | 2.6 | 100 | 96 | 4.1 | 4.0 | 7.0 | 6.7 | 40 | 33 – | 46 | 260 | 230 – | 288 |
| 6 | Antigua and Barbuda | 81 | 1.7 | 62 | 55 | 9.1 | 10.5 | 2.5 | 2.3 | 72 | 71 – | 74 | 12 | 6 – | 18 |
| 7 | Argentina | 38 372 | 1.1 | 63 | 58 | 13.1 | 13.8 | 2.8 | 2.3 | 75 | 74 – | 75 | 18 | 17 – | 20 |
| 8 | Armenia | 3 026 | −0.8 | 60 | 51 | 12.0 | 14.7 | 2.2 | 1.3 | 68 | 67 – | 69 | 32 | 26 – | 39 |
| 9 | Australia | 19 942 | 1.2 | 50 | 48 | 15.4 | 17.0 | 1.8 | 1.7 | 81 | 81 – | 81 | 5 | 5 – | 6 |
| 10 | Austria | 8 171 | 0.2 | 49 | 47 | 19.7 | 22.3 | 1.4 | 1.4 | 79 | 79 – | 80 | 5 | 4 – | 6 |
| 11 | Azerbaijan | 8 355 | 0.8 | 64 | 51 | 7.9 | 9.3 | 2.7 | 1.8 | 65 | 64 – | 67 | 90 | 73 – | 106 |
| 12 | Bahamas | 319 | 1.5 | 57 | 53 | 7.0 | 9.1 | 2.5 | 2.3 | 73 | 72 – | 74 | 13 | 10 – | 16 |
| 13 | Bahrain | 716 | 2.4 | 50 | 44 | 3.9 | 4.3 | 3.2 | 2.4 | 74 | 72 – | 75 | 11 | 10 – | 12 |
| 14 | Bangladesh | 139 215 | 2.0 | 76 | 65 | 5.1 | 5.6 | 3.9 | 3.2 | 62 | 61 – | 64 | 77 | 70 – | 84 |
| 15 | Barbados | 269 | 0.3 | 53 | 42 | 14.3 | 13.1 | 1.6 | 1.5 | 75 | 74 – | 76 | 12 | 9 – | 16 |
| 16 | Belarus | 9 811 | −0.5 | 53 | 44 | 17.8 | 18.8 | 1.5 | 1.2 | 68 | 68 – | 69 | 10 | 9 – | 11 |
| 17 | Belgium | 10 400 | 0.3 | 51 | 52 | 21.2 | 22.2 | 1.6 | 1.7 | 78 | 78 – | 79 | 5 | 4 – | 5 |
| 18 | Belize | 264 | 2.4 | 88 | 71 | 5.9 | 5.9 | 4.2 | 3.1 | 68 | 67 – | 70 | 39 | 29 – | 48 |
| 19 | Benin | 8 177 | 3.2 | 98 | 89 | 4.3 | 4.3 | 6.5 | 5.7 | 53 | 46 – | 58 | 152 | 137 – | 167 |
| 20 | Bhutan | 2 116 | 2.2 | 89 | 77 | 6.3 | 6.9 | 5.4 | 4.2 | 63 | 56 – | 69 | 80 | 64 – | 96 |
| 21 | Bolivia | 9 009 | 2.1 | 81 | 75 | 6.2 | 6.7 | 4.7 | 3.8 | 65 | 58 – | 71 | 69 | 62 – | 75 |
| 22 | Bosnia and Herzegovina | 3 909 | 1.0 | 43 | 44 | 11.8 | 18.9 | 1.5 | 1.3 | 73 | 72 – | 75 | 15 | 12 – | 19 |
| 23 | Botswana | 1 769 | 1.1 | 82 | 70 | 3.9 | 5.0 | 3.9 | 3.1 | 40 | 36 – | 44 | 116 | 99 – | 133 |
| 24 | Brazil | 183 913 | 1.5 | 61 | 52 | 7.1 | 8.7 | 2.5 | 2.3 | 70 | 70 – | 71 | 34 | 29 – | 39 |
| 25 | Brunei Darussalam | 366 | 2.4 | 56 | 49 | 4.2 | 4.6 | 3.0 | 2.4 | 77 | 76 – | 78 | 9 | 7 – | 10 |
| 26 | Bulgaria | 7 780 | −0.7 | 50 | 45 | 21.0 | 22.3 | 1.4 | 1.2 | 72 | 72 – | 73 | 15 | 14 – | 16 |
| 27 | Burkina Faso | 12 822 | 3.0 | 104 | 101 | 4.9 | 4.3 | 7.1 | 6.6 | 48 | 41 – | 53 | 192 | 173 – | 211 |
| 28 | Burundi | 7 282 | 1.8 | 100 | 93 | 4.5 | 4.2 | 6.8 | 6.8 | 45 | 38 – | 51 | 190 | 150 – | 230 |
| 29 | Cambodia | 13 798 | 2.2 | 98 | 70 | 4.7 | 5.5 | 5.1 | 4.0 | 54 | 47 – | 60 | 141 | 127 – | 155 |
| 30 | Cameroon | 16 038 | 2.1 | 93 | 83 | 5.5 | 5.6 | 5.5 | 4.5 | 50 | 44 – | 56 | 149 | 137 – | 162 |
| 31 | Canada | 31 958 | 1.0 | 48 | 45 | 16.0 | 17.5 | 1.7 | 1.5 | 80 | 80 – | 80 | 6 | 5 – | 6 |
| 32 | Cape Verde | 495 | 2.4 | 105 | 80 | 6.4 | 5.7 | 4.7 | 3.6 | 70 | 65 – | 73 | 36 | 29 – | 44 |
| 33 | Central African Republic | 3 986 | 1.8 | 89 | 89 | 6.1 | 6.1 | 5.5 | 4.9 | 41 | 35 – | 47 | 193 | 162 – | 224 |
| 34 | Chad | 9 448 | 3.3 | 98 | 101 | 5.1 | 4.7 | 6.7 | 6.7 | 46 | 39 – | 52 | 200 | 168 – | 231 |
| 35 | Chile | 16 124 | 1.3 | 57 | 50 | 9.4 | 11.3 | 2.5 | 2.0 | 77 | 77 – | 77 | 9 | 8 – | 10 |
| 36 | China | 1 315 409 | 0.8 | 48 | 42 | 9.2 | 10.8 | 1.9 | 1.7 | 72 | 71 – | 73 | 31 | 29 – | 33 |
| 37 | Colombia | 44 915 | 1.7 | 64 | 57 | 6.5 | 7.4 | 2.9 | 2.6 | 73 | 72 – | 73 | 21 | 19 – | 22 |
| 38 | Comoros | 777 | 2.8 | 93 | 81 | 4.0 | 4.3 | 5.7 | 4.7 | 64 | 57 – | 71 | 70 | 56 – | 85 |
| 39 | Congo | 3 883 | 3.2 | 97 | 100 | 4.8 | 4.5 | 6.3 | 6.3 | 54 | 48 – | 61 | 108 | 81 – | 134 |
| 40 | Cook Islands | 18 | −0.9 | 71 | 65 | 6.4 | 7.5 | 3.1 | 2.6 | 72 | 71 – | 73 | 21 | 19 – | 22 |
| 41 | Costa Rica | 4 253 | 2.3 | 66 | 53 | 7.2 | 8.1 | 2.8 | 2.2 | 77 | 77 – | 78 | 13 | 12 – | 14 |
| 42 | Côte d'Ivoire | 17 872 | 2.2 | 94 | 83 | 4.5 | 5.2 | 6.1 | 4.9 | 44 | 37 – | 50 | 194 | 155 – | 235 |
| 43 | Croatia | 4 540 | −0.3 | 47 | 49 | 19.2 | 21.9 | 1.5 | 1.3 | 75 | 75 – | 76 | 7 | 6 – | 8 |
| 44 | Cuba | 11 245 | 0.4 | 45 | 43 | 12.0 | 14.9 | 1.6 | 1.6 | 78 | 77 – | 78 | 7 | 6 – | 8 |
| 45 | Cyprus | 826 | 1.4 | 57 | 48 | 14.7 | 16.5 | 2.2 | 1.6 | 79 | 78 – | 80 | 5 | 4 – | 6 |

| | | LIFE EXPECTANCY AT BIRTH (YEARS) | | | | PROBABILITY OF DYING (PER 1000) | | | | | | | | | | | |
| --- | --- | --- | --- | --- | --- | --- | --- | --- | --- | --- | --- | --- | --- | --- | --- | --- | --- |
| | | | | | | Under age 5 years (under-5 mortality rate[b]) | | | | | | Between ages 15 and 60 years (adult mortality rate) | | | | | |
| | | Males | | Females | | Males | | Females | | Males | | Females | | Males | | Females | |
| | | 2004 | Uncertainty | 2004 | Uncertainty | 2004 | Uncertainty | 2004 | Uncertainty | 2004 | Uncertainty | 2004 | Uncertainty | | | | |
| | 1 | 42 | 31 – 52 | 42 | 29 – 55 | 258 | 183 – 338 | 256 | 176 – 328 | 509 | 311 – 760 | 448 | 212 – 716 | | | | |
| | 2 | 69 | 68 – 69 | 74 | 73 – 75 | 19 | 15 – 22 | 18 | 15 – 22 | 171 | 158 – 185 | 96 | 82 – 111 | | | | |
| | 3 | 69 | 68 – 71 | 72 | 70 – 73 | 41 | 33 – 48 | 39 | 32 – 46 | 153 | 138 – 167 | 124 | 109 – 140 | | | | |
| | 4 | 77 | 74 – 80 | 83 | 81 – 85 | 7 | 4 – 10 | 6 | 4 – 9 | 108 | 73 – 143 | 46 | 34 – 67 | | | | |
| | 5 | 38 | 32 – 44 | 42 | 34 – 49 | 276 | 246 – 305 | 243 | 215 – 270 | 591 | 458 – 754 | 504 | 324 – 697 | | | | |
| | 6 | 70 | 69 – 71 | 75 | 74 – 76 | 14 | 6 – 20 | 10 | 6 – 16 | 191 | 168 – 212 | 120 | 107 – 134 | | | | |
| | 7 | 71 | 71 – 71 | 78 | 78 – 79 | 20 | 19 – 22 | 16 | 15 – 18 | 173 | 168 – 179 | 90 | 87 – 94 | | | | |
| | 8 | 65 | 64 – 66 | 72 | 71 – 73 | 34 | 27 – 41 | 30 | 25 – 36 | 248 | 215 – 286 | 111 | 94 – 130 | | | | |
| | 9 | 78 | 78 – 79 | 83 | 83 – 83 | 6 | 5 – 7 | 5 | 4 – 5 | 86 | 83 – 88 | 50 | 48 – 52 | | | | |
| | 10 | 76 | 76 – 77 | 82 | 82 – 82 | 5 | 5 – 6 | 5 | 4 – 6 | 114 | 111 – 117 | 55 | 53 – 57 | | | | |
| | 11 | 63 | 62 – 64 | 68 | 67 – 69 | 94 | 75 – 112 | 85 | 70 – 99 | 205 | 178 – 233 | 113 | 97 – 134 | | | | |
| | 12 | 70 | 69 – 71 | 76 | 75 – 77 | 14 | 11 – 17 | 12 | 9 – 14 | 256 | 238 – 274 | 145 | 135 – 155 | | | | |
| | 13 | 73 | 71 – 74 | 75 | 73 – 76 | 11 | 10 – 12 | 11 | 10 – 12 | 112 | 98 – 127 | 82 | 67 – 97 | | | | |
| | 14 | 62 | 60 – 63 | 63 | 61 – 64 | 81 | 74 – 89 | 73 | 66 – 79 | 251 | 223 – 282 | 258 | 233 – 283 | | | | |
| | 15 | 71 | 70 – 72 | 78 | 78 – 79 | 12 | 9 – 15 | 13 | 9 – 16 | 191 | 173 – 211 | 105 | 94 – 116 | | | | |
| | 16 | 63 | 62 – 63 | 74 | 74 – 75 | 11 | 10 – 12 | 9 | 7 – 10 | 377 | 358 – 396 | 135 | 124 – 147 | | | | |
| | 17 | 75 | 75 – 76 | 81 | 81 – 82 | 5 | 5 – 6 | 4 | 4 – 5 | 122 | 119 – 125 | 65 | 63 – 67 | | | | |
| | 18 | 65 | 63 – 68 | 72 | 71 – 73 | 44 | 34 – 56 | 33 | 25 – 40 | 243 | 204 – 290 | 135 | 122 – 151 | | | | |
| | 19 | 52 | 46 – 58 | 53 | 46 – 59 | 152 | 137 – 166 | 153 | 137 – 167 | 388 | 252 – 551 | 350 | 224 – 528 | | | | |
| | 20 | 62 | 56 – 68 | 65 | 57 – 71 | 80 | 63 – 95 | 80 | 64 – 96 | 255 | 114 – 418 | 196 | 92 – 365 | | | | |
| | 21 | 63 | 56 – 70 | 66 | 59 – 72 | 70 | 63 – 76 | 68 | 62 – 74 | 248 | 106 – 426 | 184 | 87 – 346 | | | | |
| | 22 | 70 | 68 – 71 | 77 | 76 – 78 | 17 | 13 – 21 | 14 | 10 – 17 | 188 | 160 – 216 | 88 | 76 – 101 | | | | |
| | 23 | 40 | 37 – 43 | 40 | 36 – 44 | 123 | 106 – 141 | 109 | 92 – 125 | 786 | 717 – 839 | 770 | 698 – 826 | | | | |
| | 24 | 67 | 67 – 67 | 74 | 73 – 74 | 38 | 32 – 43 | 31 | 26 – 35 | 237 | 228 – 246 | 127 | 118 – 135 | | | | |
| | 25 | 76 | 74 – 77 | 78 | 78 – 79 | 10 | 8 – 11 | 8 | 6 – 9 | 107 | 89 – 125 | 81 | 70 – 93 | | | | |
| | 26 | 69 | 69 – 69 | 76 | 76 – 76 | 17 | 15 – 18 | 13 | 12 – 14 | 217 | 213 – 220 | 92 | 90 – 95 | | | | |
| | 27 | 47 | 41 – 52 | 48 | 40 – 55 | 193 | 175 – 213 | 191 | 171 – 209 | 472 | 351 – 631 | 410 | 256 – 600 | | | | |
| | 28 | 42 | 36 – 49 | 47 | 39 – 54 | 196 | 154 – 237 | 184 | 146 – 223 | 593 | 450 – 737 | 457 | 317 – 616 | | | | |
| | 29 | 51 | 45 – 56 | 58 | 50 – 64 | 154 | 138 – 169 | 127 | 115 – 140 | 430 | 293 – 580 | 276 | 154 – 466 | | | | |
| | 30 | 50 | 45 – 55 | 51 | 44 – 57 | 156 | 143 – 170 | 143 | 130 – 155 | 444 | 316 – 582 | 432 | 305 – 586 | | | | |
| | 31 | 78 | 78 – 78 | 83 | 82 – 83 | 6 | 6 – 6 | 5 | 5 – 6 | 91 | 89 – 93 | 57 | 55 – 58 | | | | |
| | 32 | 67 | 62 – 71 | 71 | 68 – 75 | 38 | 30 – 45 | 35 | 28 – 42 | 209 | 127 – 322 | 139 | 85 – 212 | | | | |
| | 33 | 40 | 35 – 46 | 41 | 35 – 48 | 201 | 169 – 233 | 185 | 155 – 214 | 667 | 530 – 781 | 624 | 490 – 745 | | | | |
| | 34 | 45 | 38 – 51 | 48 | 40 – 54 | 212 | 177 – 245 | 188 | 158 – 217 | 497 | 370 – 669 | 422 | 286 – 601 | | | | |
| | 35 | 74 | 73 – 74 | 81 | 80 – 81 | 10 | 9 – 11 | 9 | 8 – 9 | 133 | 125 – 144 | 66 | 63 – 69 | | | | |
| | 36 | 70 | 70 – 71 | 74 | 73 – 74 | 27 | 25 – 29 | 36 | 33 – 39 | 158 | 148 – 167 | 99 | 90 – 108 | | | | |
| | 37 | 68 | 68 – 69 | 77 | 77 – 78 | 24 | 21 – 26 | 17 | 16 – 19 | 226 | 216 – 237 | 93 | 86 – 100 | | | | |
| | 38 | 62 | 55 – 69 | 67 | 59 – 73 | 76 | 61 – 92 | 64 | 51 – 77 | 254 | 109 – 433 | 182 | 87 – 352 | | | | |
| | 39 | 53 | 47 – 60 | 55 | 48 – 62 | 113 | 85 – 140 | 103 | 78 – 127 | 442 | 297 – 586 | 390 | 259 – 524 | | | | |
| | 40 | 70 | 69 – 71 | 75 | 74 – 75 | 24 | 23 – 25 | 17 | 16 – 18 | 158 | 141 – 178 | 104 | 95 – 114 | | | | |
| | 41 | 75 | 75 – 76 | 80 | 79 – 80 | 14 | 13 – 15 | 11 | 10 – 13 | 124 | 119 – 128 | 71 | 68 – 75 | | | | |
| | 42 | 41 | 35 – 47 | 47 | 41 – 53 | 225 | 181 – 271 | 162 | 128 – 196 | 585 | 462 – 733 | 500 | 376 – 634 | | | | |
| | 43 | 72 | 72 – 72 | 79 | 79 – 79 | 8 | 7 – 9 | 7 | 5 – 8 | 160 | 156 – 164 | 66 | 63 – 69 | | | | |
| | 44 | 75 | 75 – 76 | 80 | 79 – 80 | 8 | 7 – 9 | 7 | 6 – 8 | 131 | 123 – 139 | 85 | 81 – 89 | | | | |
| | 45 | 77 | 76 – 78 | 82 | 80 – 83 | 5 | 4 – 6 | 5 | 4 – 7 | 94 | 84 – 104 | 47 | 38 – 56 | | | | |

## Annex Table 1 Basic indicators for all Member States

Figures computed by WHO to ensure comparability;[a] they are not necessarily the official statistics of Member States, which may use alternative rigorous methods.

| Member State | POPULATION ESTIMATES | | | | | | | | | LIFE EXPECTANCY AT BIRTH (YEARS) | | | PROBABILITY OF DYING (PER 1000) Under age 5 years (under-5 mortality rate[b]) | | |
|---|---|---|---|---|---|---|---|---|---|---|---|---|---|---|---|
| | Total population (000) | Annual growth rate (%) | Dependency ratio (per 100) | | Percentage of population aged 60+ years | | Total fertility rate | | Both sexes | | | Both sexes | | |
| | 2004 | 1994–2004 | 1994 | 2004 | 1994 | 2004 | 1994 | 2004 | 2004 | Uncertainty | | 2004 | Uncertainty | |
| 46 Czech Republic | 10 229 | −0.1 | 48 | 41 | 18.0 | 19.6 | 1.5 | 1.2 | 76 | 76 – 76 | | 5 | 4 – 5 | |
| 47 Democratic People's Republic of Korea | 22 384 | 0.8 | 47 | 47 | 7.9 | 10.9 | 2.2 | 2.0 | 66 | 58 – 74 | | 55 | 30 – 81 | |
| 48 Democratic Republic of the Congo | 55 853 | 2.5 | 99 | 100 | 4.4 | 4.3 | 6.7 | 6.7 | 44 | 38 – 51 | | 205 | 176 – 235 | |
| 49 Denmark | 5 414 | 0.4 | 48 | 51 | 20.0 | 20.7 | 1.8 | 1.8 | 78 | 77 – 78 | | 5 | 4 – 6 | |
| 50 Djibouti | 779 | 2.7 | 86 | 81 | 4.1 | 4.6 | 6.0 | 4.9 | 56 | 49 – 62 | | 126 | 106 – 144 | |
| 51 Dominica | 79 | 0.5 | 62 | 55 | 9.1 | 10.5 | 2.2 | 2.0 | 74 | 73 – 75 | | 14 | 11 – 17 | |
| 52 Dominican Republic | 8 768 | 1.5 | 70 | 59 | 5.2 | 6.1 | 3.1 | 2.7 | 67 | 66 – 68 | | 32 | 29 – 35 | |
| 53 Ecuador | 13 040 | 1.5 | 70 | 63 | 6.5 | 8.1 | 3.3 | 2.7 | 72 | 72 – 73 | | 26 | 22 – 30 | |
| 54 Egypt | 72 642 | 1.9 | 77 | 63 | 6.4 | 7.1 | 3.8 | 3.2 | 68 | 67 – 68 | | 36 | 33 – 40 | |
| 55 El Salvador | 6 762 | 2.0 | 74 | 66 | 6.8 | 7.5 | 3.4 | 2.8 | 71 | 70 – 72 | | 28 | 24 – 32 | |
| 56 Equatorial Guinea | 492 | 2.4 | 89 | 93 | 6.3 | 6.0 | 5.9 | 5.9 | 43 | 37 – 50 | | 204 | 177 – 232 | |
| 57 Eritrea | 4 232 | 3.3 | 93 | 89 | 4.0 | 3.9 | 6.1 | 5.4 | 60 | 53 – 67 | | 82 | 74 – 91 | |
| 58 Estonia | 1 335 | −1.0 | 52 | 47 | 18.9 | 21.5 | 1.5 | 1.4 | 72 | 71 – 73 | | 8 | 6 – 11 | |
| 59 Ethiopia | 75 600 | 2.6 | 95 | 91 | 4.4 | 4.6 | 6.6 | 5.7 | 50 | 43 – 56 | | 166 | 137 – 196 | |
| 60 Fiji | 841 | 1.0 | 65 | 56 | 5.0 | 6.2 | 3.3 | 2.9 | 69 | 67 – 70 | | 20 | 18 – 22 | |
| 61 Finland | 5 235 | 0.3 | 50 | 50 | 18.8 | 20.9 | 1.8 | 1.7 | 79 | 79 – 79 | | 4 | 4 – 5 | |
| 62 France | 60 257 | 0.4 | 53 | 53 | 20.3 | 20.9 | 1.7 | 1.9 | 80 | 79 – 80 | | 5 | 4 – 5 | |
| 63 Gabon | 1 362 | 2.3 | 92 | 81 | 7.2 | 6.2 | 5.0 | 3.9 | 57 | 51 – 64 | | 91 | 81 – 102 | |
| 64 Gambia | 1 478 | 3.2 | 84 | 79 | 5.2 | 5.9 | 5.5 | 4.6 | 57 | 50 – 63 | | 122 | 105 – 140 | |
| 65 Georgia | 4 518 | −1.3 | 53 | 50 | 15.9 | 18.0 | 1.8 | 1.4 | 74 | 71 – 75 | | 45 | 40 – 49 | |
| 66 Germany | 82 645 | 0.2 | 46 | 49 | 20.6 | 24.8 | 1.3 | 1.3 | 79 | 79 – 79 | | 5 | 5 – 5 | |
| 67 Ghana | 21 664 | 2.3 | 89 | 76 | 5.0 | 5.6 | 5.3 | 4.2 | 57 | 50 – 63 | | 112 | 97 – 128 | |
| 68 Greece | 11 098 | 0.5 | 47 | 48 | 21.1 | 22.9 | 1.3 | 1.2 | 79 | 79 – 79 | | 5 | 4 – 6 | |
| 69 Grenada | 102 | 0.3 | 62 | 55 | 9.1 | 10.5 | 2.6 | 2.4 | 68 | 67 – 69 | | 21 | 16 – 27 | |
| 70 Guatemala | 12 295 | 2.3 | 95 | 91 | 5.6 | 6.1 | 5.3 | 4.5 | 68 | 67 – 69 | | 45 | 40 – 50 | |
| 71 Guinea | 9 202 | 2.4 | 89 | 90 | 5.4 | 5.6 | 6.4 | 5.8 | 53 | 47 – 59 | | 155 | 140 – 170 | |
| 72 Guinea–Bissau | 1 540 | 2.9 | 96 | 102 | 5.3 | 4.8 | 7.1 | 7.1 | 47 | 40 – 53 | | 203 | 183 – 223 | |
| 73 Guyana | 750 | 0.3 | 64 | 53 | 6.9 | 7.3 | 2.5 | 2.2 | 63 | 59 – 67 | | 64 | 35 – 94 | |
| 74 Haiti | 8 407 | 1.4 | 90 | 72 | 5.8 | 6.0 | 4.6 | 3.9 | 55 | 48 – 61 | | 117 | 100 – 134 | |
| 75 Honduras | 7 048 | 2.6 | 89 | 77 | 4.7 | 5.5 | 4.7 | 3.6 | 67 | 64 – 71 | | 41 | 37 – 45 | |
| 76 Hungary | 10 124 | −0.2 | 48 | 45 | 19.3 | 20.5 | 1.6 | 1.3 | 73 | 72 – 73 | | 8 | 7 – 9 | |
| 77 Iceland | 292 | 1.0 | 55 | 51 | 15.0 | 15.6 | 2.2 | 2.0 | 81 | 80 – 81 | | 3 | 3 – 3 | |
| 78 India | 1 087 124 | 1.7 | 68 | 60 | 7.0 | 7.8 | 3.7 | 3.0 | 62 | 62 – 63 | | 85 | 77 – 94 | |
| 79 Indonesia | 220 077 | 1.3 | 61 | 52 | 6.8 | 8.2 | 2.8 | 2.3 | 67 | 66 – 68 | | 38 | 35 – 42 | |
| 80 Iran, Islamic Republic of | 68 803 | 1.2 | 90 | 52 | 6.1 | 6.4 | 3.7 | 2.1 | 70 | 69 – 71 | | 38 | 30 – 46 | |
| 81 Iraq | 28 057 | 3.0 | 88 | 79 | 4.6 | 4.5 | 5.6 | 4.7 | 55 | 50 – 61 | | 125 | 75 – 177 | |
| 82 Ireland | 4 080 | 1.3 | 57 | 45 | 15.2 | 15.0 | 1.9 | 1.9 | 78 | 77 – 79 | | 6 | 5 – 7 | |
| 83 Israel | 6 601 | 2.4 | 65 | 61 | 13.0 | 13.1 | 2.9 | 2.8 | 80 | 80 – 80 | | 6 | 5 – 6 | |
| 84 Italy | 58 033 | 0.1 | 46 | 51 | 22.1 | 25.3 | 1.2 | 1.3 | 81 | 80 – 81 | | 5 | 4 – 5 | |
| 85 Jamaica | 2 639 | 0.7 | 71 | 65 | 9.7 | 10.1 | 2.8 | 2.4 | 72 | 71 – 74 | | 20 | 16 – 24 | |
| 86 Japan | 127 923 | 0.2 | 44 | 50 | 19.9 | 25.6 | 1.5 | 1.3 | 82 | 82 – 82 | | 4 | 4 – 4 | |
| 87 Jordan | 5 561 | 3.1 | 80 | 69 | 4.2 | 5.0 | 4.9 | 3.4 | 71 | 70 – 72 | | 27 | 23 – 30 | |
| 88 Kazakhstan | 14 839 | −0.8 | 58 | 47 | 9.6 | 11.4 | 2.3 | 1.9 | 61 | 60 – 62 | | 73 | 55 – 92 | |
| 89 Kenya | 33 467 | 2.4 | 98 | 84 | 4.2 | 4.1 | 5.2 | 5.0 | 51 | 45 – 56 | | 120 | 109 – 131 | |
| 90 Kiribati | 97 | 2.2 | 69 | 60 | 5.8 | 6.5 | 4.6 | 4.1 | 65 | 64 – 66 | | 65 | 55 – 75 | |

| | LIFE EXPECTANCY AT BIRTH (YEARS) | | | | PROBABILITY OF DYING (PER 1000) | | | | | | | |
| | | | | | Under age 5 years (under-5 mortality rate[b]) | | | | Between ages 15 and 60 years (adult mortality rate) | | | |
| | Males | | Females | | Males | | Females | | Males | | Females | |
| | 2004 | Uncertainty | 2004 | Uncertainty | 2004 | Uncertainty | 2004 | Uncertainty | 2004 | Uncertainty | 2004 | Uncertainty |
|---|---|---|---|---|---|---|---|---|---|---|---|---|
| 46 | 73 | 72 – 73 | 79 | 79 – 79 | 5 | 4 – 6 | 4 | 4 – 5 | 161 | 158 – 163 | 69 | 67 – 71 |
| 47 | 65 | 57 – 72 | 68 | 59 – 75 | 56 | 31 – 82 | 54 | 29 – 81 | 231 | 87 – 402 | 168 | 68 – 341 |
| 48 | 42 | 36 – 47 | 47 | 39 – 54 | 217 | 186 – 249 | 192 | 165 – 221 | 576 | 436 – 713 | 446 | 286 – 607 |
| 49 | 75 | 75 – 76 | 80 | 80 – 80 | 5 | 5 – 7 | 5 | 4 – 6 | 117 | 110 – 125 | 72 | 68 – 75 |
| 50 | 54 | 48 – 60 | 57 | 50 – 63 | 131 | 111 – 150 | 120 | 101 – 137 | 373 | 237 – 521 | 312 | 193 – 468 |
| 51 | 72 | 71 – 73 | 76 | 75 – 77 | 13 | 11 – 14 | 15 | 11 – 20 | 204 | 187 – 221 | 122 | 103 – 143 |
| 52 | 64 | 63 – 65 | 70 | 69 – 71 | 34 | 31 – 38 | 30 | 27 – 33 | 280 | 246 – 312 | 169 | 144 – 194 |
| 53 | 70 | 69 – 70 | 75 | 75 – 76 | 29 | 24 – 33 | 24 | 20 – 28 | 210 | 197 – 223 | 128 | 119 – 137 |
| 54 | 66 | 65 – 66 | 70 | 69 – 70 | 36 | 32 – 40 | 36 | 33 – 40 | 239 | 229 – 250 | 158 | 150 – 165 |
| 55 | 68 | 67 – 69 | 74 | 73 – 75 | 30 | 25 – 34 | 26 | 22 – 30 | 244 | 211 – 278 | 138 | 127 – 152 |
| 56 | 42 | 37 – 49 | 44 | 38 – 52 | 213 | 183 – 244 | 195 | 169 – 219 | 577 | 436 – 707 | 522 | 368 – 665 |
| 57 | 58 | 52 – 65 | 62 | 55 – 68 | 89 | 79 – 98 | 75 | 67 – 83 | 345 | 196 – 498 | 281 | 170 – 427 |
| 58 | 66 | 66 – 67 | 78 | 77 – 78 | 10 | 8 – 11 | 6 | 4 – 9 | 301 | 277 – 328 | 108 | 97 – 119 |
| 59 | 49 | 42 – 55 | 51 | 44 – 58 | 175 | 141 – 209 | 158 | 131 – 183 | 451 | 315 – 620 | 389 | 260 – 559 |
| 60 | 66 | 65 – 67 | 71 | 70 – 73 | 21 | 19 – 23 | 19 | 17 – 21 | 270 | 244 – 297 | 169 | 151 – 187 |
| 61 | 75 | 75 – 75 | 82 | 82 – 82 | 5 | 4 – 6 | 3 | 3 – 4 | 137 | 134 – 141 | 62 | 60 – 65 |
| 62 | 76 | 76 – 76 | 83 | 83 – 84 | 5 | 4 – 6 | 4 | 4 – 5 | 132 | 127 – 138 | 60 | 58 – 62 |
| 63 | 55 | 49 – 61 | 59 | 53 – 66 | 102 | 91 – 114 | 80 | 70 – 90 | 411 | 270 – 557 | 344 | 218 – 482 |
| 64 | 55 | 49 – 61 | 59 | 52 – 65 | 129 | 111 – 148 | 115 | 99 – 132 | 344 | 199 – 499 | 263 | 152 – 437 |
| 65 | 70 | 68 – 72 | 77 | 75 – 79 | 51 | 46 – 56 | 38 | 34 – 42 | 161 | 127 – 196 | 60 | 48 – 83 |
| 66 | 76 | 76 – 76 | 82 | 82 – 82 | 5 | 5 – 6 | 5 | 4 – 5 | 112 | 111 – 113 | 58 | 57 – 58 |
| 67 | 56 | 50 – 62 | 58 | 51 – 63 | 113 | 98 – 131 | 111 | 95 – 125 | 349 | 208 – 509 | 319 | 209 – 477 |
| 68 | 77 | 76 – 77 | 82 | 81 – 82 | 6 | 5 – 7 | 4 | 4 – 5 | 110 | 106 – 115 | 46 | 44 – 48 |
| 69 | 66 | 65 – 67 | 69 | 68 – 70 | 24 | 18 – 30 | 19 | 14 – 24 | 256 | 234 – 277 | 218 | 200 – 237 |
| 70 | 65 | 64 – 66 | 71 | 70 – 72 | 45 | 40 – 49 | 45 | 40 – 51 | 276 | 238 – 316 | 152 | 124 – 179 |
| 71 | 52 | 47 – 58 | 55 | 47 – 61 | 160 | 144 – 175 | 150 | 135 – 165 | 364 | 228 – 523 | 319 | 188 – 494 |
| 72 | 45 | 39 – 51 | 48 | 40 – 55 | 212 | 191 – 234 | 194 | 175 – 213 | 482 | 351 – 641 | 413 | 264 – 587 |
| 73 | 62 | 59 – 66 | 64 | 60 – 68 | 64 | 36 – 93 | 64 | 34 – 96 | 291 | 242 – 354 | 258 | 202 – 328 |
| 74 | 53 | 47 – 60 | 56 | 49 – 62 | 122 | 104 – 139 | 112 | 96 – 128 | 417 | 269 – 563 | 358 | 242 – 499 |
| 75 | 65 | 61 – 69 | 70 | 67 – 73 | 42 | 37 – 46 | 40 | 36 – 43 | 258 | 180 – 352 | 159 | 103 – 229 |
| 76 | 69 | 68 – 69 | 77 | 77 – 77 | 9 | 8 – 10 | 7 | 7 – 8 | 249 | 239 – 260 | 108 | 103 – 114 |
| 77 | 79 | 78 – 80 | 83 | 82 – 83 | 3 | 3 – 4 | 2 | 2 – 2 | 79 | 70 – 89 | 52 | 48 – 55 |
| 78 | 61 | 61 – 62 | 63 | 63 – 64 | 81 | 74 – 90 | 89 | 80 – 98 | 275 | 259 – 293 | 202 | 186 – 220 |
| 79 | 65 | 65 – 66 | 68 | 67 – 69 | 41 | 37 – 45 | 36 | 33 – 39 | 239 | 222 – 256 | 200 | 186 – 216 |
| 80 | 68 | 66 – 69 | 72 | 71 – 73 | 39 | 31 – 48 | 36 | 29 – 44 | 190 | 173 – 207 | 118 | 108 – 129 |
| 81 | 51 | 45 – 57 | 61 | 56 – 66 | 130 | 82 – 183 | 120 | 69 – 170 | 452 | 336 – 539 | 201 | 173 – 235 |
| 82 | 75 | 74 – 76 | 81 | 80 – 81 | 7 | 6 – 8 | 5 | 4 – 7 | 105 | 95 – 116 | 60 | 55 – 66 |
| 83 | 78 | 78 – 78 | 82 | 82 – 82 | 6 | 5 – 6 | 6 | 5 – 6 | 91 | 88 – 93 | 48 | 46 – 51 |
| 84 | 78 | 77 – 78 | 84 | 83 – 84 | 5 | 4 – 6 | 4 | 4 – 5 | 91 | 88 – 94 | 47 | 45 – 49 |
| 85 | 70 | 68 – 72 | 74 | 73 – 75 | 21 | 16 – 25 | 19 | 16 – 23 | 188 | 159 – 222 | 120 | 104 – 135 |
| 86 | 79 | 79 – 79 | 86 | 86 – 86 | 4 | 4 – 4 | 3 | 3 – 4 | 92 | 92 – 93 | 45 | 45 – 46 |
| 87 | 69 | 68 – 70 | 73 | 73 – 74 | 28 | 24 – 31 | 26 | 23 – 29 | 187 | 169 – 207 | 119 | 111 – 128 |
| 88 | 56 | 55 – 57 | 67 | 66 – 68 | 83 | 62 – 105 | 62 | 46 – 77 | 424 | 394 – 451 | 187 | 170 – 205 |
| 89 | 51 | 45 – 56 | 50 | 45 – 56 | 129 | 118 – 142 | 110 | 99 – 120 | 477 | 350 – 618 | 502 | 389 – 627 |
| 90 | 63 | 62 – 64 | 67 | 66 – 69 | 66 | 57 – 76 | 64 | 53 – 74 | 297 | 265 – 330 | 175 | 152 – 205 |

## Annex Table 1 Basic indicators for all Member States

Figures computed by WHO to ensure comparability;[a] they are not necessarily the official statistics of Member States, which may use alternative rigorous methods.

| | | POPULATION ESTIMATES | | | | | | | | LIFE EXPECTANCY AT BIRTH (YEARS) | | PROBABILITY OF DYING (PER 1000) Under age 5 years (under-5 mortality rate[b]) | |
| | Total population (000) | Annual growth rate (%) | Dependency ratio (per 100) | | Percentage of population aged 60+ years | | Total fertility rate | | Both sexes | | Both sexes | |
| Member State | 2004 | 1994–2004 | 1994 | 2004 | 1994 | 2004 | 1994 | 2004 | 2004 | Uncertainty | 2004 | Uncertainty |
|---|---|---|---|---|---|---|---|---|---|---|---|---|
| 91 Kuwait | 2 606 | 4.1 | 48 | 36 | 2.1 | 3.0 | 3.0 | 2.3 | 77 | 76 – 79 | 12 | 9 – 15 |
| 92 Kyrgyzstan | 5 204 | 1.4 | 76 | 62 | 8.0 | 7.7 | 3.4 | 2.6 | 63 | 63 – 64 | 68 | 54 – 82 |
| 93 Lao People's Democratic Republic | 5 792 | 2.4 | 91 | 81 | 5.6 | 5.3 | 5.7 | 4.7 | 59 | 57 – 62 | 83 | 69 – 98 |
| 94 Latvia | 2 318 | –0.9 | 52 | 47 | 19.0 | 22.3 | 1.5 | 1.3 | 71 | 71 – 72 | 11 | 9 – 13 |
| 95 Lebanon | 3 540 | 1.4 | 64 | 57 | 9.5 | 10.2 | 2.9 | 2.3 | 70 | 69 – 71 | 31 | 28 – 34 |
| 96 Lesotho | 1 798 | 0.7 | 95 | 79 | 6.9 | 7.4 | 4.5 | 3.5 | 41 | 38 – 46 | 82 | 68 – 95 |
| 97 Liberia | 3 241 | 4.6 | 97 | 97 | 3.9 | 3.7 | 6.9 | 6.8 | 42 | 34 – 49 | 235 | 191 – 279 |
| 98 Libyan Arab Jamahiriya | 5 740 | 2.0 | 75 | 52 | 4.7 | 6.3 | 3.8 | 2.9 | 72 | 68 – 75 | 20 | 17 – 23 |
| 99 Lithuania | 3 443 | –0.6 | 51 | 48 | 17.3 | 20.5 | 1.7 | 1.3 | 72 | 72 – 72 | 10 | 8 – 11 |
| 100 Luxembourg | 459 | 1.4 | 46 | 49 | 18.3 | 18.3 | 1.7 | 1.7 | 79 | 78 – 79 | 6 | 5 – 7 |
| 101 Madagascar | 18 113 | 3.0 | 92 | 90 | 4.8 | 4.8 | 6.1 | 5.3 | 57 | 50 – 63 | 123 | 108 – 137 |
| 102 Malawi | 12 608 | 2.4 | 91 | 101 | 4.7 | 4.6 | 6.7 | 6.0 | 41 | 37 – 46 | 175 | 159 – 191 |
| 103 Malaysia | 24 894 | 2.3 | 66 | 59 | 5.9 | 6.8 | 3.5 | 2.8 | 72 | 71 – 72 | 12 | 11 – 14 |
| 104 Maldives | 321 | 2.8 | 99 | 81 | 5.3 | 5.1 | 5.8 | 4.1 | 67 | 66 – 68 | 46 | 31 – 58 |
| 105 Mali | 13 124 | 2.9 | 103 | 104 | 4.5 | 4.3 | 7.3 | 6.8 | 46 | 38 – 52 | 219 | 197 – 240 |
| 106 Malta | 400 | 0.7 | 51 | 46 | 15.7 | 18.3 | 2.0 | 1.5 | 79 | 78 – 79 | 6 | 5 – 7 |
| 107 Marshall Islands | 60 | 1.7 | 69 | 60 | 5.8 | 6.5 | 5.0 | 4.4 | 62 | 60 – 64 | 59 | 43 – 74 |
| 108 Mauritania | 2 980 | 2.9 | 89 | 87 | 5.4 | 5.3 | 6.1 | 5.7 | 58 | 50 – 64 | 125 | 107 – 144 |
| 109 Mauritius | 1 233 | 1.1 | 51 | 46 | 8.5 | 9.4 | 2.2 | 2.0 | 72 | 71 – 72 | 15 | 12 – 19 |
| 110 Mexico | 105 699 | 1.5 | 69 | 58 | 6.2 | 7.6 | 3.0 | 2.3 | 74 | 74 – 74 | 28 | 27 – 28 |
| 111 Micronesia, Federated States of | 110 | 0.4 | 89 | 74 | 5.6 | 4.9 | 4.7 | 4.3 | 70 | 68 – 72 | 23 | 16 – 30 |
| 112 Monaco | 35 | 1.1 | 53 | 53 | 20.3 | 20.9 | 1.7 | 1.8 | 82 | 80 – 83 | 4 | 3 – 6 |
| 113 Mongolia | 2 614 | 1.0 | 77 | 54 | 5.8 | 5.7 | 3.1 | 2.4 | 65 | 64 – 66 | 52 | 42 – 64 |
| 114 Morocco | 31 020 | 1.6 | 71 | 57 | 6.3 | 6.8 | 3.4 | 2.7 | 71 | 70 – 72 | 43 | 35 – 51 |
| 115 Mozambique | 19 424 | 2.4 | 92 | 90 | 5.0 | 5.2 | 6.1 | 5.4 | 45 | 40 – 51 | 152 | 133 – 170 |
| 116 Myanmar | 50 004 | 1.3 | 68 | 54 | 6.8 | 7.4 | 3.6 | 2.3 | 59 | 51 – 66 | 105 | 72 – 138 |
| 117 Namibia | 2 009 | 2.3 | 91 | 84 | 5.1 | 5.2 | 5.5 | 3.8 | 54 | 49 – 58 | 63 | 53 – 75 |
| 118 Nauru | 13 | 2.5 | 69 | 60 | 5.8 | 6.5 | 4.3 | 3.8 | 61 | 56 – 67 | 30 | 24 – 36 |
| 119 Nepal | 26 591 | 2.3 | 83 | 76 | 5.4 | 5.7 | 4.8 | 3.6 | 61 | 60 – 62 | 76 | 68 – 84 |
| 120 Netherlands | 16 226 | 0.5 | 46 | 48 | 17.7 | 18.9 | 1.6 | 1.7 | 79 | 79 – 79 | 5 | 5 – 6 |
| 121 New Zealand | 3 989 | 1.0 | 53 | 51 | 15.4 | 16.5 | 2.0 | 2.0 | 80 | 79 – 80 | 6 | 5 – 7 |
| 122 Nicaragua | 5 376 | 2.1 | 93 | 75 | 4.4 | 4.8 | 4.4 | 3.2 | 69 | 69 – 70 | 38 | 32 – 44 |
| 123 Niger | 13 499 | 3.5 | 103 | 104 | 3.5 | 3.3 | 8.2 | 7.8 | 41 | 32 – 50 | 259 | 208 – 309 |
| 124 Nigeria | 128 709 | 2.4 | 96 | 91 | 4.7 | 4.8 | 6.5 | 5.7 | 46 | 40 – 51 | 197 | 176 – 218 |
| 125 Niue | 1 | –2.1 | 71 | 65 | 6.4 | 7.5 | 3.4 | 2.8 | 71 | 68 – 73 | 36 | 36 – 36 |
| 126 Norway | 4 598 | 0.6 | 55 | 53 | 20.2 | 19.8 | 1.9 | 1.8 | 80 | 79 – 80 | 4 | 4 – 5 |
| 127 Oman | 2 534 | 1.8 | 76 | 60 | 3.1 | 4.0 | 6.0 | 3.6 | 74 | 70 – 77 | 13 | 11 – 14 |
| 128 Pakistan | 154 794 | 2.3 | 90 | 74 | 5.5 | 5.8 | 5.5 | 4.1 | 62 | 60 – 64 | 101 | 86 – 116 |
| 129 Palau | 20 | 1.6 | 69 | 60 | 5.8 | 6.5 | 1.6 | 1.4 | 68 | 67 – 69 | 27 | 20 – 35 |
| 130 Panama | 3 175 | 2.0 | 63 | 58 | 7.4 | 8.6 | 2.8 | 2.7 | 76 | 75 – 76 | 24 | 21 – 26 |
| 131 Papua New Guinea | 5 772 | 2.4 | 79 | 76 | 4.0 | 3.9 | 4.9 | 3.9 | 60 | 58 – 62 | 93 | 75 – 110 |
| 132 Paraguay | 6 017 | 2.5 | 83 | 71 | 5.2 | 5.6 | 4.4 | 3.8 | 72 | 71 – 73 | 24 | 20 – 28 |
| 133 Peru | 27 562 | 1.6 | 69 | 61 | 6.4 | 7.6 | 3.5 | 2.8 | 71 | 70 – 72 | 29 | 25 – 33 |
| 134 Philippines | 81 617 | 2.0 | 75 | 65 | 5.1 | 6.0 | 4.0 | 3.1 | 68 | 68 – 69 | 34 | 29 – 39 |
| 135 Poland | 38 559 | 0.0 | 52 | 42 | 15.6 | 16.7 | 1.8 | 1.2 | 75 | 75 – 75 | 8 | 7 – 8 |

| | LIFE EXPECTANCY AT BIRTH (YEARS) | | | | PROBABILITY OF DYING (PER 1000) | | | | | | | |
| | | | | | Under age 5 years (under-5 mortality rate[b]) | | | | Between ages 15 and 60 years (adult mortality rate) | | | |
| | Males | | Females | | Males | | Females | | Males | | Females | |
| | 2004 | Uncertainty | 2004 | Uncertainty | 2004 | Uncertainty | 2004 | Uncertainty | 2004 | Uncertainty | 2004 | Uncertainty |
|---|---|---|---|---|---|---|---|---|---|---|---|---|
| 91 | 76 | 76 – 77 | 78 | 76 – 80 | 12 | 10 – 15 | 11 | 8 – 15 | 72 | 66 – 78 | 54 | 44 – 59 |
| 92 | 59 | 59 – 60 | 67 | 67 – 68 | 72 | 57 – 87 | 63 | 50 – 76 | 336 | 316 – 355 | 162 | 145 – 178 |
| 93 | 58 | 56 – 61 | 60 | 58 – 62 | 88 | 72 – 103 | 78 | 65 – 93 | 331 | 275 – 386 | 300 | 267 – 335 |
| 94 | 66 | 66 – 66 | 76 | 76 – 77 | 11 | 9 – 13 | 11 | 9 – 13 | 300 | 293 – 307 | 115 | 110 – 120 |
| 95 | 68 | 67 – 69 | 72 | 72 – 73 | 35 | 32 – 38 | 26 | 23 – 29 | 198 | 174 – 222 | 136 | 121 – 151 |
| 96 | 39 | 36 – 43 | 44 | 40 – 48 | 87 | 73 – 101 | 76 | 64 – 89 | 845 | 772 – 892 | 728 | 650 – 795 |
| 97 | 39 | 33 – 46 | 44 | 35 – 52 | 249 | 205 – 296 | 220 | 176 – 261 | 596 | 451 – 747 | 477 | 310 – 656 |
| 98 | 70 | 66 – 73 | 75 | 72 – 77 | 20 | 17 – 23 | 19 | 16 – 22 | 186 | 118 – 276 | 109 | 70 – 164 |
| 99 | 66 | 66 – 67 | 78 | 78 – 78 | 10 | 9 – 12 | 9 | 7 – 10 | 304 | 298 – 310 | 102 | 98 – 107 |
| 100 | 76 | 75 – 76 | 81 | 80 – 82 | 6 | 5 – 8 | 5 | 5 – 6 | 118 | 109 – 127 | 59 | 52 – 67 |
| 101 | 55 | 49 – 61 | 59 | 51 – 65 | 128 | 113 – 143 | 117 | 103 – 131 | 338 | 198 – 510 | 270 | 150 – 444 |
| 102 | 41 | 37 – 46 | 41 | 36 – 47 | 179 | 161 – 195 | 172 | 156 – 187 | 663 | 560 – 768 | 638 | 526 – 748 |
| 103 | 69 | 68 – 70 | 74 | 74 – 75 | 14 | 12 – 16 | 11 | 10 – 13 | 200 | 182 – 220 | 109 | 98 – 120 |
| 104 | 66 | 65 – 67 | 68 | 67 – 68 | 47 | 32 – 60 | 44 | 31 – 56 | 186 | 159 – 215 | 140 | 126 – 156 |
| 105 | 44 | 37 – 50 | 47 | 39 – 53 | 230 | 205 – 252 | 208 | 187 – 228 | 490 | 356 – 670 | 414 | 253 – 605 |
| 106 | 76 | 76 – 77 | 81 | 81 – 82 | 7 | 6 – 8 | 5 | 4 – 6 | 82 | 78 – 87 | 48 | 44 – 51 |
| 107 | 60 | 58 – 62 | 64 | 62 – 66 | 66 | 48 – 82 | 52 | 38 – 66 | 327 | 297 – 356 | 275 | 250 – 295 |
| 108 | 55 | 49 – 62 | 60 | 52 – 66 | 134 | 115 – 155 | 115 | 99 – 132 | 325 | 166 – 493 | 246 | 128 – 421 |
| 109 | 69 | 68 – 69 | 75 | 75 – 75 | 17 | 13 – 20 | 14 | 11 – 17 | 217 | 201 – 234 | 112 | 106 – 119 |
| 110 | 72 | 72 – 72 | 77 | 77 – 77 | 31 | 30 – 31 | 25 | 24 – 25 | 161 | 160 – 163 | 94 | 93 – 94 |
| 111 | 68 | 67 – 70 | 71 | 70 – 73 | 26 | 18 – 33 | 19 | 14 – 26 | 202 | 177 – 228 | 169 | 146 – 191 |
| 112 | 78 | 77 – 80 | 85 | 83 – 87 | 5 | 4 – 7 | 3 | 3 – 6 | 105 | 85 – 124 | 45 | 32 – 58 |
| 113 | 61 | 60 – 62 | 69 | 68 – 70 | 60 | 47 – 72 | 45 | 36 – 55 | 303 | 277 – 330 | 185 | 163 – 210 |
| 114 | 69 | 68 – 70 | 73 | 72 – 74 | 47 | 39 – 56 | 38 | 31 – 45 | 157 | 146 – 169 | 102 | 90 – 113 |
| 115 | 44 | 39 – 50 | 46 | 41 – 52 | 154 | 135 – 173 | 150 | 131 – 168 | 627 | 502 – 739 | 549 | 427 – 665 |
| 116 | 56 | 49 – 63 | 63 | 54 – 69 | 116 | 82 – 153 | 93 | 63 – 122 | 334 | 174 – 510 | 219 | 110 – 399 |
| 117 | 52 | 48 – 56 | 55 | 51 – 60 | 70 | 59 – 81 | 57 | 46 – 69 | 548 | 467 – 629 | 489 | 411 – 568 |
| 118 | 58 | 52 – 65 | 65 | 61 – 70 | 35 | 28 – 43 | 24 | 19 – 29 | 448 | 283 – 596 | 303 | 184 – 417 |
| 119 | 61 | 60 – 62 | 61 | 60 – 62 | 74 | 66 – 81 | 79 | 70 – 87 | 297 | 274 – 320 | 285 | 264 – 306 |
| 120 | 77 | 77 – 77 | 81 | 81 – 82 | 6 | 5 – 6 | 5 | 4 – 5 | 89 | 87 – 91 | 63 | 62 – 65 |
| 121 | 77 | 77 – 78 | 82 | 82 – 82 | 7 | 6 – 8 | 6 | 5 – 7 | 95 | 92 – 98 | 62 | 59 – 65 |
| 122 | 67 | 67 – 68 | 71 | 71 – 72 | 41 | 35 – 47 | 35 | 30 – 40 | 214 | 199 – 228 | 151 | 135 – 168 |
| 123 | 42 | 33 – 50 | 41 | 31 – 50 | 256 | 205 – 308 | 262 | 211 – 310 | 506 | 351 – 714 | 478 | 252 – 725 |
| 124 | 45 | 40 – 51 | 46 | 39 – 52 | 198 | 179 – 220 | 195 | 174 – 215 | 513 | 377 – 648 | 478 | 338 – 634 |
| 125 | 68 | 65 – 70 | 74 | 71 – 76 | 50 | 50 – 50 | 20 | 20 – 20 | 178 | 139 – 222 | 138 | 107 – 178 |
| 126 | 77 | 77 – 78 | 82 | 82 – 82 | 4 | 4 – 5 | 4 | 4 – 5 | 93 | 88 – 99 | 57 | 55 – 59 |
| 127 | 71 | 68 – 75 | 77 | 74 – 79 | 13 | 11 – 15 | 12 | 10 – 14 | 164 | 106 – 244 | 92 | 58 – 137 |
| 128 | 62 | 60 – 63 | 63 | 61 – 65 | 102 | 86 – 117 | 100 | 85 – 115 | 222 | 199 – 249 | 198 | 173 – 223 |
| 129 | 67 | 66 – 67 | 70 | 69 – 71 | 27 | 19 – 34 | 28 | 20 – 37 | 224 | 213 – 234 | 206 | 186 – 228 |
| 130 | 73 | 73 – 74 | 78 | 77 – 79 | 26 | 24 – 29 | 22 | 19 – 24 | 139 | 129 – 151 | 82 | 75 – 91 |
| 131 | 58 | 56 – 60 | 61 | 59 – 63 | 98 | 79 – 116 | 87 | 71 – 103 | 322 | 293 – 352 | 265 | 240 – 293 |
| 132 | 70 | 69 – 70 | 74 | 74 – 75 | 25 | 21 – 29 | 23 | 19 – 27 | 176 | 164 – 188 | 127 | 115 – 137 |
| 133 | 69 | 68 – 70 | 73 | 72 – 74 | 31 | 27 – 35 | 27 | 23 – 31 | 184 | 164 – 208 | 134 | 118 – 152 |
| 134 | 65 | 64 – 65 | 72 | 71 – 72 | 40 | 34 – 46 | 28 | 24 – 32 | 269 | 257 – 281 | 149 | 137 – 159 |
| 135 | 71 | 71 – 71 | 79 | 79 – 79 | 8 | 8 – 9 | 7 | 6 – 8 | 198 | 193 – 203 | 79 | 76 – 82 |

## Annex Table 1 Basic indicators for all Member States

Figures computed by WHO to ensure comparability;[a] they are not necessarily the official statistics of Member States, which may use alternative rigorous methods.

| | | POPULATION ESTIMATES | | | | | | | LIFE EXPECTANCY AT BIRTH (YEARS) | | PROBABILITY OF DYING (PER 1000) | | |
| --- | --- | --- | --- | --- | --- | --- | --- | --- | --- | --- | --- | --- | --- |
| | | | | | | | | | | | Under age 5 years (under-5 mortality rate[b]) | | |
| | Member State | Total population (000) | Annual growth rate (%) | Dependency ratio (per 100) | | Percentage of population aged 60+ years | | Total fertility rate | | Both sexes | | Both sexes | | |
| | | 2004 | 1994–2004 | 1994 | 2004 | 1994 | 2004 | 1994 | 2004 | 2004 | Uncertainty | 2004 | Uncertainty | |
| 136 | Portugal | 10 441 | 0.4 | 49 | 49 | 20.1 | 22.1 | 1.5 | 1.5 | 78 | 77 – 78 | 5 | 5 – 6 | |
| 137 | Qatar | 777 | 4.2 | 39 | 31 | 2.2 | 2.6 | 3.9 | 2.9 | 76 | 74 – 78 | 12 | 9 – 15 | |
| 138 | Republic of Korea | 47 645 | 0.7 | 42 | 39 | 8.9 | 13.3 | 1.7 | 1.2 | 77 | 77 – 76 | 6 | 5 – 6 | |
| 139 | Republic of Moldova | 4 218 | −0.3 | 56 | 41 | 13.0 | 13.7 | 1.9 | 1.2 | 67 | 67 – 68 | 28 | 21 – 35 | |
| 140 | Romania | 21 790 | −0.5 | 49 | 44 | 17.1 | 19.2 | 1.4 | 1.3 | 72 | 72 – 72 | 20 | 19 – 21 | |
| 141 | Russian Federation | 143 899 | −0.3 | 50 | 41 | 16.5 | 17.3 | 1.4 | 1.3 | 65 | 64 – 68 | 16 | 14 – 17 | |
| 142 | Rwanda | 8 882 | 4.9 | 110 | 87 | 3.5 | 3.9 | 6.7 | 5.6 | 46 | 39 – 51 | 203 | 183 – 223 | |
| 143 | Saint Kitts and Nevis | 42 | 0.5 | 62 | 55 | 9.1 | 10.5 | 2.6 | 2.4 | 71 | 70 – 71 | 21 | 18 – 25 | |
| 144 | Saint Lucia | 159 | 0.9 | 75 | 58 | 9.4 | 9.8 | 3.0 | 2.2 | 74 | 73 – 75 | 14 | 13 – 17 | |
| 145 | Saint Vincent and the Grenadines | 118 | 0.5 | 78 | 57 | 8.6 | 8.9 | 2.7 | 2.2 | 69 | 68 – 70 | 22 | 18 – 27 | |
| 146 | Samoa | 184 | 1.0 | 77 | 83 | 6.3 | 6.5 | 4.7 | 4.3 | 68 | 67 – 69 | 30 | 24 – 36 | |
| 147 | San Marino | 28 | 0.9 | 46 | 51 | 22.1 | 25.3 | 1.2 | 1.2 | 82 | 80 – 83 | 4 | 4 – 4 | |
| 148 | Sao Tome and Principe | 153 | 2.0 | 101 | 79 | 6.5 | 5.8 | 4.8 | 3.9 | 59 | 51 – 65 | 118 | 89 – 148 | |
| 149 | Saudi Arabia | 23 950 | 2.8 | 78 | 68 | 3.4 | 4.5 | 5.4 | 3.9 | 71 | 67 – 74 | 27 | 20 – 34 | |
| 150 | Senegal | 11 386 | 2.5 | 98 | 86 | 4.8 | 4.8 | 6.0 | 4.9 | 55 | 49 – 61 | 137 | 120 – 154 | |
| 151 | Serbia and Montenegro | 10 510 | 0.0 | 50 | 48 | 16.8 | 18.4 | 1.9 | 1.6 | 73 | 72 – 73 | 15 | 13 – 16 | |
| 152 | Seychelles | 80 | 0.7 | 51 | 46 | 8.5 | 9.4 | 2.4 | 2.1 | 72 | 71 – 73 | 14 | 10 – 17 | |
| 153 | Sierra Leone | 5 336 | 2.6 | 83 | 86 | 5.6 | 5.5 | 6.5 | 6.5 | 39 | 29 – 46 | 283 | 241 – 327 | |
| 154 | Singapore | 4 273 | 2.4 | 39 | 40 | 9.1 | 11.8 | 1.7 | 1.3 | 80 | 79 – 80 | 3 | 3 – 4 | |
| 155 | Slovakia | 5 401 | 0.1 | 51 | 41 | 15.1 | 16.0 | 1.7 | 1.2 | 74 | 74 – 75 | 8 | 7 – 11 | |
| 156 | Slovenia | 1 967 | 0.0 | 45 | 42 | 17.6 | 20.2 | 1.3 | 1.2 | 77 | 77 – 77 | 4 | 4 – 5 | |
| 157 | Solomon Islands | 466 | 2.8 | 88 | 77 | 4.2 | 4.1 | 5.0 | 4.2 | 68 | 64 – 72 | 56 | 48 – 64 | |
| 158 | Somalia | 7 964 | 2.3 | 87 | 88 | 4.3 | 4.2 | 6.7 | 6.3 | 44 | 37 – 51 | 225 | 203 – 247 | |
| 159 | South Africa | 47 208 | 1.4 | 65 | 58 | 5.2 | 6.6 | 3.2 | 2.8 | 48 | 45 – 51 | 67 | 57 – 78 | |
| 160 | Spain | 42 646 | 0.7 | 46 | 44 | 20.5 | 21.3 | 1.2 | 1.3 | 80 | 80 – 80 | 5 | 4 – 5 | |
| 161 | Sri Lanka | 20 570 | 1.0 | 56 | 46 | 8.7 | 10.5 | 2.3 | 1.9 | 71 | 70 – 73 | 14 | 12 – 16 | |
| 162 | Sudan | 35 523 | 2.2 | 83 | 76 | 5.0 | 5.6 | 5.2 | 4.3 | 58 | 51 – 64 | 91 | 82 – 101 | |
| 163 | Suriname | 446 | 0.8 | 65 | 58 | 7.7 | 8.9 | 2.7 | 2.6 | 67 | 66 – 69 | 39 | 34 – 44 | |
| 164 | Swaziland | 1 034 | 1.0 | 97 | 82 | 4.3 | 5.3 | 5.1 | 3.8 | 37 | 34 – 42 | 156 | 137 – 176 | |
| 165 | Sweden | 9 008 | 0.2 | 57 | 54 | 22.1 | 23.0 | 1.9 | 1.7 | 81 | 80 – 81 | 4 | 3 – 4 | |
| 166 | Switzerland | 7 240 | 0.4 | 47 | 48 | 19.2 | 21.4 | 1.5 | 1.4 | 81 | 81 – 81 | 5 | 4 – 6 | |
| 167 | Syrian Arab Republic | 18 582 | 2.6 | 93 | 68 | 4.3 | 4.7 | 4.4 | 3.3 | 72 | 71 – 73 | 16 | 15 – 18 | |
| 168 | Tajikistan | 6 430 | 1.2 | 91 | 77 | 5.9 | 5.2 | 4.7 | 3.7 | 63 | 61 – 66 | 118 | 84 – 147 | |
| 169 | Thailand | 63 694 | 1.0 | 50 | 45 | 7.3 | 10.2 | 2.0 | 1.9 | 70 | 70 – 71 | 21 | 18 – 24 | |
| 170 | The former Yugoslav Republic of Macedonia | 2 030 | 0.4 | 50 | 45 | 13.0 | 15.3 | 1.9 | 1.5 | 72 | 72 – 73 | 14 | 13 – 15 | |
| 171 | Timor–Leste | 887 | 0.5 | 78 | 80 | 3.7 | 5.0 | 4.6 | 7.8 | 63 | 56 – 69 | 80 | 69 – 92 | |
| 172 | Togo | 5 988 | 3.2 | 95 | 88 | 4.7 | 4.8 | 6.1 | 5.2 | 54 | 48 – 59 | 140 | 122 – 157 | |
| 173 | Tonga | 102 | 0.6 | 81 | 73 | 7.5 | 8.7 | 4.4 | 3.4 | 71 | 70 – 71 | 25 | 20 – 29 | |
| 174 | Trinidad and Tobago | 1 301 | 0.4 | 60 | 41 | 8.8 | 10.5 | 1.9 | 1.6 | 70 | 69 – 71 | 20 | 17 – 23 | |
| 175 | Tunisia | 9 995 | 1.2 | 68 | 49 | 7.9 | 8.6 | 2.8 | 1.9 | 72 | 71 – 73 | 25 | 23 – 28 | |
| 176 | Turkey | 72 220 | 1.6 | 61 | 54 | 7.2 | 7.9 | 2.8 | 2.4 | 71 | 70 – 72 | 32 | 29 – 35 | |
| 177 | Turkmenistan | 4 766 | 1.5 | 79 | 60 | 6.2 | 6.3 | 3.7 | 2.7 | 60 | 59 – 61 | 103 | 92 – 113 | |
| 178 | Tuvalu | 10 | 0.6 | 71 | 65 | 6.4 | 7.5 | 4.4 | 3.7 | 61 | 58 – 64 | 51 | 37 – 64 | |
| 179 | Uganda | 27 821 | 3.2 | 109 | 112 | 4.1 | 3.9 | 7.1 | 7.1 | 49 | 44 – 55 | 138 | 124 – 151 | |
| 180 | Ukraine | 46 989 | −1.0 | 52 | 45 | 18.3 | 21.0 | 1.5 | 1.1 | 67 | 67 – 68 | 18 | 16 – 20 | |

| | LIFE EXPECTANCY AT BIRTH (YEARS) | | | | PROBABILITY OF DYING (PER 1000) | | | | | | | |
| | | | | | Under age 5 years (under-5 mortality rate[b]) | | | | Between ages 15 and 60 years (adult mortality rate) | | | |
| | Males | | Females | | Males | | Females | | Males | | Females | |
| | 2004 | Uncertainty | 2004 | Uncertainty | 2004 | Uncertainty | 2004 | Uncertainty | 2004 | Uncertainty | 2004 | Uncertainty |
|---|---|---|---|---|---|---|---|---|---|---|---|---|
| 136 | 74 | 74 – 75 | 81 | 81 – 81 | 6 | 4 – 7 | 5 | 5 – 6 | 144 | 137 – 152 | 61 | 59 – 63 |
| 137 | 76 | 75 – 78 | 75 | 74 – 77 | 12 | 10 – 15 | 11 | 9 – 15 | 75 | 66 – 85 | 70 | 56 – 85 |
| 138 | 73 | 73 – 74 | 80 | 79 – 80 | 5 | 4 – 5 | 7 | 6 – 7 | 151 | 146 – 156 | 55 | 54 – 58 |
| 139 | 64 | 63 – 64 | 71 | 71 – 71 | 32 | 24 – 40 | 24 | 18 – 30 | 300 | 287 – 313 | 150 | 141 – 159 |
| 140 | 68 | 68 – 68 | 76 | 75 – 76 | 22 | 21 – 23 | 18 | 17 – 18 | 232 | 229 – 234 | 100 | 99 – 102 |
| 141 | 59 | 58 – 64 | 72 | 71 – 72 | 18 | 16 – 19 | 14 | 13 – 15 | 485 | 455 – 507 | 180 | 168 – 180 |
| 142 | 44 | 38 – 49 | 47 | 40 – 53 | 211 | 190 – 230 | 195 | 176 – 215 | 518 | 399 – 672 | 435 | 289 – 608 |
| 143 | 69 | 68 – 70 | 72 | 71 – 73 | 21 | 17 – 24 | 22 | 19 – 25 | 197 | 182 – 213 | 145 | 120 – 175 |
| 144 | 71 | 71 – 72 | 77 | 76 – 78 | 15 | 13 – 18 | 13 | 12 – 15 | 209 | 194 – 224 | 116 | 102 – 132 |
| 145 | 66 | 65 – 67 | 73 | 72 – 74 | 26 | 23 – 29 | 19 | 14 – 25 | 301 | 266 – 338 | 174 | 155 – 191 |
| 146 | 66 | 64 – 67 | 70 | 69 – 71 | 42 | 36 – 49 | 17 | 13 – 21 | 235 | 218 – 252 | 203 | 187 – 219 |
| 147 | 79 | 76 – 79 | 84 | 82 – 86 | 4 | 4 – 8 | 3 | 3 – 3 | 66 | 54 – 86 | 34 | 27 – 37 |
| 148 | 57 | 49 – 64 | 60 | 52 – 67 | 122 | 92 – 152 | 114 | 86 – 143 | 301 | 155 – 498 | 236 | 118 – 419 |
| 149 | 68 | 64 – 73 | 74 | 70 – 76 | 29 | 22 – 37 | 24 | 18 – 31 | 196 | 117 – 296 | 120 | 77 – 183 |
| 150 | 54 | 48 – 60 | 57 | 50 – 63 | 141 | 125 – 159 | 132 | 116 – 148 | 358 | 215 – 529 | 288 | 164 – 464 |
| 151 | 70 | 70 – 70 | 75 | 75 – 76 | 17 | 15 – 19 | 13 | 11 – 14 | 191 | 183 – 200 | 98 | 94 – 102 |
| 152 | 67 | 67 – 68 | 78 | 76 – 79 | 14 | 11 – 18 | 13 | 10 – 17 | 232 | 209 – 254 | 83 | 66 – 105 |
| 153 | 37 | 29 – 44 | 40 | 30 – 48 | 296 | 250 – 340 | 269 | 232 – 313 | 579 | 428 – 778 | 497 | 284 – 745 |
| 154 | 77 | 76 – 79 | 82 | 81 – 82 | 4 | 4 – 4 | 3 | 3 – 3 | 92 | 80 – 106 | 51 | 48 – 56 |
| 155 | 70 | 70 – 71 | 78 | 78 – 79 | 9 | 7 – 11 | 8 | 6 – 10 | 203 | 193 – 214 | 76 | 72 – 81 |
| 156 | 73 | 72 – 73 | 81 | 81 – 81 | 5 | 4 – 6 | 4 | 4 – 4 | 158 | 150 – 167 | 67 | 64 – 71 |
| 157 | 66 | 62 – 70 | 70 | 66 – 73 | 60 | 51 – 68 | 52 | 44 – 59 | 193 | 125 – 265 | 143 | 83 – 207 |
| 158 | 43 | 36 – 50 | 45 | 37 – 52 | 222 | 199 – 243 | 228 | 207 – 251 | 524 | 372 – 658 | 428 | 254 – 622 |
| 159 | 47 | 44 – 50 | 49 | 46 – 53 | 72 | 62 – 83 | 62 | 52 – 74 | 667 | 602 – 733 | 598 | 519 – 669 |
| 160 | 77 | 76 – 77 | 83 | 83 – 84 | 5 | 4 – 5 | 4 | 4 – 4 | 113 | 107 – 120 | 45 | 44 – 47 |
| 161 | 68 | 66 – 70 | 75 | 74 – 76 | 16 | 14 – 19 | 12 | 10 – 13 | 232 | 183 – 278 | 119 | 104 – 133 |
| 162 | 56 | 49 – 62 | 60 | 53 – 67 | 98 | 89 – 108 | 84 | 75 – 93 | 390 | 255 – 538 | 304 | 187 – 450 |
| 163 | 65 | 63 – 66 | 70 | 69 – 72 | 42 | 37 – 48 | 36 | 32 – 41 | 261 | 224 – 301 | 159 | 135 – 183 |
| 164 | 36 | 33 – 40 | 39 | 35 – 43 | 163 | 141 – 184 | 150 | 132 – 168 | 823 | 744 – 882 | 741 | 656 – 816 |
| 165 | 78 | 78 – 78 | 83 | 83 – 83 | 4 | 3 – 4 | 3 | 3 – 4 | 82 | 80 – 84 | 51 | 49 – 52 |
| 166 | 78 | 78 – 79 | 83 | 83 – 84 | 5 | 5 – 6 | 5 | 4 – 5 | 87 | 83 – 91 | 49 | 48 – 51 |
| 167 | 70 | 69 – 71 | 74 | 74 – 75 | 19 | 17 – 20 | 14 | 13 – 15 | 186 | 171 – 201 | 125 | 115 – 134 |
| 168 | 62 | 60 – 64 | 64 | 62 – 67 | 120 | 84 – 147 | 115 | 85 – 147 | 166 | 130 – 219 | 139 | 121 – 174 |
| 169 | 67 | 67 – 68 | 73 | 73 – 74 | 23 | 19 – 26 | 20 | 17 – 23 | 265 | 243 – 287 | 154 | 135 – 174 |
| 170 | 69 | 69 – 70 | 76 | 75 – 76 | 16 | 15 – 18 | 12 | 11 – 13 | 198 | 186 – 210 | 84 | 78 – 91 |
| 171 | 61 | 54 – 67 | 66 | 58 – 72 | 91 | 78 – 104 | 69 | 60 – 79 | 267 | 123 – 430 | 184 | 84 – 357 |
| 172 | 52 | 46 – 58 | 56 | 49 – 61 | 151 | 134 – 171 | 128 | 111 – 143 | 401 | 264 – 551 | 327 | 213 – 485 |
| 173 | 71 | 70 – 72 | 70 | 70 – 71 | 32 | 26 – 36 | 17 | 14 – 21 | 140 | 135 – 144 | 194 | 187 – 201 |
| 174 | 67 | 66 – 68 | 73 | 73 – 74 | 24 | 20 – 28 | 15 | 13 – 18 | 257 | 229 – 287 | 156 | 140 – 173 |
| 175 | 70 | 69 – 71 | 74 | 73 – 75 | 29 | 26 – 31 | 22 | 20 – 24 | 166 | 153 – 178 | 110 | 99 – 124 |
| 176 | 69 | 68 – 70 | 73 | 72 – 74 | 33 | 29 – 36 | 31 | 28 – 34 | 180 | 168 – 193 | 112 | 98 – 125 |
| 177 | 56 | 55 – 56 | 65 | 64 – 66 | 117 | 105 – 128 | 88 | 79 – 97 | 350 | 327 – 374 | 166 | 145 – 188 |
| 178 | 61 | 57 – 64 | 62 | 59 – 65 | 50 | 36 – 62 | 52 | 38 – 65 | 325 | 237 – 433 | 277 | 213 – 387 |
| 179 | 48 | 43 – 53 | 51 | 45 – 57 | 144 | 130 – 157 | 132 | 119 – 144 | 525 | 398 – 654 | 446 | 326 – 592 |
| 180 | 62 | 62 – 62 | 73 | 73 – 74 | 21 | 19 – 23 | 15 | 14 – 17 | 386 | 370 – 402 | 144 | 130 – 158 |

### Annex Table 1 Basic indicators for all Member States

Figures computed by WHO to ensure comparability;[a] they are not necessarily the official statistics of Member States, which may use alternative rigorous methods.

| | Member State | POPULATION ESTIMATES | | | | | | | | | LIFE EXPECTANCY AT BIRTH (YEARS) | | PROBABILITY OF DYING (PER 1000) | | |
|---|---|---|---|---|---|---|---|---|---|---|---|---|---|---|---|
| | | Total population (000) | Annual growth rate (%) | Dependency ratio (per 100) | | Percentage of population aged 60+ years | | Total fertility rate | | Both sexes | | Under age 5 years (under-5 mortality rate[b]) Both sexes | | |
| | | 2004 | 1994–2004 | 1994 | 2004 | 1994 | 2004 | 1994 | 2004 | 2004 | Uncertainty | 2004 | Uncertainty | |
| 181 | United Arab Emirates | 4 284 | 6.4 | 42 | 31 | 1.9 | 1.7 | 3.6 | 2.5 | 77 | 77 – 78 | 8 | 6 – 9 | |
| 182 | United Kingdom | 59 479 | 0.3 | 54 | 52 | 20.9 | 21.0 | 1.8 | 1.7 | 79 | 79 – 79 | 6 | 5 – 6 | |
| 183 | United Republic of Tanzania | 37 627 | 2.3 | 92 | 86 | 4.5 | 5.0 | 5.8 | 4.9 | 48 | 46 – 51 | 126 | 116 – 136 | |
| 184 | United States of America | 295 410 | 1.0 | 53 | 50 | 16.3 | 16.5 | 2.0 | 2.0 | 78 | 77 – 78 | 8 | 7 – 8 | |
| 185 | Uruguay | 3 439 | 0.7 | 60 | 60 | 16.9 | 17.4 | 2.5 | 2.3 | 75 | 75 – 76 | 14 | 13 – 15 | |
| 186 | Uzbekistan | 26 209 | 1.5 | 81 | 63 | 6.3 | 6.3 | 3.6 | 2.7 | 66 | 65 – 67 | 69 | 62 – 75 | |
| 187 | Vanuatu | 207 | 2.1 | 89 | 78 | 5.2 | 5.1 | 4.8 | 4.0 | 68 | 65 – 72 | 40 | 29 – 51 | |
| 188 | Venezuela, Bolivarian Republic of | 26 282 | 2.0 | 68 | 58 | 6.1 | 7.4 | 3.1 | 2.7 | 75 | 74 – 75 | 19 | 17 – 20 | |
| 189 | Viet Nam | 83 123 | 1.5 | 74 | 56 | 7.4 | 7.5 | 3.0 | 2.3 | 71 | 70 – 72 | 23 | 20 – 26 | |
| 190 | Yemen | 20 329 | 3.4 | 111 | 96 | 3.8 | 3.7 | 7.4 | 6.0 | 59 | 52 – 65 | 111 | 97 – 125 | |
| 191 | Zambia | 11 479 | 2.1 | 98 | 96 | 4.3 | 4.6 | 6.3 | 5.5 | 40 | 36 – 45 | 182 | 162 – 204 | |
| 192 | Zimbabwe | 12 936 | 1.1 | 92 | 79 | 4.6 | 5.4 | 4.5 | 3.4 | 36 | 33 – 39 | 129 | 115 – 146 | |

[a]See explanatory notes for sources and methods.

[b]Under-five mortality rate is the probability (expressed as per 1000 live births) of a child born in a specific year dying before reaching five years of age, if subjected to current age-specific mortality rate.

| | LIFE EXPECTANCY AT BIRTH (YEARS) | | | | PROBABILITY OF DYING (PER 1000) | | | | | | | |
|---|---|---|---|---|---|---|---|---|---|---|---|---|
| | | | | | Under age 5 years (under-5 mortality rate[b]) | | | | Between ages 15 and 60 years (adult mortality rate) | | | |
| | Males | | Females | | Males | | Females | | Males | | Females | |
| | 2004 | Uncertainty | 2004 | Uncertainty | 2004 | Uncertainty | 2004 | Uncertainty | 2004 | Uncertainty | 2004 | Uncertainty |
| 181 | 76 | 76 – 77 | 79 | 79 – 80 | 8 | 7 – 10 | 7 | 6 – 8 | 89 | 79 – 99 | 67 | 60 – 73 |
| 182 | 76 | 76 – 77 | 81 | 81 – 81 | 6 | 6 – 7 | 5 | 5 – 6 | 102 | 99 – 104 | 63 | 61 – 64 |
| 183 | 47 | 45 – 49 | 49 | 47 – 52 | 134 | 124 – 145 | 117 | 107 – 126 | 551 | 509 – 597 | 524 | 470 – 576 |
| 184 | 75 | 75 – 76 | 80 | 80 – 80 | 8 | 8 – 9 | 7 | 7 – 7 | 137 | 130 – 145 | 81 | 80 – 83 |
| 185 | 71 | 71 – 72 | 79 | 79 – 80 | 16 | 14 – 18 | 12 | 11 – 13 | 172 | 163 – 183 | 87 | 83 – 90 |
| 186 | 63 | 63 – 64 | 69 | 68 – 70 | 80 | 72 – 88 | 57 | 51 – 62 | 223 | 209 – 237 | 141 | 125 – 157 |
| 187 | 67 | 63 – 71 | 69 | 66 – 73 | 40 | 29 – 51 | 40 | 29 – 50 | 212 | 144 – 280 | 170 | 115 – 227 |
| 188 | 72 | 71 – 73 | 78 | 77 – 78 | 20 | 18 – 22 | 17 | 15 – 19 | 185 | 171 – 198 | 97 | 90 – 104 |
| 189 | 69 | 68 – 69 | 74 | 73 – 74 | 24 | 21 – 27 | 22 | 19 – 25 | 197 | 182 – 212 | 122 | 111 – 134 |
| 190 | 57 | 51 – 63 | 61 | 54 – 67 | 118 | 103 – 132 | 104 | 91 – 117 | 298 | 152 – 474 | 225 | 110 – 403 |
| 191 | 40 | 36 – 45 | 40 | 35 – 45 | 190 | 169 – 213 | 173 | 153 – 194 | 683 | 578 – 777 | 656 | 545 – 766 |
| 192 | 37 | 35 – 40 | 34 | 30 – 38 | 136 | 125 – 148 | 121 | 105 – 142 | 857 | 802 – 904 | 849 | 791 – 902 |

## Annex Table 2 Selected indicators of health expenditure ratios, 1999–2003

Figures computed by WHO to assure comparability;[a] they are not necessarily the official statistics of Member States. which may use alternative methods.

| Member State | Total expenditure on health as % of gross domestic product | | | | | General government expenditure on health as % of total expenditure on health[b] | | | | | Private expenditure on health as % of total expenditure on health[b] | | | | | General government expenditure on health as % of total government expenditure | | | | |
|---|---|---|---|---|---|---|---|---|---|---|---|---|---|---|---|---|---|---|---|---|
| | 1999 | 2000 | 2001 | 2002 | 2003 | 1999 | 2000 | 2001 | 2002 | 2003 | 1999 | 2000 | 2001 | 2002 | 2003 | 1999 | 2000 | 2001 | 2002 | 2003 |
| Afghanistan | 3.2 | 2.8 | 3.2 | 6.7 | 6.5 | 1.5 | 1.5 | 1.9 | 41.1 | 39.5 | 98.5 | 98.5 | 98.1 | 58.9 | 60.5 | 1.6 | 1.6 | 1.6 | 7.4 | 7.3 |
| Albania | 6.9 | 6.5 | 6.6 | 6.8 | 6.5 | 45.2 | 42.4 | 42.2 | 41.7 | 41.7 | 54.8 | 57.6 | 57.8 | 58.3 | 58.3 | 8.9 | 8.6 | 8.8 | 9 | 9.2 |
| Algeria | 3.7 | 3.5 | 3.8 | 4.2 | 4.1 | 71.9 | 73.3 | 77.4 | 78.9 | 80.8 | 28.1 | 26.7 | 22.6 | 21.1 | 19.2 | 9 | 9 | 9.5 | 9.6 | 10 |
| Andorra | 7.3 | 7.5 | 7 | 7.2 | 7.1 | 67.2 | 65.4 | 68.8 | 68.8 | 68.6 | 32.8 | 34.6 | 31.3 | 31.2 | 31.4 | 31.8 | 30.6 | 28.9 | 30.6 | 33.7 |
| Angola | 3.2 | 2.5 | 3.3 | 2.4 | 2.8 | 45.3 | 82.2 | 84.6 | 80.9 | 84.2 | 54.7 | 17.8 | 15.4 | 19.1 | 15.8 | 2.4 | 3.4 | 5.5 | 4.1 | 5.3 |
| Antigua and Barbuda | 4.5 | 4.5 | 4.6 | 5.4 | 4.5 | 72.2 | 72 | 70.8 | 72.4 | 70.6 | 27.8 | 28 | 29.2 | 27.6 | 29.4 | 11.8 | 12.1 | 10.8 | 12.1 | 10.8 |
| Argentina | 9.1 | 8.9 | 9.5 | 8.6 | 8.9 | 56.5 | 55.4 | 53.6 | 52.1 | 48.6 | 43.5 | 44.6 | 46.4 | 47.9 | 51.4 | 15 | 14.7 | 14.3 | 15.2 | 14.7 |
| Armenia | 6 | 6.3 | 6.5 | 5.8 | 6 | 22.9 | 15.2 | 20.5 | 20 | 20.2 | 77.1 | 84.8 | 79.5 | 80 | 79.8 | 5.1 | 3.9 | 5.7 | 5.3 | 5.4 |
| Australia | 8.7 | 9 | 9.2 | 9.3 | 9.5 | 69.5 | 68.9 | 67.8 | 68.1 | 67.5 | 30.5 | 31.1 | 32.2 | 31.9 | 32.5 | 16.9 | 16.8 | 16.9 | 17.7 | 17.7 |
| Austria | 7.6 | 7.5 | 7.4 | 7.5 | 7.5 | 67.7 | 68.1 | 67 | 67.8 | 67.6 | 32.3 | 31.9 | 33 | 32.2 | 32.4 | 9.7 | 10 | 9.8 | 10 | 10 |
| Azerbaijan | 4.7 | 4.1 | 3.9 | 3.7 | 3.6 | 21 | 21.3 | 22.3 | 21.5 | 23.8 | 79 | 78.7 | 77.7 | 78.5 | 76.2 | 4.2 | 4.2 | 4.3 | 2.9 | 2.8 |
| Bahamas | 6.6 | 6.5 | 6.5 | 6.5 | 6.4 | 46.8 | 47.2 | 47.5 | 48.6 | 47.5 | 53.2 | 52.8 | 52.5 | 51.4 | 52.5 | 14.4 | 14.3 | 13.6 | 14.6 | 13.9 |
| Bahrain | 4.7 | 3.9 | 4.2 | 4.2 | 4.1 | 69.2 | 67 | 67.6 | 67.8 | 69.2 | 30.8 | 33 | 32.4 | 32.2 | 30.8 | 11.2 | 10 | 10.1 | 8.7 | 8.8 |
| Bangladesh | 3.2 | 3.2 | 3.2 | 3.3 | 3.4 | 27.2 | 25.6 | 25.8 | 29.6 | 31.3 | 72.8 | 74.4 | 74.2 | 70.4 | 68.7 | 4.7 | 4.3 | 4.7 | 5.4 | 5.8 |
| Barbados | 6.1 | 6.2 | 6.7 | 6.9 | 6.9 | 65.4 | 65.8 | 67.6 | 68.4 | 69.4 | 34.6 | 34.2 | 32.4 | 31.6 | 30.6 | 12 | 12 | 12.2 | 12.3 | 11.1 |
| Belarus | 6.1 | 6.1 | 6.6 | 6.4 | 5.5 | 81 | 80.1 | 75.5 | 73.9 | 71.2 | 19 | 19.9 | 24.5 | 26.1 | 28.8 | 10.4 | 10.7 | 10.7 | 10.1 | 8.3 |
| Belgium | 8.5 | 8.5 | 8.7 | 8.9 | 9.4 | 69.4 | 69.3 | 70.8 | 70.3 | 67.2 | 30.6 | 30.7 | 29.2 | 29.7 | 32.8 | 11.8 | 12.1 | 12.5 | 12.5 | 12.4 |
| Belize | 4.8 | 4.5 | 4.8 | 4.6 | 4.5 | 48.6 | 48 | 45.1 | 47.4 | 49.3 | 51.4 | 52 | 54.9 | 52.6 | 50.7 | 5.5 | 5.3 | 5 | 5.3 | 5 |
| Benin | 4.8 | 4.7 | 5 | 4.7 | 4.4 | 43.8 | 44.5 | 46.9 | 43.5 | 43.1 | 56.2 | 55.5 | 53.1 | 56.5 | 56.9 | 11.1 | 10 | 9.8 | 8 | 9.8 |
| Bhutan | 4.5 | 4.2 | 5.2 | 3.6 | 3.1 | 88.5 | 87.7 | 89.8 | 85.2 | 83.5 | 11.5 | 12.3 | 10.2 | 14.8 | 16.5 | 8.7 | 7.2 | 11.2 | 8.3 | 7.6 |
| Bolivia | 6.2 | 6.1 | 6.4 | 6.6 | 6.7 | 58.1 | 60.1 | 59.3 | 62.8 | 64 | 41.9 | 39.9 | 40.7 | 37.2 | 36 | 10.5 | 9.9 | 10.4 | 11.6 | 11.9 |
| Bosnia and Herzegovina | 10.7 | 9.7 | 9.1 | 9 | 9.5 | 56.7 | 52 | 48.8 | 49.2 | 50.7 | 43.3 | 48 | 51.2 | 50.8 | 49.3 | 8.9 | 7.8 | 7.9 | 8.6 | 11.4 |
| Botswana | 5.2 | 5.4 | 4.8 | 5.1 | 5.6 | 54.3 | 57.2 | 50.4 | 54 | 58.2 | 45.7 | 42.8 | 49.6 | 46 | 41.8 | 6.7 | 7.4 | 6 | 6.4 | 7.5 |
| Brazil | 7.8 | 7.6 | 7.8 | 7.7 | 7.6 | 42.8 | 41 | 42.9 | 44.8 | 45.3 | 57.2 | 59 | 57.1 | 55.2 | 54.7 | 9.3 | 8.5 | 9.2 | 9.7 | 10.3 |
| Brunei Darussalam | 3.7 | 3.4 | 3.5 | 3.5 | 3.5 | 73.1 | 83.5 | 77 | 78.5 | 80 | 26.9 | 16.5 | 23 | 21.5 | 20 | 4.7 | 5.1 | 4.5 | 4.7 | 5.2 |
| Bulgaria | 6 | 6.2 | 7.2 | 7.9 | 7.5 | 65.4 | 59.2 | 56.1 | 56.6 | 54.5 | 34.6 | 40.8 | 43.9 | 43.4 | 45.5 | 9.8 | 8.6 | 9.6 | 11.3 | 10.1 |
| Burkina Faso | 5.4 | 5.2 | 5 | 5.4 | 5.6 | 44 | 42.4 | 39.5 | 44.2 | 46.8 | 56 | 57.6 | 60.5 | 55.8 | 53.2 | 10 | 9.4 | 10.5 | 12.8 | 12.7 |
| Burundi | 3 | 3.1 | 3.1 | 3.1 | 3.1 | 19.9 | 17.9 | 21.6 | 21 | 23.3 | 80.1 | 82.1 | 78.4 | 79 | 76.7 | 2.8 | 2 | 2.2 | 2 | 2 |
| Cambodia | 10.8 | 11 | 10.8 | 10.9 | 10.9 | 10.1 | 14.2 | 14.9 | 17.1 | 19.3 | 89.9 | 85.8 | 85.1 | 82.9 | 80.7 | 7.5 | 10.4 | 9.3 | 9.9 | 11.8 |
| Cameroon | 4.9 | 4.4 | 4.5 | 4.6 | 4.2 | 24.4 | 28 | 27.6 | 27.6 | 28.9 | 75.6 | 72 | 72.4 | 72.4 | 71.1 | 7.2 | 9.6 | 8 | 8.4 | 8 |
| Canada | 9 | 8.9 | 9.4 | 9.6 | 9.9 | 70.3 | 70.3 | 70.1 | 69.7 | 69.9 | 29.7 | 29.7 | 29.9 | 30.3 | 30.1 | 14.6 | 15.1 | 15.5 | 16.1 | 16.7 |
| Cape Verde | 4.5 | 4.6 | 5 | 5 | 4.6 | 73.9 | 73.5 | 75.8 | 75.1 | 73.2 | 26.1 | 26.5 | 24.2 | 24.9 | 26.8 | 9 | 9.6 | 12.4 | 11.1 | 11.1 |
| Central African Republic | 3.6 | 4 | 3.9 | 4 | 4 | 38 | 41.1 | 38.6 | 41.2 | 38.6 | 62 | 58.9 | 61.4 | 58.8 | 61.4 | 6.7 | 10 | 11.5 | 11.2 | 12.4 |
| Chad | 6.1 | 6.7 | 6.8 | 6.3 | 6.5 | 33.6 | 42 | 40.9 | 35.5 | 39.9 | 66.4 | 58 | 59.1 | 64.5 | 60.1 | 11.9 | 13.1 | 13.8 | 9.4 | 10.5 |
| Chile | 7.1 | 6.1 | 6.2 | 6.2 | 6.1 | 39 | 46.4 | 48.1 | 48 | 48.8 | 61 | 53.6 | 51.9 | 52 | 51.2 | 10 | 10.7 | 11.6 | 11.8 | 12.7 |
| China[c] | 4.9 | 5.1 | 5.2 | 5.5 | 5.6 | 40.9 | 38.3 | 35.6 | 35.8 | 36.2 | 59.1 | 61.7 | 64.4 | 64.2 | 63.8 | 12.5 | 11.1 | 9.5 | 9.4 | 9.7 |
| Colombia | 9.3 | 7.7 | 7.7 | 7.5 | 7.6 | 76.3 | 80.9 | 80.2 | 82.2 | 84.1 | 23.7 | 19.1 | 19.8 | 17.8 | 15.9 | 23.2 | 21.4 | 18.6 | 19 | 20.5 |
| Comoros | 3.2 | 2.7 | 2.3 | 2.9 | 2.7 | 60.8 | 54.9 | 47.7 | 58 | 54.1 | 39.2 | 45.1 | 52.3 | 42 | 45.9 | 10.5 | 9.5 | 5 | 6.4 | 6.4 |
| Congo | 2.4 | 1.8 | 2 | 1.9 | 2 | 63.8 | 66.5 | 67 | 66.9 | 64.2 | 36.2 | 33.5 | 33 | 33.1 | 35.8 | 4.9 | 4.8 | 4.2 | 3.7 | 4.3 |
| Cook Islands | 3.6 | 4 | 3.8 | 3.6 | 3.8 | 87.1 | 88 | 87.7 | 87 | 87.9 | 12.9 | 12 | 12.3 | 13 | 12.1 | 7.7 | 8.2 | 8.6 | 8.6 | 9.6 |
| Costa Rica | 6 | 6.3 | 6.8 | 7.2 | 7.3 | 78 | 79 | 78.5 | 79.6 | 78.8 | 22 | 21 | 21.5 | 20.4 | 21.2 | 21 | 21.7 | 21.4 | 22.2 | 22.8 |
| Côte d'Ivoire[d] | 5.1 | 4.7 | 3.9 | 3.8 | 3.6 | 17.4 | 19.8 | 18.3 | 31.6 | 27.6 | 82.6 | 80.2 | 81.7 | 68.4 | 72.4 | 4.5 | 5.2 | 4.3 | 6.2 | 5 |
| Croatia | 8.7 | 9.3 | 8.4 | 7.8 | 7.8 | 86.3 | 86.8 | 85.8 | 82.8 | 83.6 | 13.7 | 13.2 | 14.2 | 17.2 | 16.4 | 13.7 | 14.9 | 14.2 | 13.2 | 13.8 |
| Cuba | 6.9 | 7 | 7.1 | 7.2 | 7.3 | 85.5 | 85.8 | 86 | 86.5 | 86.8 | 14.5 | 14.2 | 14 | 13.5 | 13.2 | 11.1 | 10.8 | 11.4 | 11.2 | 11.2 |
| Cyprus[e] | 5.7 | 5.8 | 5.9 | 6.1 | 6.4 | 42.7 | 41.6 | 42.3 | 44.9 | 49.1 | 57.3 | 58.4 | 57.7 | 55.1 | 50.9 | 6.5 | 6.4 | 6.4 | 6.8 | 7 |
| Czech Republic | 6.6 | 6.6 | 6.9 | 7.2 | 7.5 | 91.5 | 91.4 | 91.4 | 91.1 | 90 | 8.5 | 8.6 | 8.6 | 8.9 | 10 | 14.1 | 14.3 | 13.9 | 13.9 | 12.7 |
| Democratic People's Republic of Korea | 4.8 | 5.9 | 5.8 | 5.8 | 5.8 | 89.2 | 91.4 | 91.2 | 91.3 | 91.2 | 10.8 | 8.6 | 8.8 | 8.7 | 8.8 | 6.8 | 8.1 | 7.8 | 7.5 | 7.3 |
| Democratic Republic of Congo | 3.2 | 3.7 | 3.1 | 3.3 | 4 | 7.7 | 5.3 | 6.8 | 13.1 | 18.3 | 92.3 | 94.7 | 93.2 | 86.9 | 81.7 | 2.6 | 2.6 | 4.7 | 4.2 | 5.4 |
| Denmark | 8.5 | 8.4 | 8.6 | 8.8 | 9 | 82.2 | 82.4 | 82.7 | 82.9 | 83 | 17.8 | 17.6 | 17.3 | 17.1 | 17 | 12.5 | 12.6 | 13 | 13.2 | 13.5 |
| Djibouti | 5.1 | 5.4 | 5.3 | 5.5 | 5.7 | 65.2 | 65.7 | 64.7 | 65 | 66.9 | 34.8 | 34.3 | 35.3 | 35 | 33.1 | 10.2 | 10.7 | 11.6 | 10.8 | 10.5 |
| Dominica | 6.2 | 6.2 | 5.9 | 6.3 | 6.3 | 74.3 | 73.6 | 71.3 | 71.3 | 71.3 | 25.7 | 26.4 | 28.7 | 28.7 | 28.7 | 12.8 | 9.5 | 11.3 | 11.9 | 11.6 |
| Dominican Republic | 6 | 6.8 | 6.9 | 7.3 | 7 | 30.3 | 32.1 | 31.9 | 32.3 | 33.2 | 69.7 | 67.9 | 68.1 | 67.7 | 66.8 | 10.5 | 13.1 | 12 | 12.4 | 12.8 |
| Ecuador | 4.7 | 4.1 | 4.8 | 5 | 5.1 | 39.4 | 31.2 | 33.5 | 38.4 | 38.6 | 60.6 | 68.8 | 66.5 | 61.6 | 61.4 | 9.8 | 6.4 | 8.5 | 9.7 | 8.7 |
| Egypt | 5 | 5.2 | 5.4 | 5.9 | 5.8 | 33.9 | 36.5 | 39.9 | 42.7 | 42.6 | 66.1 | 63.5 | 60.1 | 57.3 | 57.4 | 5.6 | 6.3 | 7.1 | 8.4 | 8.2 |
| El Salvador | 8 | 8 | 7.7 | 8 | 8.1 | 43.5 | 45.1 | 42.4 | 44.7 | 46.1 | 56.5 | 54.9 | 57.6 | 55.3 | 53.9 | 25.1 | 25 | 21.2 | 22.8 | 22 |

| Member State | External resources for health as % of total expenditure on health | | | | | Social security expenditure on health as % of general government expenditure on health | | | | | Out-of-pocket expenditure as % of private expenditure on health | | | | | Private prepaid plans as % of private expenditure on health | | | | |
|---|---|---|---|---|---|---|---|---|---|---|---|---|---|---|---|---|---|---|---|---|
| | 1999 | 2000 | 2001 | 2002 | 2003 | 1999 | 2000 | 2001 | 2002 | 2003 | 1999 | 2000 | 2001 | 2002 | 2003 | 1999 | 2000 | 2001 | 2002 | 2003 |
| Afghanistan | 3 | 3.2 | 4.2 | 46.8 | 45.6 | 0 | 0 | 0 | 0 | 0 | 98.2 | 98 | 97.3 | 75.9 | 76.5 | 0 | 0 | 0 | 0 | 0 |
| Albania | 6.8 | 8.6 | 4.9 | 3.7 | 3.4 | 19.2 | 16.7 | 18.1 | 20.3 | 25.1 | 99.7 | 99.8 | 99.8 | 99.8 | 99.8 | 0 | 0 | 0 | 0 | 0 |
| Algeria | 0.1 | 0.1 | 0.1 | 0 | 0 | 40.8 | 35.5 | 33.3 | 29.1 | 28.4 | 97 | 96.7 | 96 | 95.7 | 95.3 | 2.9 | 3.1 | 3.8 | 4.1 | 4.4 |
| Andorra | 0 | 0 | 0 | 0 | 0 | 87.5 | 88.1 | 86.2 | 88 | 89.2 | 77.9 | 77.5 | 70 | 70.6 | 71.1 | 19.9 | 20.3 | 26.7 | 26.5 | 26.3 |
| Angola | 5.7 | 17.5 | 16.7 | 8.3 | 6.7 | 0 | 0 | 0 | 0 | 0 | 100 | 100 | 100 | 100 | 100 | 0 | 0 | 0 | 0 | 0 |
| Antigua and Barbuda | 3.8 | 3.8 | 3.4 | 1 | 2.2 | 0 | 0 | 0 | 0 | 0 | 100 | 100 | 100 | 100 | 100 | n/a | n/a | n/a | n/a | n/a |
| Argentina | 0.3 | 0.3 | 0.3 | 0.3 | 0.2 | 58.7 | 59.3 | 58.5 | 57.9 | 56.8 | 64 | 63.3 | 62.4 | 60.3 | 55.6 | 31.9 | 32.6 | 31.1 | 32.7 | 38.2 |
| Armenia | 19 | 13 | 21.9 | 22.2 | 17.2 | 0 | 0 | 0 | 0 | 0 | 82.2 | 91 | 79.6 | 79.4 | 80.6 | n/a | n/a | 0.1 | 0.1 | n/a |
| Australia | 0 | 0 | 0 | 0 | 0 | 0 | 0 | 0 | 0 | 0 | 62.5 | 65.2 | 65.9 | 67.6 | 67.8 | 21.8 | 21.9 | 23.7 | 23.3 | 23.9 |
| Austria | 0 | 0 | 0 | 0 | 0 | 63.5 | 64 | 65.4 | 65.5 | 65.8 | 62.9 | 63.8 | 58.9 | 59.8 | 59.2 | 22.9 | 23 | 22.9 | 23.6 | 23.5 |
| Azerbaijan | 1 | 2.1 | 4.1 | 1.9 | 1.9 | 0 | 0 | 0 | 0 | 0 | 96.3 | 96 | 96.1 | 96.2 | 96.8 | 0 | 0 | 0 | 0 | 0 |
| Bahamas | 0 | 0 | 0.2 | 0.2 | 0.2 | 1.8 | 1.8 | 1.7 | 1.6 | 1.7 | 40.3 | 40.3 | 40.3 | 40.3 | 40.5 | 58.6 | 58.6 | 58.6 | 58.6 | 58.4 |
| Bahrain | 0 | 0 | 0 | 0 | 0 | 0.4 | 0.5 | 0.5 | 0.5 | 0.5 | 72.1 | 68.7 | 65.8 | 62.4 | 61.2 | 22.7 | 25.4 | 24.2 | 24.1 | 22 |
| Bangladesh | 12.2 | 12.9 | 13.3 | 12.9 | 12.4 | 0 | 0 | 0 | 0 | 0 | 88.8 | 86.5 | 86 | 85.9 | 85.8 | 0 | 0 | 0 | 0.1 | 0.1 |
| Barbados | 4.2 | 4 | 4.4 | 4.2 | 2.7 | 0 | 0 | 0 | 0 | 0 | 77.2 | 77.3 | 76.9 | 77.2 | 77.2 | 22.8 | 22.7 | 23.1 | 22.8 | 22.8 |
| Belarus | 0.1 | 0.1 | 0.2 | 0.1 | n/a | 3.8 | 4.1 | 3.7 | 3.9 | 6.1 | 70.2 | 70.4 | 74.7 | 79.7 | 80.5 | 0.6 | 0.3 | 0.1 | 0.2 | 0.2 |
| Belgium | 0 | 0 | 0 | 0 | 0 | 87.3 | 87.6 | 87.4 | 88.8 | 88.4 | 80.9 | 80.2 | 79.5 | 80.5 | 66.6 | 6.6 | 6.4 | 6.7 | 6.6 | 6 |
| Belize | 3.1 | 2.9 | 8.5 | 8 | 7.3 | 0 | 0 | 12.5 | 21.6 | 22.8 | 100 | 100 | 100 | 100 | 100 | 0 | 0 | 0 | 0 | 0 |
| Benin | 14.6 | 16.8 | 12.2 | 8.5 | 11.5 | n/a | n/a | n/a | n/a | n/a | 91 | 91 | 90.6 | 90.3 | 90.3 | 8.4 | 8.4 | 8.7 | 9 | 9 |
| Bhutan | 32.5 | 31.2 | 45.7 | 23.9 | 18.6 | 0 | 0 | 0 | 0 | 0 | 100 | 100 | 100 | 100 | 100 | 0 | 0 | 0 | 0 | 0 |
| Bolivia | 5.7 | 6 | 7.1 | 7.4 | 7.3 | 60.9 | 62 | 65.2 | 65 | 65 | 83.8 | 81.6 | 77.9 | 78.9 | 79.3 | 5.5 | 8.1 | 12 | 10.8 | 10.6 |
| Bosnia and Herzegovina | 3.9 | 5.2 | 3 | 1.8 | 1.5 | 79 | 78 | 79 | 83.5 | 77.5 | 100 | 100 | 100 | 100 | 100 | n/a | n/a | n/a | n/a | n/a |
| Botswana | 2.2 | 1.8 | 2.9 | 3.4 | 2.9 | n/a | n/a | n/a | n/a | n/a | 30.3 | 31.3 | 31.5 | 29.7 | 28.8 | 22.7 | 20.6 | 20 | 19.6 | 21.8 |
| Brazil | 0.5 | 0.5 | 0.5 | 0.5 | 0.3 | 0 | 0 | 0 | 0 | 0 | 67.1 | 64.9 | 64.1 | 64.2 | 64.2 | 32.9 | 35.1 | 35.9 | 35.8 | 35.8 |
| Brunei Darussalam | n/a | n/a | n/a | n/a | n/a | 0 | 0 | 0 | 0 | 0 | 100 | 100 | 100 | 100 | 100 | 0 | 0 | 0 | 0 | 0 |
| Bulgaria | 0.5 | 2 | 1.5 | 1.3 | 1 | 9.9 | 13 | 35.8 | 40.6 | 51.6 | 99 | 99 | 99.2 | 98.4 | 98.4 | 0 | 0 | 0.1 | 0.9 | 0.9 |
| Burkina Faso | 10.2 | 9.9 | 10.1 | 7 | 7.4 | 0.3 | 0.8 | 1.2 | 0.7 | 1 | 98.1 | 98.1 | 98.1 | 98.1 | 98.1 | 0.9 | 0.9 | 0.9 | 0.9 | 0.9 |
| Burundi | 10.7 | 8 | 10.6 | 10.3 | 14.1 | n/a | n/a | n/a | n/a | n/a | 100 | 100 | 100 | 100 | 100 | n/a | n/a | n/a | n/a | n/a |
| Cambodia | 13.4 | 18.8 | 19.7 | 11.5 | 18.5 | 0 | 0 | 0 | 0 | 0 | 90.1 | 85.4 | 84.6 | 85.2 | 86.2 | 0 | 0 | 0 | 0 | 0 |
| Cameroon | 5.2 | 6 | 6.9 | 2.3 | 3.2 | 0.1 | 0.1 | 0.1 | 0.1 | 0.1 | 94.2 | 93.3 | 93.4 | 93.6 | 98.3 | n/a | n/a | n/a | n/a | n/a |
| Canada | 0 | 0 | 0 | 0 | 0 | 1.9 | 2 | 2 | 2 | 2.1 | 55 | 53.6 | 51.1 | 50.4 | 49.6 | 37.9 | 39 | 41.6 | 42.1 | 42.3 |
| Cape Verde | 8.4 | 13.5 | 15.1 | 15.2 | 10 | 36.9 | 36.1 | 35.1 | 33.6 | 35.5 | 99.7 | 99.6 | 99.5 | 99.8 | 99.7 | 0.3 | 0.4 | 0.5 | 0.2 | 0.3 |
| Central African Republic | 20 | 20 | 15.4 | 13.4 | 2.9 | n/a | n/a | n/a | n/a | n/a | 95.1 | 95.5 | 95.5 | 95.5 | 95.3 | n/a | n/a | n/a | n/a | n/a |
| Chad | 29.1 | 36.6 | 33.8 | 17 | 11.8 | n/a | n/a | n/a | n/a | n/a | 96.7 | 96.5 | 96.6 | 96.5 | 96.3 | 0.3 | 0.4 | 0.4 | 0.4 | 0.4 |
| Chile | 0.1 | 0.1 | 0.1 | 0 | 0 | 77.2 | 31.1 | 31.6 | 32.2 | 32.1 | 60.6 | 47.1 | 48 | 47.3 | 46.2 | 39.4 | 52.9 | 52 | 52.7 | 53.8 |
| China[c] | 0.3 | 0.2 | 0.2 | 0.1 | 0.1 | 54.2 | 57.2 | 55.1 | 54.8 | 53.4 | 94.5 | 95.6 | 93.1 | 90 | 87.6 | 1.7 | 1 | 1.9 | 3.3 | 5.8 |
| Colombia | 0.3 | 0.3 | 0.2 | 0 | 0 | 63.2 | 60.2 | 66.3 | 63.9 | 66 | 72.4 | 59 | 59.1 | 55.9 | 47.2 | 27.6 | 41 | 40.9 | 44.1 | 52.8 |
| Comoros | 47.6 | 35.9 | 26.2 | 43 | 40.5 | 0 | 0 | 0 | 0 | 0 | 100 | 100 | 100 | 100 | 100 | 0 | 0 | 0 | 0 | 0 |
| Congo | 2.8 | 2.4 | 2.5 | 2.4 | 2.2 | 0 | 0 | 0 | 0 | 0 | 100 | 100 | 100 | 100 | 100 | n/a | n/a | n/a | n/a | n/a |
| Cook Islands | 35.9 | 28.4 | 25.8 | 6.8 | 12.2 | 0 | 0 | 0 | 0 | 0 | 100 | 100 | 100 | 100 | 100 | 0 | 0 | 0 | 0 | 0 |
| Costa Rica | 1 | 1 | 1.9 | 1.6 | 2.7 | 90.7 | 89.6 | 87.5 | 88.4 | 88.6 | 97.5 | 97.4 | 97.8 | 97.8 | 88.7 | 2.5 | 2.6 | 2.2 | 2.2 | 2.1 |
| Côte d'Ivoire[d] | 2.7 | 2.9 | 3.5 | 3.7 | 3.4 | n/a | n/a | n/a | n/a | n/a | 94 | 93.4 | 92.1 | 90.3 | 90.5 | 6 | 6.6 | 7.9 | 9.7 | 9.5 |
| Croatia | 0.9 | 1 | 1 | 1 | 0.6 | 97.5 | 97.6 | 97.7 | 97.9 | 96.1 | 100 | 100 | 100 | 100 | 100 | 0 | 0 | 0 | 0 | 0 |
| Cuba | 0.2 | 0.2 | 0.3 | 0.2 | 0.2 | 0 | 0 | 0 | 0 | 0 | 76 | 75.6 | 75.2 | 75.2 | 75.2 | 0 | 0 | 0 | 0 | 0 |
| Cyprus[e] | 0 | 0 | 2.8 | 2.6 | 2.3 | 9.5 | 10.9 | 11.9 | 12.5 | 10.7 | 95.3 | 95.3 | 95.6 | 95.7 | 96 | 4.7 | 4.7 | 4.4 | 4.3 | 4 |
| Czech Republic | 0 | 0 | 0 | 0 | 0 | 89.4 | 89.4 | 90.4 | 87.4 | 85.4 | 100 | 100 | 100 | 93.6 | 83.9 | 0 | 0 | 0 | 2.5 | 2.5 |
| Democratic People's Republic of Korea | 0.2 | 0.2 | 0.3 | 17.3 | 19.1 | 0 | 0 | 0 | 0 | 0 | 100 | 100 | 100 | 100 | 100 | 0 | 0 | 0 | 0 | 0 |
| Democratic Republic of Congo | 6 | 4.9 | 6.6 | 12.7 | 15.1 | 0 | 0 | 0 | 0 | 0 | 100 | 100 | 100 | 100 | 100 | n/a | n/a | n/a | n/a | n/a |
| Denmark | 0 | 0 | 0 | 0 | 0 | 0 | 0 | 0 | 0 | 0 | 90.4 | 91 | 92 | 92.8 | 92.5 | 9.6 | 9 | 8 | 7.2 | 7.5 |
| Djibouti | 22.2 | 26.4 | 31.2 | 31.6 | 31.5 | 11.6 | 12.1 | 12 | 13.3 | 12.9 | 100 | 100 | 100 | 100 | 100 | n/a | n/a | n/a | n/a | n/a |
| Dominica | 2.1 | 1.2 | 0.9 | 0.5 | 0.4 | 0 | 0 | 0 | 0 | 0 | 100 | 100 | 100 | 100 | 100 | n/a | n/a | n/a | n/a | n/a |
| Dominican Republic | 3 | 2.2 | 1.5 | 2 | 1.5 | 20.3 | 22.4 | 20.5 | 19.9 | 17.4 | 80.4 | 77.4 | 73.3 | 70.6 | 70.8 | 9.4 | 12.8 | 17.3 | 20 | 20.7 |
| Ecuador | 3.2 | 4.1 | 1.8 | 1 | 0.9 | 31.7 | 28 | 32.2 | 32 | 31.9 | 84.2 | 85.3 | 87.6 | 88.4 | 88.1 | 5.4 | 4.8 | 3 | 2.3 | 2.2 |
| Egypt | 1.3 | 1.1 | 1.3 | 0.8 | 0.9 | 32.8 | 32.7 | 30.2 | 24.7 | 27.1 | 93.7 | 93.8 | 93.7 | 93.9 | 93.2 | 0.4 | 0.4 | 0.4 | 0.4 | 0.3 |
| El Salvador | 1.5 | 0.9 | 0.8 | 0.7 | 1 | 44 | 44.2 | 36.3 | 44.5 | 44.1 | 90.2 | 95.6 | 93.6 | 93.9 | 93.5 | 9.6 | 4.2 | 6.4 | 6.1 | 6.3 |

## Annex Table 2 Selected indicators of health expenditure ratios, 1999–2003

Figures computed by WHO to assure comparability;[a] they are not necessarily the official statistics of Member States. which may use alternative methods.

| Member State | Total expenditure on health as % of gross domestic product | | | | | General government expenditure on health as % of total expenditure on health[b] | | | | | Private expenditure on health as % of total expenditure on health[b] | | | | | General government expenditure on health as % of total government expenditure | | | | |
|---|---|---|---|---|---|---|---|---|---|---|---|---|---|---|---|---|---|---|---|---|
| | 1999 | 2000 | 2001 | 2002 | 2003 | 1999 | 2000 | 2001 | 2002 | 2003 | 1999 | 2000 | 2001 | 2002 | 2003 | 1999 | 2000 | 2001 | 2002 | 2003 |
| Equatorial Guinea | 2.8 | 2 | 1.7 | 1.8 | 1.5 | 60.8 | 67.6 | 70.2 | 72.2 | 67.5 | 39.2 | 32.4 | 29.8 | 27.8 | 32.5 | 9.9 | 11 | 10.1 | 8.8 | 7 |
| Eritrea | 3.8 | 4.5 | 4.6 | 4.5 | 4.4 | 70.3 | 66.9 | 59.2 | 50.9 | 45.5 | 29.7 | 33.1 | 40.8 | 49.1 | 54.5 | 2.9 | 4.4 | 4.6 | 3.9 | 4 |
| Estonia | 6 | 5.5 | 5.1 | 5 | 5.3 | 81 | 77.5 | 78.6 | 77.1 | 77.1 | 19 | 22.5 | 21.4 | 22.9 | 22.9 | 11.4 | 11.1 | 10.7 | 10.6 | 11.2 |
| Ethiopia | 5.4 | 5.7 | 5.8 | 6 | 5.9 | 53 | 54.6 | 53.2 | 56.9 | 58.4 | 47 | 45.4 | 46.8 | 43.1 | 41.6 | 8.9 | 9.3 | 10.5 | 9.9 | 9.6 |
| Fiji | 3.7 | 3.9 | 3.8 | 4.1 | 3.7 | 65.2 | 65.2 | 66.4 | 66.4 | 61.3 | 34.8 | 34.8 | 33.6 | 33.6 | 38.7 | 7.3 | 8.1 | 7.9 | 8.3 | 7.8 |
| Finland | 6.9 | 6.6 | 6.9 | 7.2 | 7.4 | 75.3 | 75.1 | 75.9 | 76.3 | 76.5 | 24.7 | 24.9 | 24.1 | 23.7 | 23.5 | 10 | 10.2 | 10.7 | 11 | 11.2 |
| France | 9.3 | 9.3 | 9.4 | 9.7 | 10.1 | 76 | 75.8 | 75.9 | 76.1 | 76.3 | 24 | 24.2 | 24.1 | 23.9 | 23.7 | 13.3 | 13.5 | 13.7 | 13.8 | 14.2 |
| Gabon | 4.5 | 4.2 | 4.2 | 4.4 | 4.4 | 68.4 | 73.1 | 73 | 69.8 | 66.6 | 31.6 | 26.9 | 27 | 30.2 | 33.4 | 10.9 | 13.9 | 9.9 | 10.7 | 12.8 |
| Gambia | 7 | 7.9 | 7.8 | 7.5 | 8.1 | 32.3 | 40.5 | 40.1 | 40.9 | 40 | 67.7 | 59.5 | 59.9 | 59.1 | 60 | 10 | 14.4 | 9.4 | 12 | 13.9 |
| Georgia | 2.9 | 4.3 | 4.4 | 4.5 | 4 | 35.4 | 28.4 | 30 | 28.8 | 23.9 | 64.6 | 71.6 | 70 | 71.2 | 76.1 | 4.8 | 6.4 | 6.6 | 6.6 | 4.7 |
| Germany | 10.6 | 10.6 | 10.8 | 10.9 | 11.1 | 78.5 | 78.6 | 78.4 | 78.6 | 78.2 | 21.5 | 21.4 | 21.6 | 21.4 | 21.8 | 17.1 | 18.2 | 17.4 | 17.6 | 17.6 |
| Ghana | 5.5 | 5.4 | 4.8 | 4.7 | 4.5 | 35.3 | 35.3 | 28.8 | 30.5 | 31.8 | 64.7 | 64.7 | 71.2 | 69.5 | 68.2 | 7.8 | 6.8 | 4.2 | 5.4 | 5 |
| Greece | 9.6 | 9.9 | 10.2 | 9.8 | 9.9 | 53.4 | 52.6 | 54.2 | 51.6 | 51.3 | 46.6 | 47.4 | 45.8 | 48.4 | 48.7 | 10.4 | 10 | 10.9 | 10.1 | 10.1 |
| Grenada | 5.5 | 7.2 | 7.6 | 7.1 | 6.7 | 73.3 | 74 | 77.9 | 72.9 | 73.6 | 26.7 | 26 | 22.1 | 27.1 | 26.4 | 14.7 | 13.2 | 15.1 | 10.7 | 12.4 |
| Guatemala | 4.7 | 5.5 | 5.4 | 5.2 | 5.4 | 48.3 | 39.8 | 38.1 | 36.9 | 39.7 | 51.7 | 60.2 | 61.9 | 63.1 | 60.3 | 17 | 16.2 | 15.4 | 14.1 | 15.3 |
| Guinea | 4.7 | 4.8 | 4.8 | 5.2 | 5.4 | 13.4 | 13.5 | 18.3 | 14.7 | 16.6 | 86.6 | 86.5 | 81.7 | 85.3 | 83.4 | 3.9 | 3.9 | 4.7 | 4.2 | 4.9 |
| Guinea-Bissau | 4.8 | 4.1 | 4.3 | 6.2 | 5.6 | 29.7 | 23.7 | 21.3 | 40.8 | 45.8 | 70.3 | 76.3 | 78.7 | 59.2 | 54.2 | 4.6 | 2.2 | 2.1 | 6.6 | 6.9 |
| Guyana | 4.3 | 5.5 | 5.3 | 5 | 4.8 | 82.8 | 84.5 | 82.6 | 83.1 | 82.6 | 17.2 | 15.5 | 17.4 | 16.9 | 17.4 | 8 | 10.8 | 12.3 | 12.2 | 11.6 |
| Haiti | 6.8 | 6.8 | 7.1 | 7.5 | 7.5 | 36.3 | 36 | 37.7 | 39.4 | 38.1 | 63.7 | 64 | 62.3 | 60.6 | 61.9 | 18.5 | 20.7 | 23.8 | 23.8 | 23.8 |
| Honduras | 5.7 | 6.4 | 6.5 | 6.9 | 7.1 | 50.8 | 55.9 | 54.7 | 55.3 | 56.5 | 49.2 | 44.1 | 45.3 | 44.7 | 43.5 | 12.2 | 15.1 | 14.1 | 15.6 | 16.8 |
| Hungary | 7.4 | 7.1 | 7.4 | 7.8 | 8.4 | 72.4 | 70.7 | 69 | 70.2 | 72.4 | 27.6 | 29.3 | 31 | 29.8 | 27.6 | 10.7 | 10.6 | 10.5 | 10.4 | 12.1 |
| Iceland | 9.4 | 9.3 | 9.3 | 10 | 10.5 | 83.6 | 82.6 | 82.7 | 83.2 | 83.5 | 16.4 | 17.4 | 17.3 | 16.8 | 16.5 | 18.1 | 17.8 | 17.5 | 18.2 | 18.3 |
| India | 5.1 | 5 | 5 | 4.9 | 4.8 | 24.6 | 24.6 | 24.2 | 23.7 | 24.8 | 75.4 | 75.4 | 75.8 | 76.3 | 75.2 | 4.5 | 4.3 | 4.2 | 3.9 | 3.9 |
| Indonesia | 2.6 | 2.5 | 3.1 | 3.2 | 3.1 | 30.4 | 28.1 | 35.6 | 34.5 | 35.9 | 69.6 | 71.9 | 64.4 | 65.5 | 64.1 | 3.8 | 3.5 | 4.7 | 5.1 | 5.1 |
| Iran, Islamic Republic of | 6.2 | 5.8 | 6.3 | 5.8 | 6.5 | 41.1 | 43.2 | 44.5 | 37.7 | 47.3 | 58.9 | 56.8 | 55.5 | 62.3 | 52.7 | 10.9 | 11.7 | 11.5 | 8 | 10.3 |
| Iraq[f] | 1.9 | 1.7 | 1.6 | 1.6 | 2.7 | 39.6 | 29.1 | 27.1 | 16.8 | 51.8 | 60.4 | 70.9 | 72.9 | 83.2 | 48.2 | 1.2 | 1.3 | 1.2 | 0.7 | 4.2 |
| Ireland | 6.2 | 6.2 | 6.8 | 7 | 7.3 | 73.7 | 73.9 | 75.3 | 77.5 | 78.9 | 26.3 | 26.1 | 24.7 | 22.5 | 21.1 | 13.4 | 14.6 | 15.4 | 16.3 | 17.2 |
| Israel | 8.6 | 8.6 | 9.2 | 9.3 | 8.9 | 69.5 | 67.9 | 67.7 | 67.2 | 68.2 | 30.5 | 32.1 | 32.3 | 32.8 | 31.8 | 11.3 | 11.5 | 11.6 | 11.4 | 11.4 |
| Italy | 7.7 | 8.1 | 8.2 | 8.4 | 8.4 | 72 | 73.5 | 75.8 | 75.4 | 75.1 | 28 | 26.5 | 24.2 | 24.6 | 24.9 | 11.4 | 12.6 | 12.7 | 13.1 | 12.8 |
| Jamaica | 5.4 | 6.2 | 5.4 | 4.9 | 5.3 | 50.3 | 52.6 | 45.7 | 51.1 | 50.6 | 49.7 | 47.4 | 54.3 | 48.9 | 49.4 | 5.6 | 6.6 | 4.3 | 4.5 | 4.5 |
| Japan | 7.4 | 7.6 | 7.8 | 7.9 | 7.9 | 81.1 | 81.3 | 81.7 | 81.5 | 81 | 18.9 | 18.7 | 18.3 | 18.5 | 19 | 15.9 | 16.1 | 16.9 | 16.8 | 16.8 |
| Jordan[g] | 8.8 | 9.2 | 9.4 | 9.3 | 9.4 | 48 | 45.2 | 45.7 | 46.3 | 45.2 | 52 | 54.8 | 54.3 | 53.7 | 54.8 | 10.1 | 9.8 | 9.8 | 9.9 | 8.9 |
| Kazakhstan | 4.3 | 4.1 | 3.4 | 3.5 | 3.5 | 51.9 | 50.9 | 56.4 | 53.2 | 57.3 | 48.1 | 49.1 | 43.6 | 46.8 | 42.7 | 8.8 | 9.3 | 8.4 | 9 | 9 |
| Kenya | 4.6 | 4.3 | 4.2 | 4.5 | 4.3 | 41.1 | 46.5 | 42.8 | 44 | 38.7 | 58.9 | 53.5 | 57.2 | 56 | 61.3 | 4.1 | 11.1 | 8 | 9.2 | 7.2 |
| Kiribati | 7.6 | 10.7 | 11.5 | 11.3 | 13.1 | 98.9 | 99.1 | 99.2 | 99.1 | 92.4 | 1.1 | 0.9 | 0.8 | 0.9 | 7.6 | 6.8 | 9.8 | 10.5 | 10.4 | 7.8 |
| Kuwait | 3.6 | 3.1 | 3.6 | 3.9 | 3.5 | 77.2 | 78.2 | 77.7 | 78.1 | 77.5 | 22.8 | 21.8 | 22.3 | 21.9 | 22.5 | 6.4 | 8.8 | 6.2 | 6.6 | 6.1 |
| Kyrgyzstan | 4.9 | 4.4 | 4.5 | 5.1 | 5.3 | 48 | 46.8 | 43 | 41.3 | 40.8 | 52 | 53.2 | 57 | 58.7 | 59.2 | 7.8 | 8.2 | 8.7 | 8.7 | 9 |
| Lao People's Democratic Republic | 2.4 | 2.5 | 2.7 | 2.9 | 3.2 | 41.5 | 38.7 | 40.5 | 44.5 | 38.5 | 58.5 | 61.3 | 59.5 | 55.5 | 61.5 | 6 | 4.8 | 5.4 | 7.6 | 6.2 |
| Latvia | 6.4 | 6 | 6.2 | 6.3 | 6.4 | 59 | 55 | 51.2 | 52.1 | 51.3 | 41 | 45 | 48.8 | 47.9 | 48.7 | 9.1 | 8.9 | 9.1 | 9.3 | 9.4 |
| Lebanon | 11.3 | 11.7 | 11.7 | 10.6 | 10.2 | 27.5 | 28.5 | 30.2 | 30.1 | 29.3 | 72.5 | 71.5 | 69.8 | 69.9 | 70.7 | 9.5 | 7.9 | 10.2 | 8.8 | 8.4 |
| Lesotho | 5.4 | 5.8 | 5.6 | 6.5 | 5.2 | 80.9 | 82.6 | 82 | 83.1 | 79.7 | 19.1 | 17.4 | 18 | 16.9 | 20.3 | 9.1 | 9.7 | 10.1 | 10.9 | 9.5 |
| Liberia | 6.3 | 4.8 | 4.1 | 3.9 | 4.7 | 67.7 | 57.7 | 50.3 | 47.7 | 56.7 | 32.3 | 42.3 | 49.7 | 52.3 | 43.3 | 18.1 | 13 | 12.4 | 10.5 | 17.6 |
| Libyan Arab Jamahiriya | 3.6 | 3.2 | 5.5 | 5 | 4.1 | 50.7 | 58.1 | 73.2 | 65.5 | 62.9 | 49.3 | 41.9 | 26.8 | 34.5 | 37.1 | 5.5 | 6 | 9.2 | 7.9 | 5.9 |
| Lithuania | 6.3 | 6.5 | 6.3 | 6.5 | 6.6 | 74.9 | 69.7 | 72.6 | 74.9 | 76 | 25.1 | 30.3 | 27.4 | 25.1 | 24 | 12.2 | 14.6 | 15.2 | 14.2 | 14.7 |
| Luxembourg | 6.2 | 6 | 6.3 | 7.1 | 6.8 | 89.8 | 90.3 | 90.8 | 91.1 | 90.8 | 10.2 | 9.7 | 9.2 | 8.9 | 9.2 | 13.4 | 14 | 14.7 | 14.8 | 13.7 |
| Madagascar | 2.2 | 2.1 | 1.9 | 2.8 | 2.7 | 53.7 | 53 | 64.7 | 63 | 63.4 | 46.3 | 47 | 35.3 | 37 | 36.6 | 6.9 | 6.5 | 7 | 11.4 | 9.3 |
| Malawi | 9.8 | 8.6 | 10.5 | 9.4 | 9.3 | 36.9 | 30.2 | 45.2 | 34 | 35.2 | 63.1 | 69.8 | 54.8 | 66 | 64.8 | 12.2 | 7.5 | 11.7 | 9.1 | 9.1 |
| Malaysia | 3.2 | 3.3 | 3.7 | 3.7 | 3.8 | 51.2 | 52.4 | 55.8 | 55.4 | 58.2 | 48.8 | 47.6 | 44.2 | 44.6 | 41.8 | 6.5 | 6.5 | 6.4 | 6.6 | 6.9 |
| Maldives | 5.6 | 5.9 | 6 | 5.8 | 6.2 | 85.2 | 86.9 | 87.5 | 87.7 | 89 | 14.8 | 13.1 | 12.5 | 12.3 | 11 | 13.2 | 13.7 | 13.8 | 13.3 | 13.8 |
| Mali | 4 | 4.7 | 4.3 | 4.5 | 4.8 | 42.9 | 49.5 | 50.1 | 52.6 | 57.4 | 57.1 | 50.5 | 49.9 | 47.4 | 42.6 | 6.6 | 8.5 | 8.2 | 9 | 9.2 |
| Malta | 7 | 8 | 8 | 9.1 | 9.3 | 75.6 | 76.5 | 77.8 | 79.7 | 80.1 | 24.4 | 23.5 | 22.2 | 20.3 | 19.9 | 11.9 | 14.2 | 13.8 | 15.3 | 15.5 |
| Marshall Islands | 15.9 | 14.7 | 12.4 | 12 | 13.1 | 97.2 | 96.9 | 96.3 | 96.3 | 96.7 | 2.8 | 3.1 | 3.7 | 3.7 | 3.3 | 17.9 | 13.7 | 12.1 | 11.5 | 14.4 |
| Mauritania | 2.7 | 2.5 | 2.9 | 3.9 | 4.2 | 64.2 | 63.3 | 67.9 | 74.2 | 76.8 | 35.8 | 36.7 | 32.1 | 25.8 | 23.2 | 8.6 | 6.5 | 6.8 | 9.2 | 14.3 |
| Mauritius | 3.1 | 3.3 | 3.5 | 3.6 | 3.7 | 62 | 58.7 | 60.5 | 60.7 | 60.8 | 38 | 41.3 | 39.5 | 39.3 | 39.2 | 7.2 | 6.6 | 9 | 9.4 | 9.2 |
| Mexico | 5.6 | 5.6 | 6 | 6 | 6.2 | 47.8 | 46.6 | 44.8 | 44.9 | 46.4 | 52.2 | 53.4 | 55.2 | 55.1 | 53.6 | 12.2 | 11.4 | 11.9 | 11.6 | 11.7 |

| Member State | External resources for health as % of total expenditure on health | | | | | Social security expenditure on health as % of general government expenditure on health | | | | | Out-of-pocket expenditure as % of private expenditure on health | | | | | Private prepaid plans as % of private expenditure on health | | | | |
|---|---|---|---|---|---|---|---|---|---|---|---|---|---|---|---|---|---|---|---|---|
| | 1999 | 2000 | 2001 | 2002 | 2003 | 1999 | 2000 | 2001 | 2002 | 2003 | 1999 | 2000 | 2001 | 2002 | 2003 | 1999 | 2000 | 2001 | 2002 | 2003 |
| Equatorial Guinea | 9.2 | 7.7 | 5.9 | 3.6 | 5.5 | 0 | 0 | 0 | 0 | 0 | 91.8 | 83.9 | 81.3 | 80.5 | 80.5 | 0 | 0 | 0 | 0 | 0 |
| Eritrea | 20.2 | 30.6 | 24.1 | 22.5 | 19.6 | 0 | 0 | 0 | 0 | 0 | 100 | 100 | 100 | 100 | 100 | 0 | 0 | 0 | 0 | 0 |
| Estonia | 3.6 | 0.9 | 0 | 0 | 0.1 | 82.1 | 86 | 86.1 | 86 | 84.9 | 74.4 | 88.5 | 88.9 | 87.6 | 88.3 | n/a | n/a | n/a | n/a | n/a |
| Ethiopia | 22.6 | 19.3 | 23.4 | 21.7 | 26 | 0.4 | 0.4 | 0.4 | 0.4 | 0.4 | 79.7 | 79.1 | 79.8 | 79.3 | 78.7 | 0.4 | 0.5 | 0.5 | 0.5 | 0.5 |
| Fiji | 11.1 | 10.9 | 10.3 | 5.7 | 13.4 | 0 | 0 | 0 | 0 | 0 | 100 | 100 | 100 | 100 | 100 | 0 | 0 | 0 | 0 | 0 |
| Finland | 0 | 0 | 0 | 0 | 0 | 19.8 | 20.4 | 20.8 | 21.1 | 21.5 | 82.2 | 82 | 81.8 | 81.7 | 81.2 | 10.8 | 10.5 | 10.4 | 10 | 10.2 |
| France | 0 | 0 | 0 | 0 | 0 | 96.7 | 96.6 | 96.5 | 96.6 | 96.7 | 43 | 43.4 | 43.3 | 42.5 | 42.2 | 52.6 | 52.2 | 52.5 | 53.2 | 53.5 |
| Gabon | 2.4 | 1 | 1.6 | 0.7 | 0.7 | 1.7 | 1.6 | 1.7 | 1.7 | 1.7 | 100 | 100 | 100 | 100 | 100 | n/a | n/a | n/a | n/a | n/a |
| Gambia | 29.8 | 35.8 | 30.8 | 18.5 | 21.8 | 0 | 0 | 0 | 0 | 0 | 68.1 | 69.3 | 69.6 | 69.2 | 67 | n/a | n/a | n/a | n/a | n/a |
| Georgia | 6.8 | 8.6 | 4.4 | 10.7 | 5.3 | 48.8 | 44 | 42.8 | 46.5 | 59.2 | 99.5 | 98.9 | 96.9 | 98.2 | 98.2 | 0.5 | 1.1 | 3.1 | 1.8 | 1.8 |
| Germany | 0 | 0 | 0 | 0 | 0 | 87.2 | 87.3 | 87.1 | 87.2 | 87.4 | 50.8 | 49.6 | 49.7 | 48.2 | 47.9 | 38 | 38.7 | 38.6 | 39.9 | 40.2 |
| Ghana | 6.4 | 12.8 | 20.7 | 14.4 | 15.8 | n/a | n/a | n/a | n/a | n/a | 100 | 100 | 100 | 100 | 100 | 0 | 0 | 0 | 0 | 0 |
| Greece | n/a | n/a | n/a | n/a | n/a | 35.4 | 32.3 | 33.2 | 36.6 | 32 | 69.5 | 94.7 | 95.2 | 95 | 95.4 | 4.1 | 5.3 | 4.8 | 5 | 4.6 |
| Grenada | n/a | n/a | n/a | 10.5 | 10.3 | 0 | 0 | 0 | 0 | 0 | 100 | 100 | 100 | 100 | 100 | n/a | n/a | n/a | n/a | n/a |
| Guatemala | 2.4 | 3.4 | 2.5 | 2.2 | 3.8 | 54.8 | 52.3 | 51 | 52 | 50.5 | 85.6 | 89.7 | 90 | 90.5 | 91.9 | 5.4 | 4.2 | 4.2 | 4.2 | 3.9 |
| Guinea | 5.5 | 5.8 | 10.5 | 6.3 | 7.3 | 1.8 | 1.8 | 1.5 | 1.7 | 1.5 | 99.4 | 99.4 | 99.4 | 99.5 | 99.4 | 0 | 0 | 0 | 0 | 0 |
| Guinea-Bissau | 22.4 | 16 | 15.8 | 35.5 | 26.8 | 1.2 | 2.1 | 3 | 1.5 | 2.2 | 85.1 | 83.7 | 85.2 | 84.1 | 80.2 | 0 | 0 | 0 | 0 | 0 |
| Guyana | 4.5 | 2.9 | 2.2 | 2.6 | 3.2 | 0 | 0 | 0 | 0 | 0 | 100 | 100 | 100 | 100 | 100 | n/a | n/a | n/a | n/a | n/a |
| Haiti | 27.3 | 27.9 | 23.6 | 15.6 | 12.4 | 0 | 0 | 0 | 0 | 0 | 68.9 | 68.9 | 71 | 69.5 | 69.5 | n/a | n/a | n/a | n/a | n/a |
| Honduras | 13.1 | 8.8 | 6 | 7.2 | 3 | 16.6 | 14.3 | 14.2 | 12.9 | 11.6 | 85.6 | 85.4 | 85.4 | 85.5 | 85.5 | 7.2 | 7.3 | 7.2 | 7.2 | 7.1 |
| Hungary | 0 | 0 | 0 | 0 | 0.4 | 83.8 | 83.9 | 83.3 | 81.3 | 83.4 | 90 | 89.8 | 89.3 | 88.2 | 88.9 | 0.3 | 0.6 | 1 | 1.3 | 2.1 |
| Iceland | 0 | 0 | 0 | 0 | 0 | 26.8 | 29.2 | 28.2 | 32.5 | 36.5 | 100 | 100 | 100 | 100 | 100 | 0 | 0 | 0 | 0 | 0 |
| India | 1.2 | 2.2 | 2 | 1.3 | 1.6 | 4.4 | 4.4 | 4.4 | 4.4 | 4.2 | 96.6 | 96.4 | 96.3 | 96.2 | 97 | 0.6 | 0.7 | 0.8 | 0.9 | 0.9 |
| Indonesia | 8.5 | 7.3 | 2.8 | 1.8 | 1.4 | 6.8 | 6.8 | 8 | 9.9 | 9.9 | 73.6 | 72.2 | 75.1 | 75.3 | 74.3 | 5.1 | 4.7 | 4.1 | 5.1 | 5.4 |
| Iran, Islamic Republic of | 0 | 0.1 | 0.3 | 0.1 | 0.1 | 39.2 | 38 | 36.6 | 42.6 | 30.9 | 95.3 | 95 | 94.7 | 95 | 94.8 | 3.9 | 4.2 | 4.5 | 4.3 | 4.4 |
| Iraqᶠ | 1 | 0.9 | 1.5 | 0.6 | 3.8 | n/a | n/a | n/a | n/a | n/a | 100 | 100 | 100 | 100 | 100 | n/a | n/a | n/a | n/a | n/a |
| Ireland | 0 | 0 | 0 | 0 | 0 | 1.1 | 1.2 | 1 | 0.9 | 0.8 | 53 | 52 | 48.3 | 60.1 | 61.9 | 30.2 | 29.2 | 25.7 | 24.5 | 29.6 |
| Israel | 3.1 | 4.3 | 5.3 | 4.9 | 3.4 | 63.1 | 60.7 | 62.7 | 59.7 | 61.9 | 94.8 | 86 | 82.9 | 84.6 | 89.1 | 0 | 0 | 0 | 0 | 0 |
| Italy | 0 | 0 | 0 | 0 | 0 | 0.1 | 0.1 | 0.3 | 0.1 | 0.2 | 86.7 | 86.2 | 83.9 | 83.2 | 83.3 | 3.4 | 3.4 | 3.7 | 3.7 | 3.8 |
| Jamaica | 2.6 | 1.8 | 3.4 | 4.7 | 1.2 | 0 | 0 | 0 | 0 | 0 | 69.5 | 65 | 66.2 | 61.8 | 64.7 | 25.1 | 30 | 28.8 | 32.5 | 30.8 |
| Japan | 0 | 0 | 0 | 0 | 0 | 81.2 | 80.9 | 80.5 | 80.5 | 80.5 | 90.6 | 90.1 | 89.9 | 93.3 | 90.1 | 1.5 | 1.7 | 1.5 | 1.7 | 1.7 |
| Jordanᵍ | 6.3 | 5 | 5.2 | 3.4 | 4.2 | 0.8 | 0.9 | 0.7 | 0.7 | 0.7 | 73.5 | 74.7 | 74.5 | 73.9 | 74 | 5.3 | 5.5 | 7.3 | 7.4 | 8.1 |
| Kazakhstan | 0.8 | 0.7 | 0.7 | 0.8 | 1.2 | 0 | 0 | 0 | 0 | 0 | 100 | 100 | 100 | 100 | 100 | n/a | n/a | n/a | n/a | n/a |
| Kenya | 13.3 | 13.2 | 17.2 | 16.4 | 15.3 | 16.7 | 11.7 | 14.8 | 9.2 | 10 | 79.3 | 80.1 | 80.5 | 80 | 82.6 | 7.4 | 7.1 | 6.8 | 6.9 | 6 |
| Kiribati | n/a | 1.5 | 2.8 | 1.7 | 0.8 | 0 | 0 | 0 | 0 | 0 | 100 | 100 | 100 | 100 | 100 | 0 | 0 | 0 | 0 | 0 |
| Kuwait | 0 | 0 | 0 | 0 | 0 | 0 | 0 | 0 | 0 | 0 | 96.4 | 94.9 | 95 | 93.8 | 91.2 | 3.6 | 5.1 | 5 | 6.2 | 8.8 |
| Kyrgyzstan | 15.9 | 16.3 | 14.3 | 9.9 | 17.3 | 7.1 | 10.4 | 9.4 | 10.6 | 15.2 | 100 | 100 | 100 | 100 | 100 | n/a | n/a | n/a | n/a | n/a |
| Lao People's Democratic Republic | 34.5 | 22.5 | 10.1 | 9.5 | 30 | 0.2 | 0.5 | 0.5 | 0.6 | 1 | 66.3 | 69.6 | 70.3 | 70.6 | 75.5 | 12.6 | 13 | 12.2 | 11.8 | 9.8 |
| Latvia | 0.7 | 0.5 | 0.5 | 0.4 | 0.4 | 50.1 | 57 | 52 | 49.6 | 82.7 | 100 | 100 | 99.4 | 99.4 | 94.3 | 0 | 0 | 0.6 | 0.6 | 5.7 |
| Lebanon | 0.7 | 0.2 | 0.2 | 0.1 | 0.1 | 45.5 | 45.2 | 41.8 | 45.3 | 46 | 82.3 | 80.9 | 80.8 | 79.7 | 79.4 | 15.4 | 16.6 | 16.6 | 17.6 | 17.8 |
| Lesotho | 3.6 | 10.8 | 16.2 | 6.4 | 8.2 | 0 | 0 | 0 | 0 | 0 | 20 | 20 | 19.4 | 18.6 | 18.2 | n/a | n/a | n/a | n/a | n/a |
| Liberia | 55.7 | 43.6 | 31.2 | 25.5 | 32.3 | 0 | 0 | 0 | 0 | 0 | 98.5 | 98.5 | 98.5 | 98.5 | 98.5 | 0 | 0 | 0 | 0 | 0 |
| Libyan Arab Jamahiriya | 0 | 0 | 0 | 0 | 0 | 0 | 0 | 0 | 0 | 0 | 100 | 100 | 100 | 100 | 100 | 0 | 0 | 0 | 0 | 0 |
| Lithuania | 0 | 1.7 | 1.6 | 1.5 | 1.3 | 89.8 | 88.3 | 84.3 | 76.7 | 74.6 | 99.6 | 86.2 | 97 | 98.2 | 96.6 | 0.1 | 0.3 | 0.2 | 0.5 | 0.5 |
| Luxembourg | 0 | 0 | 0 | 0 | 0 | 93.1 | 82.6 | 78.9 | 86 | 88.1 | 72 | 72.6 | 72.7 | 78.3 | 77.3 | 13.6 | 11.3 | 10.2 | 9.8 | 10 |
| Madagascar | 40.5 | 43.3 | 39.1 | 31.6 | 22 | n/a | n/a | n/a | n/a | n/a | 89.7 | 90.5 | 87.1 | 91.6 | 91.7 | 10.3 | 9.5 | 12.9 | 8.4 | 8.3 |
| Malawi | 26.1 | 18.5 | 31 | 23 | 25.1 | 0 | 0 | 0 | 0 | 0 | 42.3 | 41.7 | 42 | 42.5 | 42.7 | 1.7 | 1.6 | 1.7 | 1.6 | 1.6 |
| Malaysia | 1 | 0.8 | 0 | 0 | 0.1 | 0.6 | 0.6 | 0.8 | 0.8 | 0.8 | 75 | 75.4 | 73.5 | 73.6 | 73.8 | 12.2 | 11.9 | 14.1 | 14.2 | 13.7 |
| Maldives | 7.7 | 3.3 | 1.8 | 3.4 | 0.4 | 21.3 | 20.5 | 24.9 | 23.8 | 22.9 | 100 | 100 | 100 | 100 | 100 | 0 | 0 | 0 | 0 | 0 |
| Mali | 18.8 | 24.1 | 20.8 | 3.4 | 13.7 | 24 | 21.8 | 22.9 | 27.7 | 26 | 89.3 | 88.6 | 89.1 | 89.2 | 89.3 | 0 | 0 | 0 | 0 | 0 |
| Malta | 0 | 0 | 0 | 0 | 0 | 77.9 | 70 | 71 | 62.1 | 64.1 | 89.7 | 90.4 | 89.6 | 89.7 | 89.9 | 10.3 | 9.6 | 10.4 | 10.3 | 10.1 |
| Marshall Islands | 22.7 | 24.4 | 47.6 | 22.9 | 16.4 | 32.5 | 53.9 | 54.9 | 51.9 | 17.4 | 100 | 100 | 100 | 100 | 100 | n/a | n/a | n/a | n/a | n/a |
| Mauritania | 5.5 | 5.7 | 4.9 | 2.5 | 4.7 | 0 | 0 | 0 | 0 | 0 | 100 | 100 | 100 | 100 | 100 | 0 | 0 | 0 | 0 | 0 |
| Mauritius | 1.2 | 1.1 | 1.6 | 1.4 | 1 | 6.5 | 7.8 | 8.3 | 8.3 | 8.7 | 100 | 100 | 100 | 100 | 100 | n/a | n/a | n/a | n/a | n/a |
| Mexico | 1.2 | 1 | 0.9 | 0.8 | 0.4 | 69.1 | 67.6 | 66.3 | 66 | 66.9 | 95.9 | 95.3 | 95 | 94.6 | 94.2 | 4.1 | 4.7 | 5 | 5.4 | 5.8 |

## Annex Table 2 Selected indicators of health expenditure ratios, 1999–2003

Figures computed by WHO to assure comparability;[a] they are not necessarily the official statistics of Member States. which may use alternative methods.

| Member State | Total expenditure on health as % of gross domestic product | | | | | General government expenditure on health as % of total expenditure on health[b] | | | | | Private expenditure on health as % of total expenditure on health[b] | | | | | General government expenditure on health as % of total government expenditure | | | | |
|---|---|---|---|---|---|---|---|---|---|---|---|---|---|---|---|---|---|---|---|---|
| | 1999 | 2000 | 2001 | 2002 | 2003 | 1999 | 2000 | 2001 | 2002 | 2003 | 1999 | 2000 | 2001 | 2002 | 2003 | 1999 | 2000 | 2001 | 2002 | 2003 |
| Micronesia, Federated States of | 6.8 | 6.5 | 6.5 | 6.4 | 6.4 | 88 | 86.8 | 87 | 88.2 | 88 | 12 | 13.2 | 13 | 11.8 | 12 | 7.9 | 8 | 8.9 | 8.8 | 8.8 |
| Monaco | 9.3 | 9.4 | 9.4 | 9.2 | 9.7 | 69.4 | 70.7 | 71.9 | 73.1 | 75.9 | 30.6 | 29.3 | 28.1 | 26.9 | 24.1 | 11.6 | 14 | 13.6 | 14.3 | 17.5 |
| Mongolia | 5.4 | 7 | 7.3 | 6.7 | 6.7 | 73.3 | 65.9 | 66.3 | 69.8 | 63.8 | 26.7 | 34.1 | 33.7 | 30.2 | 36.2 | 10.9 | 10.6 | 10.6 | 11.5 | 10.3 |
| Morocco[h] | 4.6 | 4.7 | 4.9 | 5 | 5.1 | 30.2 | 30.7 | 32.4 | 32.4 | 33.1 | 69.8 | 69.3 | 67.6 | 67.6 | 66.9 | 4.4 | 4.2 | 4.5 | 5.3 | 6 |
| Mozambique | 4.7 | 5.5 | 4.8 | 5.1 | 4.7 | 63 | 67.8 | 66.2 | 67.6 | 61.7 | 37 | 32.2 | 33.8 | 32.4 | 38.3 | 12.1 | 12.9 | 10.7 | 11.5 | 10.9 |
| Myanmar | 1.8 | 2.2 | 2.1 | 2.8 | 2.8 | 11 | 13.7 | 12.5 | 18.5 | 19.4 | 89 | 86.3 | 87.5 | 81.5 | 80.6 | 0.8 | 1.2 | 1.3 | 2.3 | 2.5 |
| Namibia | 7 | 7 | 6.4 | 5.9 | 6.4 | 73.3 | 68.9 | 69.4 | 68.6 | 70 | 26.7 | 31.1 | 30.6 | 31.4 | 30 | 13.1 | 12.3 | 11.1 | 11 | 12.4 |
| Nauru | 16 | 13.8 | 12.2 | 12.9 | 12.3 | 89.1 | 88.9 | 88.7 | 88.8 | 88.5 | 10.9 | 11.1 | 11.3 | 11.2 | 11.5 | 9.2 | 9.2 | 9.1 | 9.2 | 8.8 |
| Nepal | 5.1 | 4.9 | 5.4 | 5.6 | 5.3 | 25.4 | 24.9 | 31.4 | 32.2 | 27.8 | 74.6 | 75.1 | 68.6 | 67.8 | 72.2 | 7.4 | 7 | 8.7 | 9.5 | 7.9 |
| Netherlands | 8.4 | 8.3 | 8.7 | 9.3 | 9.8 | 62.7 | 63.1 | 62.8 | 62.5 | 62.4 | 37.3 | 36.9 | 37.2 | 37.5 | 37.6 | 11.2 | 11.5 | 11.5 | 12 | 12.4 |
| New Zealand | 7.7 | 7.8 | 7.9 | 8.2 | 8.1 | 77.5 | 78 | 76.4 | 77.9 | 78.3 | 22.5 | 22 | 23.6 | 22.1 | 21.7 | 14.9 | 15.6 | 16.1 | 17.3 | 17.2 |
| Nicaragua | 5.8 | 7.1 | 7.7 | 7.9 | 7.7 | 54 | 52.5 | 48.6 | 49.4 | 48.4 | 46 | 47.5 | 51.4 | 50.6 | 51.6 | 11.2 | 13.1 | 12.9 | 15.2 | 11.7 |
| Niger | 4.5 | 4.4 | 4.3 | 4.3 | 4.7 | 49.7 | 52.4 | 53.1 | 52.8 | 53 | 50.3 | 47.6 | 46.9 | 47.2 | 47 | 12.5 | 12.3 | 12 | 11.5 | 12.4 |
| Nigeria | 5.4 | 4.3 | 5.3 | 5 | 5 | 29.1 | 33.5 | 31.4 | 25.6 | 25.5 | 70.9 | 66.5 | 68.6 | 74.4 | 74.5 | 5.4 | 4.2 | 3.2 | 3.1 | 3.2 |
| Niue[i] | 8 | 7.7 | 38.2 | 10.3 | 9.7 | 97 | 96.8 | 99.4 | 98.5 | 98.4 | 3 | 3.2 | 0.6 | 1.5 | 1.6 | 6.7 | 6.1 | 30.6 | 8.9 | 9.3 |
| Norway | 9.4 | 8.5 | 8.9 | 9.9 | 10.3 | 82.6 | 82.5 | 83.6 | 83.5 | 83.7 | 17.4 | 17.5 | 16.4 | 16.5 | 16.3 | 16.1 | 16.4 | 16.7 | 17.4 | 17.6 |
| Oman | 3.6 | 3.1 | 3.1 | 3.3 | 3.2 | 83.2 | 81 | 82.2 | 82.8 | 83 | 16.8 | 19 | 17.8 | 17.2 | 17 | 7.9 | 7.3 | 6.8 | 7.2 | 7 |
| Pakistan | 3.7 | 2.8 | 2.6 | 2.6 | 2.4 | 32.6 | 33 | 32.3 | 34.7 | 27.7 | 67.4 | 67 | 67.7 | 65.3 | 72.3 | 4 | 3.4 | 3.4 | 3.1 | 2.6 |
| Palau | 9.5 | 9.9 | 9.7 | 9.4 | 9.7 | 88.5 | 89.1 | 89 | 87.3 | 86.7 | 11.5 | 10.9 | 11 | 12.7 | 13.3 | 13.9 | 14.8 | 13.3 | 11.8 | 15.2 |
| Panama[j] | 6.9 | 7.8 | 7.7 | 8 | 7.6 | 66.3 | 68.1 | 67.1 | 69 | 66.4 | 33.7 | 31.9 | 32.9 | 31 | 33.6 | 18.9 | 21.3 | 19.8 | 20.2 | 16.2 |
| Papua New Guinea | 3.5 | 3.6 | 3.7 | 3.5 | 3.4 | 89.3 | 88.3 | 89.5 | 89.8 | 88.9 | 10.7 | 11.7 | 10.5 | 10.2 | 11.1 | 10.3 | 10.5 | 11 | 11.4 | 10.9 |
| Paraguay | 7.2 | 8.4 | 8.4 | 8.3 | 7.3 | 44.9 | 40.2 | 35.2 | 33.3 | 31.5 | 55.1 | 59.8 | 64.8 | 66.7 | 68.5 | 16.7 | 17.5 | 15.9 | 15 | 14.2 |
| Peru | 4.9 | 4.7 | 4.6 | 4.4 | 4.4 | 53.1 | 53 | 51 | 48.6 | 48.3 | 46.9 | 47 | 49 | 51.4 | 51.7 | 12.3 | 12.1 | 12.1 | 12.1 | 10.7 |
| Philippines | 3.5 | 3.4 | 3.2 | 3 | 3.2 | 44.2 | 47.6 | 44.2 | 40 | 43.7 | 55.8 | 52.4 | 55.8 | 60 | 56.3 | 6.5 | 7.1 | 5.9 | 4.9 | 5.9 |
| Poland | 5.9 | 5.7 | 6 | 6.6 | 6.5 | 71.1 | 70 | 71.9 | 71.2 | 69.9 | 28.9 | 30 | 28.1 | 28.8 | 30.1 | 8.7 | 8.9 | 9.7 | 10.2 | 9.8 |
| Portugal | 8.7 | 9.2 | 9.4 | 9.3 | 9.6 | 67.6 | 69.5 | 70.6 | 70.5 | 69.7 | 32.4 | 30.5 | 29.4 | 29.5 | 30.3 | 13 | 14.1 | 14.3 | 14.3 | 14.1 |
| Qatar | 3.6 | 2.8 | 2.9 | 3.3 | 2.7 | 73.6 | 75 | 74.1 | 73.6 | 73.9 | 26.4 | 25 | 25.9 | 26.4 | 26.1 | 6.9 | 6.7 | 6.8 | 6.8 | 6.7 |
| Republic of Korea | 4.8 | 4.7 | 5.4 | 5.3 | 5.6 | 44.4 | 46.2 | 51.9 | 50.3 | 49.4 | 55.6 | 53.8 | 48.1 | 49.7 | 50.6 | 9 | 9.1 | 11.2 | 10.7 | 8.9 |
| Republic of Moldova | 6.8 | 6.5 | 6.4 | 7.1 | 7.2 | 45.8 | 51.3 | 51.1 | 57.2 | 54.5 | 54.2 | 48.7 | 48.9 | 42.8 | 45.5 | 8.5 | 9.8 | 11.2 | 12.9 | 11.8 |
| Romania | 5.4 | 5.4 | 5.5 | 5.9 | 6.1 | 62.6 | 65.5 | 64.6 | 63.9 | 62.9 | 37.4 | 34.5 | 35.4 | 36.1 | 37.1 | 9.6 | 9.9 | 10.3 | 10.5 | 10.9 |
| Russian Federation | 5.6 | 5.8 | 5.7 | 5.9 | 5.6 | 57.8 | 56.1 | 58.8 | 59.4 | 59 | 42.2 | 43.9 | 41.2 | 40.6 | 41 | 8.8 | 9.4 | 9.6 | 9.6 | 9.3 |
| Rwanda | 4.6 | 4.3 | 4.1 | 4.2 | 3.7 | 47.7 | 34.6 | 38.8 | 47 | 43.5 | 52.3 | 65.4 | 61.2 | 53 | 56.5 | 9.9 | 8 | 7.7 | 10.2 | 7.2 |
| Saint Kitts and Nevis | 5.5 | 5.6 | 5.4 | 5.4 | 5.3 | 60.1 | 63.7 | 64.2 | 63.3 | 63.8 | 39.9 | 36.3 | 35.8 | 36.7 | 36.2 | 10.4 | 10.4 | 10.9 | 9.7 | 11.4 |
| Saint Lucia | 4.6 | 4.8 | 5.1 | 5 | 5 | 68.8 | 69.8 | 68.9 | 68.4 | 68.2 | 31.2 | 30.2 | 31.1 | 31.6 | 31.8 | 10.2 | 10.7 | 11.8 | 10.6 | 10.3 |
| Saint Vincent and the Grenadines | 5.7 | 5.7 | 5.7 | 6.2 | 6.1 | 60.8 | 63.9 | 64.3 | 66.8 | 67.5 | 39.2 | 36.1 | 35.7 | 33.2 | 32.5 | 8.5 | 10.8 | 10.1 | 10.7 | 11 |
| Samoa | 6.3 | 6.2 | 5.7 | 5.8 | 5.4 | 75.3 | 75 | 74.5 | 78.4 | 79 | 24.7 | 25 | 25.5 | 21.6 | 21 | 20.3 | 21.3 | 22 | 24.5 | 20.1 |
| San Marino | 7.3 | 7.4 | 7.7 | 7.7 | 7.5 | 77.8 | 77.4 | 79.4 | 79.2 | 78.7 | 22.2 | 22.6 | 20.6 | 20.8 | 21.3 | 18.2 | 18 | 15.2 | 20.4 | 21 |
| Sao Tome and Principe | 10 | 8.6 | 10.5 | 9 | 8.6 | 87.3 | 85.9 | 85.8 | 85 | 83.9 | 12.7 | 14.1 | 14.2 | 15 | 16.1 | 12.5 | 11.2 | 10.9 | 11.3 | 11.1 |
| Saudi Arabia | 4.3 | 4.2 | 4.7 | 4.5 | 4 | 76.1 | 76.8 | 78.6 | 78.2 | 75.9 | 23.9 | 23.2 | 21.4 | 21.8 | 24.1 | 10.7 | 9.8 | 9.9 | 10.6 | 9.4 |
| Senegal | 4.5 | 4.4 | 4.7 | 5 | 5.1 | 36.2 | 36.4 | 38.5 | 39.8 | 41.8 | 63.8 | 63.6 | 61.5 | 60.2 | 58.2 | 7.8 | 8.1 | 8 | 9.5 | 9.3 |
| Serbia-Montenegro[k] | 9.6 | 7.7 | 7.3 | 7.9 | 9.6 | 59.5 | 63.3 | 67.2 | 72.9 | 75.5 | 40.5 | 36.7 | 32.8 | 27.1 | 24.5 | 12.4 | 13.5 | 12.4 | 12.2 | 16 |
| Seychelles | 5.3 | 5.2 | 5.1 | 5.1 | 5.9 | 74.8 | 75 | 74.7 | 74.9 | 73.2 | 25.2 | 25 | 25.3 | 25.1 | 26.8 | 6.9 | 6.8 | 8.1 | 7 | 10.2 |
| Sierra Leone | 3.1 | 3.8 | 3.4 | 3.5 | 3.5 | 46.1 | 55.5 | 53.7 | 63.6 | 58.3 | 53.9 | 44.5 | 46.3 | 36.4 | 41.7 | 6.9 | 7.6 | 6.4 | 7.9 | 7.9 |
| Singapore | 4.1 | 3.6 | 4.3 | 4.3 | 4.5 | 38.4 | 35.4 | 36.2 | 32.4 | 36.1 | 61.6 | 64.6 | 63.8 | 67.6 | 63.9 | 8.2 | 6.7 | 7 | 6.6 | 7.7 |
| Slovakia | 5.8 | 5.5 | 5.6 | 5.7 | 5.9 | 89.6 | 89.4 | 89.3 | 89.1 | 88.3 | 10.4 | 10.6 | 10.7 | 10.9 | 11.7 | 10.9 | 9.7 | 11.4 | 11.5 | 13.2 |
| Slovenia | 7.7 | 8.6 | 9 | 8.9 | 8.8 | 75.5 | 77.7 | 76.9 | 76.5 | 76.3 | 24.5 | 22.3 | 23.1 | 23.5 | 23.7 | 14 | 13.7 | 14.2 | 14 | 13.8 |
| Solomon Islands | 4.7 | 5.1 | 5.1 | 4.9 | 4.8 | 93 | 93 | 93.5 | 93.2 | 93.4 | 7 | 7 | 6.5 | 6.8 | 6.6 | 11.1 | 11.4 | 11.5 | 13.2 | 9.4 |
| Somalia | 2.7 | 2.6 | 2.6 | n/a | n/a | 45 | 44.8 | 44.6 | n/a | n/a | 55 | 55.2 | 55.4 | n/a | n/a | 4.2 | 4.2 | 4.2 | n/a | n/a |
| South Africa | 8.7 | 8.1 | 8.4 | 8.4 | 8.4 | 41.1 | 42.4 | 41.2 | 40.6 | 38.6 | 58.9 | 57.6 | 58.8 | 59.4 | 61.4 | 10.7 | 10.9 | 11.2 | 11.6 | 10.2 |
| Spain[l] | 7.5 | 7.4 | 7.5 | 7.6 | 7.7 | 72 | 71.6 | 71.2 | 71.3 | 71.3 | 28 | 28.4 | 28.8 | 28.7 | 28.7 | 13.4 | 13.3 | 13.4 | 13.4 | 13.7 |
| Sri Lanka | 3.5 | 3.6 | 3.6 | 3.6 | 3.5 | 48.4 | 48.5 | 46.6 | 45 | 45 | 51.6 | 51.5 | 53.4 | 55 | 55 | 6.8 | 6.5 | 6.1 | 6.4 | 6.5 |
| Sudan | 4.3 | 3.8 | 4 | 4 | 4.3 | 25.5 | 34.4 | 37.1 | 38.1 | 43.2 | 74.5 | 65.6 | 62.9 | 61.9 | 56.8 | 9 | 8.6 | 9.5 | 8.8 | 9.1 |
| Suriname | 7.6 | 8 | 7.9 | 8.1 | 7.9 | 51.3 | 48.8 | 47.8 | 46.3 | 45.8 | 48.7 | 51.2 | 52.2 | 53.7 | 54.2 | 10.7 | 9.7 | 10.8 | 10.4 | 10.4 |
| Swaziland | 6.4 | 6.1 | 6 | 5.9 | 5.8 | 59 | 58.6 | 57.8 | 59.3 | 57.3 | 41 | 41.4 | 42.2 | 40.7 | 42.7 | 11.8 | 11.6 | 11.3 | 10.9 | 10.9 |
| Sweden | 8.4 | 8.4 | 8.8 | 9.2 | 9.4 | 85.7 | 84.9 | 84.9 | 85.1 | 85.2 | 14.3 | 15.1 | 15.1 | 14.9 | 14.8 | 12 | 12.5 | 13.1 | 13.4 | 13.6 |

| Member State | External resources for health as % of total expenditure on health | | | | | Social security expenditure on health as % of general government expenditure on health | | | | | Out-of-pocket expenditure as % of private expenditure on health | | | | | Private prepaid plans as % of private expenditure on health | | | | |
|---|---|---|---|---|---|---|---|---|---|---|---|---|---|---|---|---|---|---|---|---|
| | 1999 | 2000 | 2001 | 2002 | 2003 | 1999 | 2000 | 2001 | 2002 | 2003 | 1999 | 2000 | 2001 | 2002 | 2003 | 1999 | 2000 | 2001 | 2002 | 2003 |
| Micronesia, Federated States of | 11.8 | 11.7 | 11.7 | 11.9 | n/a | 0 | 0 | 0 | 0 | 0 | 35.7 | 35.7 | 35.7 | 40 | 40 | 0 | 0 | 0 | 0 | 0 |
| Monaco | 0 | 0 | 0 | 0 | 0 | 98 | 98.1 | 98.2 | 98.3 | 98.6 | 84.8 | 81.8 | 81.8 | 84.6 | 85.3 | 15.2 | 18.2 | 18.2 | 15.4 | 14.7 |
| Mongolia | 18.4 | 22.5 | 21.1 | 12.8 | 3.2 | 26.1 | 24.1 | 31.5 | 37.4 | 37.8 | 55.7 | 42.6 | 41.9 | 84.6 | 91.1 | 0 | 0 | 0 | 0 | 0 |
| Morocco[h] | 1.8 | 1.8 | 1.7 | 0.5 | 1 | 0 | 0 | 0 | 0 | 0 | 76.7 | 76.6 | 76.4 | 76.3 | 76.1 | 23.3 | 23.4 | 23.6 | 23.7 | 23.9 |
| Mozambique | 39.6 | 42.9 | 47.6 | 38.3 | 40.8 | 0 | 0 | 0 | 0 | 0 | 38.5 | 39 | 34.3 | 32 | 38.8 | 0.6 | 0.6 | 0.6 | 0.6 | 0.5 |
| Myanmar | 3.1 | 1.9 | 1.9 | 1 | 2.2 | 2.1 | 2 | 3.4 | 1.2 | 1.3 | 99.8 | 99.7 | 99.7 | 99.7 | 99.7 | 0 | 0 | 0 | 0 | 0 |
| Namibia | 2.4 | 3.8 | 4 | 4.3 | 5.3 | 1.2 | 1.8 | 2 | 2 | 1.9 | 21.3 | 18.2 | 20.1 | 20.4 | 19.2 | 74.7 | 77.3 | 75.1 | 74.9 | 76 |
| Nauru | n/a | n/a | n/a | n/a | n/a | 0 | 0 | 0 | 0 | 0 | 100 | 100 | 100 | 100 | 100 | 0 | 0 | 0 | 0 | 0 |
| Nepal | 8.9 | 13.1 | 12.1 | 8.4 | 9.9 | 0 | 0 | 0 | 0 | 0 | 92.5 | 92.2 | 92.2 | 92.2 | 92.2 | 0 | 0 | 0 | 0 | 0 |
| Netherlands | 0 | 0 | 0 | 0 | 0 | 93.8 | 93.9 | 93.8 | 93.8 | 93 | 24.1 | 24.3 | 23.4 | 21.4 | 20.8 | 44.5 | 43 | 43.6 | 45.6 | 45.7 |
| New Zealand | 0 | 0 | 0 | 0 | 0 | 0 | 0 | 0 | 0 | 0 | 70.7 | 69.9 | 72 | 72.6 | 72.1 | 27.6 | 28.5 | 26.5 | 25.9 | 26.5 |
| Nicaragua | 10 | 8.4 | 7.7 | 9.3 | 11.2 | 31.5 | 27 | 31.3 | 29.2 | 26.6 | 93.8 | 92 | 93.1 | 96 | 95.7 | 4.9 | 7 | 6 | 4 | 4.1 |
| Niger | 28.6 | 46.6 | 23.1 | 22.7 | 32.8 | 2.6 | 2.8 | 2.6 | 2.4 | 2.2 | 88.9 | 88 | 88.2 | 88.8 | 89.2 | 6.4 | 7.4 | 7.3 | 7 | 7.2 |
| Nigeria | 13.8 | 16.2 | 5.6 | 6.1 | 5.3 | 0 | 0 | 0 | 0 | 0 | 94.8 | 92.7 | 91.4 | 90.4 | 91.2 | 3.4 | 5.1 | 6.5 | 6.7 | 6.7 |
| Niue[i] | n/a | n/a | 75.6 | 5.2 | 9.2 | 0 | 0 | 0 | 0 | 0 | 100 | 100 | 100 | 100 | 100 | 0 | 0 | 0 | 0 | 0 |
| Norway | 0 | 0 | 0 | 0 | 0 | 16.5 | 17.1 | 17.2 | 18.2 | 17.9 | 95.4 | 95.5 | 95.7 | 95.4 | 95.4 | 0 | 0 | 0 | 0 | 0 |
| Oman | 0 | 0.1 | 0 | 0 | 0 | 0 | 0 | 0 | 0 | 0 | 59.8 | 59.6 | 56.1 | 57 | 56.1 | 26.8 | 27 | 29.2 | 28.7 | 29.3 |
| Pakistan | 2.2 | 3.5 | 3.5 | 2 | 2.5 | 33.7 | 41.3 | 42.5 | 42.1 | 53.3 | 98.6 | 98.1 | 98 | 98 | 98 | n/a | n/a | n/a | n/a | n/a |
| Palau | 15.9 | 15 | 16.3 | 10.4 | 15.8 | 0 | 0 | 0 | 0 | 0 | 100 | 100 | 100 | 100 | 100 | 0 | 0 | 0 | 0 | 0 |
| Panama[j] | 1.1 | 1 | 0.5 | 1 | 0.2 | 51.5 | 50 | 53.5 | 52.3 | 55.5 | 81.9 | 81.3 | 82.3 | 81.6 | 82.2 | 18.1 | 18.7 | 17.7 | 18.4 | 17.8 |
| Papua New Guinea | 26.2 | 24.2 | 25 | 37.7 | 28.3 | 0 | 0 | 0 | 0 | 0 | 87 | 88.8 | 87.6 | 87.1 | 87.2 | 9.8 | 8.7 | 9.9 | 10.4 | 10.1 |
| Paraguay | 5.2 | 2.8 | 1.6 | 3.2 | 1.8 | 48.1 | 53 | 47.7 | 36.2 | 39.8 | 85.6 | 88.6 | 87 | 80.2 | 74.6 | 13.4 | 10.9 | 13.2 | 10.3 | 11.7 |
| Peru | 1.4 | 1.2 | 4.6 | 4.6 | 3.2 | 43.5 | 42.9 | 42.9 | 42.9 | 42.4 | 82.6 | 79.4 | 79.4 | 78.9 | 79 | 13.6 | 17.2 | 17.2 | 17.8 | 17.6 |
| Philippines | 3.7 | 3.5 | 3.7 | 2.8 | 3.8 | 11.4 | 14.7 | 18 | 22.6 | 21.8 | 77.6 | 77.2 | 78.6 | 78 | 78.2 | 11 | 11.1 | 10.1 | 10.7 | 10.5 |
| Poland | 0 | 0 | 0 | 0 | n/a | 83.5 | 82.6 | 83.8 | 86.2 | 86 | 100 | 100 | 100 | 88.2 | 87.8 | n/a | n/a | n/a | n/a | n/a |
| Portugal | 0 | 0 | 0 | 0 | 0 | 7.1 | 6.5 | 6.5 | 6.4 | 6.5 | 95.3 | 95.7 | 95.6 | 95.6 | 95.7 | 4.3 | 4.3 | 4.4 | 4.4 | 4.3 |
| Qatar | 0 | 0 | 0 | 0 | 0 | 0 | 0 | 0 | 0 | 0 | 88.4 | 86.7 | 86.7 | 88.7 | 87.5 | n/a | n/a | n/a | n/a | n/a |
| Republic of Korea | 0 | 0 | 0 | 0 | 0 | 78.7 | 79.6 | 81.4 | 81 | 81.7 | 85.9 | 83.5 | 83.2 | 84 | 82.8 | 3.7 | 5.3 | 4.4 | 3.8 | 4.1 |
| Republic of Moldova | 16.1 | 32.6 | 8.3 | 2.8 | 2.5 | 0 | 0 | 0 | 0 | 1.1 | 99.6 | 98 | 96.9 | 96 | 96.1 | n/a | n/a | n/a | n/a | n/a |
| Romania | 3 | 5.5 | 7 | 3.7 | 3.8 | 86 | 89.4 | 89.5 | 84.3 | 85.8 | 90.1 | 92 | 94.6 | 88.7 | 90.4 | 9.9 | 8 | 5.4 | 5.5 | 4.7 |
| Russian Federation | 0.8 | 0.2 | 0.2 | 0.2 | 0.2 | 39.4 | 40.6 | 40.7 | 41.7 | 43.7 | 67.8 | 71.1 | 71.9 | 70.8 | 71.1 | 6.3 | 6.9 | 6.2 | 6.9 | 6.6 |
| Rwanda | 43 | 48.9 | 38.2 | 46.9 | 54.5 | 5.1 | 6.8 | 8.3 | 9 | 9.8 | 41.4 | 35.6 | 39.2 | 43.8 | 41.7 | 3.8 | 5.6 | 6.5 | 7.5 | 7.1 |
| Saint Kitts and Nevis | 5.7 | 5.2 | 5 | 4.8 | 5.7 | 0 | 0 | 0 | 0 | 0 | 100 | 100 | 100 | 100 | 100 | n/a | n/a | n/a | n/a | n/a |
| Saint Lucia | 0.5 | 0.5 | 0.6 | 0.1 | 0.1 | 5.2 | 4.9 | 4.9 | 4.8 | 5 | 100 | 100 | 100 | 100 | 100 | n/a | n/a | n/a | n/a | n/a |
| Saint Vincent and the Grenadines | 0.2 | 0.2 | 0.2 | 0.1 | 0.1 | 0 | 0 | 0 | 0 | 0 | 100 | 100 | 100 | 100 | 100 | n/a | n/a | n/a | n/a | n/a |
| Samoa | 14.7 | 14.5 | 15.2 | 18.3 | 18.9 | 0.9 | 2.4 | 0.7 | 0.6 | 1.4 | 80.5 | 83.3 | 81.3 | 79.3 | 77.9 | 0 | 0 | 0 | 0 | 0 |
| San Marino | 0 | 0 | 0 | 0 | 0 | 97.6 | 94.5 | 96 | 95.5 | 92.6 | 96.5 | 96.7 | 96.7 | 96.8 | 96.8 | 3.5 | 3.3 | 3.3 | 3.2 | 3.2 |
| Sao Tome and Principe | 59.9 | 62.5 | 62.9 | 74.9 | 56 | 0 | 0 | 0 | 0 | 0 | 100 | 100 | 100 | 100 | 100 | 0 | 0 | 0 | 0 | 0 |
| Saudi Arabia | 0 | 0 | 0 | 0 | 0 | n/a | n/a | n/a | n/a | n/a | 32.5 | 30.3 | 30.7 | 30.3 | 28.6 | 39 | 40.8 | 40.1 | 40.4 | 41.6 |
| Senegal | 12.6 | 14 | 19.2 | 10.3 | 15.4 | 19 | 19.2 | 18.8 | 16.6 | 15.8 | 96.7 | 96.6 | 96.5 | 95.4 | 95.3 | 2.1 | 2.2 | 2.2 | 3.3 | 3.4 |
| Serbia-Montenegro[k] | 1.1 | 1.9 | 1.2 | 0.5 | 0.5 | 96.3 | 93.8 | 94.5 | 94.7 | 89.8 | 100 | 100 | 100 | 100 | 85.3 | 0 | 0 | 0 | 0 | 14.7 |
| Seychelles | 1.3 | 0.6 | 0.4 | 0.5 | 2 | 5.3 | 5.2 | 5.1 | 4.8 | 3.3 | 62.5 | 61.8 | 62.5 | 62.5 | 62.5 | 0 | 0 | 0 | 0 | 0 |
| Sierra Leone | 8.8 | 11.8 | 14.8 | 5.8 | 15.5 | 0 | 0 | 0 | 0 | 0 | 100 | 100 | 100 | 100 | 100 | 0 | 0 | 0 | 0 | 0 |
| Singapore | 0 | 0 | 0 | 0 | 0 | 19 | 23.3 | 20.9 | 23.1 | 21.5 | 97.4 | 97.1 | 97.1 | 97.1 | 97.1 | 0 | 0 | 0 | 0 | 0 |
| Slovakia | 0.1 | 0 | 0 | 0 | 0 | 94.2 | 94.4 | 95.1 | 96.4 | 93.5 | 100 | 100 | 100 | 100 | 100 | 0 | 0 | 0 | 0 | 0 |
| Slovenia | 0 | 0.1 | 0.1 | 0.1 | 0.1 | 87.5 | 79.5 | 78.3 | 79.7 | 82.6 | 39.3 | 38.6 | 41.7 | 40.9 | 41.1 | 60.7 | 61.4 | 58.3 | 58.3 | 58.9 |
| Solomon Islands | 7.1 | 16.5 | 16.5 | 40.9 | 68.5 | 0 | 0 | 0 | 0 | 0 | 50.2 | 51.6 | 49.2 | 49.7 | 53.1 | 0 | 0 | 0 | 0 | 0 |
| Somalia | 6.1 | 9 | 9.3 | n/a | n/a | 0 | 0 | 0 | n/a | n/a | 100 | 100 | 100 | n/a | n/a | 0 | 0 | 0 | n/a | n/a |
| South Africa | 0.1 | 0.4 | 0.4 | 0.4 | 0.5 | 3.5 | 3.3 | 3.1 | 3.8 | 4.6 | 17.1 | 18.9 | 17.8 | 16.8 | 17.1 | 77.4 | 75.6 | 76.7 | 77.7 | 77.7 |
| Spain[l] | 0 | 0 | 0 | 0 | 0 | 41.1 | 41.4 | 41.7 | 7.3 | 7 | 83.3 | 83.1 | 83.1 | 82.6 | 82 | 13.4 | 13.7 | 13.9 | 14.3 | 14.9 |
| Sri Lanka | 2.7 | 2.7 | 3.1 | 1.9 | 2.3 | 0.2 | 0.3 | 0.4 | 0.3 | 0.3 | 86.6 | 86.4 | 87.1 | 88.9 | 88.9 | 3 | 3.9 | 3.4 | 3.2 | 3.2 |
| Sudan | 3.7 | 2.4 | 2.8 | 2.9 | 2.2 | 36.8 | 38.7 | 45.5 | 42.1 | 44.7 | 96.2 | 95.9 | 95.8 | 95.9 | 96.3 | n/a | n/a | n/a | n/a | n/a |
| Suriname | 11.4 | 10.9 | 13.5 | 7.3 | 7 | 35.3 | 40.7 | 35 | 35.9 | 35.3 | 49.5 | 44 | 52.7 | 45.4 | 51.8 | 0.7 | 0.8 | 0.7 | 0.7 | 0.7 |
| Swaziland | 10.3 | 5.5 | 5.2 | 5.1 | 5.5 | 0 | 0 | 0 | 0 | 0 | 40.9 | 42.4 | 41.8 | 41.7 | 42.4 | 18.6 | 18.9 | 20 | 20 | 19.6 |
| Sweden | 0 | 0 | 0 | 0 | 0 | 0 | 0 | 0 | 0 | 0 | 93.8 | 91.1 | 92.2 | 91.6 | 92.1 | 1 | 1.2 | 1.5 | 1.4 | 2.3 |

## Annex Table 2 Selected indicators of health expenditure ratios, 1999–2003

Figures computed by WHO to assure comparability;[a] they are not necessarily the official statistics of Member States. which may use alternative methods.

| Member State | Total expenditure on health as % of gross domestic product | | | | | General government expenditure on health as % of total expenditure on health[b] | | | | | Private expenditure on health as % of total expenditure on health[b] | | | | | General government expenditure on health as % of total government expenditure | | | | |
|---|---|---|---|---|---|---|---|---|---|---|---|---|---|---|---|---|---|---|---|---|
| | 1999 | 2000 | 2001 | 2002 | 2003 | 1999 | 2000 | 2001 | 2002 | 2003 | 1999 | 2000 | 2001 | 2002 | 2003 | 1999 | 2000 | 2001 | 2002 | 2003 |
| Switzerland | 10.5 | 10.4 | 10.9 | 11.1 | 11.5 | 55.3 | 55.6 | 57.1 | 57.9 | 58.5 | 44.7 | 44.4 | 42.9 | 42.1 | 41.5 | 16.7 | 17.1 | 17.9 | 18.2 | 19.4 |
| Syrian Arab Republic | 5.5 | 5.1 | 5 | 5 | 5.1 | 41 | 43 | 45 | 45.8 | 48.2 | 59 | 57 | 55 | 54.2 | 51.8 | 7.2 | 7.3 | 6.7 | 6.5 | 6.3 |
| Tajikistan | 3.8 | 3.3 | 3.3 | 3.3 | 4.4 | 27.6 | 28.2 | 28.9 | 27.7 | 20.8 | 72.4 | 71.8 | 71.1 | 72.3 | 79.2 | 6.3 | 4.9 | 5.3 | 4.8 | 4.8 |
| Thailand | 3.5 | 3.4 | 3.3 | 3.4 | 3.3 | 54.8 | 56.1 | 56.3 | 60.2 | 61.6 | 45.2 | 43.9 | 43.7 | 39.8 | 38.4 | 10.5 | 10.8 | 10.3 | 11.8 | 13.6 |
| The former Yugoslav Republic of Macedonia | 6.3 | 6 | 6.1 | 6.8 | 7.1 | 85.2 | 84.6 | 83.1 | 84.7 | 84.5 | 14.8 | 15.4 | 16.9 | 15.3 | 15.5 | 15.1 | 15 | 12.3 | 14 | 17.1 |
| Timor-Leste[m] | 10 | 8.4 | 7.9 | 7.7 | 9.6 | 68.3 | 75.3 | 72.6 | 72.6 | 75.9 | 31.7 | 24.7 | 27.4 | 27.4 | 24.1 | 8.7 | 8.1 | 8.5 | 8.6 | 7.7 |
| Togo[n] | 5.4 | 4.6 | 5.4 | 4.9 | 5.6 | 40 | 29 | 25.2 | 18.7 | 24.8 | 60 | 71 | 74.8 | 81.3 | 75.2 | 12.4 | 7.5 | 8.6 | 6.9 | 9.3 |
| Tonga | 6.8 | 6.8 | 7.3 | 6.5 | 6.5 | 75.4 | 74.7 | 75.7 | 74.2 | 85.1 | 24.6 | 25.3 | 24.3 | 25.8 | 14.9 | 14.6 | 13.2 | 11.9 | 17.1 | 21.2 |
| Trinidad and Tobago | 3.8 | 3.7 | 3.6 | 3.9 | 3.9 | 43.3 | 40.3 | 39.9 | 37.3 | 37.8 | 56.7 | 59.7 | 60.1 | 62.7 | 62.2 | 6.4 | 6.3 | 5.8 | 5.7 | 5.9 |
| Tunisia | 5.5 | 5.6 | 5.7 | 5.6 | 5.4 | 49.4 | 48.5 | 49.6 | 47.4 | 45.7 | 50.6 | 51.5 | 50.4 | 52.6 | 54.3 | 7.2 | 6.9 | 7.6 | 6.9 | 7.2 |
| Turkey | 6.4 | 6.6 | 7.5 | 7.2 | 7.6 | 61.1 | 62.9 | 68.2 | 69.5 | 71.6 | 38.9 | 37.1 | 31.8 | 30.5 | 28.4 | 10.3 | 9.8 | 10.3 | 12.1 | 13.9 |
| Turkmenistan | 3.5 | 4.5 | 4 | 3.6 | 3.9 | 69.9 | 72.6 | 69 | 64.3 | 67.4 | 30.1 | 27.4 | 31 | 35.7 | 32.6 | 12.7 | 12.7 | 12.7 | 12.7 | 12.7 |
| Tuvalu[o] | 9.3 | 11.5 | 7.5 | 31.6 | 6.1 | 88.7 | 90.8 | 86.9 | 96.8 | 83.3 | 11.3 | 9.2 | 13.1 | 3.2 | 16.7 | 5.9 | 5 | 4.2 | 33.5 | 6 |
| Uganda | 6.3 | 6.6 | 7.3 | 7.6 | 7.3 | 30.6 | 26.8 | 27.3 | 31.1 | 30.4 | 69.4 | 73.2 | 72.7 | 68.9 | 69.6 | 9.4 | 9 | 9.6 | 10.8 | 10.7 |
| Ukraine | 5.5 | 5 | 5 | 5.4 | 5.7 | 53.1 | 58 | 61 | 62.4 | 65.9 | 46.9 | 42 | 39 | 37.6 | 34.1 | 8.6 | 8.4 | 8.9 | 9.4 | 10.2 |
| United Arab Emirates | 3.8 | 3.2 | 3.7 | 3.4 | 3.3 | 77.5 | 76.6 | 78.3 | 75 | 74.7 | 22.5 | 23.4 | 21.7 | 25 | 25.3 | 7.9 | 7.6 | 7.7 | 7.8 | 8 |
| United Kingdom | 7.2 | 7.3 | 7.5 | 7.7 | 8 | 80.6 | 80.9 | 83 | 83.4 | 85.7 | 19.4 | 19.1 | 17 | 16.6 | 14.3 | 14.5 | 14.8 | 15.3 | 15.4 | 15.8 |
| United Republic of Tanzania | 4.3 | 4.4 | 4.5 | 4.5 | 4.3 | 43.4 | 48.1 | 48.5 | 51.6 | 55.4 | 56.6 | 51.9 | 51.5 | 48.4 | 44.6 | 12.4 | 12.6 | 12.8 | 12.8 | 12.7 |
| United States of America | 13.1 | 13.3 | 14 | 14.7 | 15.2 | 43.8 | 44 | 44.8 | 44.8 | 44.6 | 56.2 | 56 | 55.2 | 55.2 | 55.4 | 16.7 | 17.1 | 17.7 | 18.2 | 18.5 |
| Uruguay | 10.6 | 10.5 | 10.8 | 10.3 | 9.8 | 34.8 | 33.4 | 33.8 | 31.3 | 27.2 | 65.2 | 66.6 | 66.2 | 68.7 | 72.8 | 10.6 | 10.3 | 9.4 | 8 | 6.3 |
| Uzbekistan | 6 | 5.7 | 5.7 | 5.6 | 5.5 | 48.4 | 45.6 | 45.4 | 44.3 | 43 | 51.6 | 54.4 | 54.6 | 55.7 | 57 | 7 | 6.6 | 7.1 | 6.8 | 7.6 |
| Vanuatu | 4.2 | 3.9 | 3.8 | 4.1 | 3.9 | 75.4 | 72.8 | 74.3 | 75.2 | 73.8 | 24.6 | 27.2 | 25.7 | 24.8 | 26.2 | 11.5 | 10.1 | 11.1 | 12 | 12.9 |
| Venezuela, Bolivarian Republic of | 6.2 | 6.2 | 5.2 | 5 | 4.5 | 51.8 | 54.4 | 43.4 | 46.1 | 44.3 | 48.2 | 45.6 | 56.6 | 53.9 | 55.7 | 13.1 | 11.5 | 7.2 | 7.8 | 6.4 |
| Viet Nam | 4.9 | 5.3 | 5.5 | 5.1 | 5.4 | 32.7 | 28 | 29.2 | 28.1 | 27.8 | 67.3 | 72 | 70.8 | 71.9 | 72.2 | 6.7 | 6 | 6.7 | 5.1 | 5.6 |
| Yemen | 4.2 | 4.6 | 5 | 4.9 | 5.5 | 37.2 | 42.9 | 42.8 | 38.4 | 40.9 | 62.8 | 57.1 | 57.2 | 61.6 | 59.1 | 5.9 | 6.4 | 6.5 | 5.6 | 6 |
| Zambia | 5.7 | 5.5 | 5.8 | 6 | 5.4 | 48.8 | 50.6 | 56.5 | 56.7 | 51.4 | 51.2 | 49.4 | 43.5 | 43.3 | 48.6 | 9.5 | 9.1 | 10.2 | 10.6 | 11.8 |
| Zimbabwe | 8.1 | 7.8 | 9.1 | 8.4 | 7.9 | 48.9 | 48.3 | 38.6 | 37.7 | 35.9 | 51.1 | 51.7 | 61.4 | 62.3 | 64.1 | 10 | 7.4 | 9.3 | 9.8 | 9.2 |

Afghanistan, Democratic People's Republic of Korea, Equatorial Guinea, Gabon, Guinea Bissau, Iraq, Liberia, Libya, Sao Tome and Principe, Somalia, Sudan and Turkmenistan: estimates for these countries should be read with caution as these are derived from limited sources (mostly macro data that are publicly accessible).

Burkina Faso, China, Djibouti, Georgia, Guinea, India, Malaysia, Mauritius, Mongolia, Niue, Philippines, Russia, Rwanda, Samoa, Singapore, Sri Lanka, Tonga, Yemen: new NHA reports, surveys, and/or country consultations provided new bases for the estimates.

For OECD countries, data are updated from the *OECD health data*. For Japan the 2003 ratios have been estimated by WHO. USA figures do not as yet reflect introduction of estimates of investments in medical equipment and software and expanded estimates of investments in medical sector structures.

[a]See explanatory notes for sources and methods.
[b]In some cases the sum of the ratios of general government and private expenditures on health may not add to 100 because of rounding.
[c]The estimates do not include expenditures of Hong Kong and Macao Special Administrative Regions.
[d]The series was adjusted for the removal of social security expenditure on health, which could not be confirmed due to incomplete information.
[e]Expenditures on health by the social security funds have increased due to a reclassification. (Note, however, that this estimate is likely to increase further due to changes in the social security scheme.)
[f]The estimates do not include expenditures of Northern Iraq.
[g]The public expenditure on health includes contributions from the United Nations Relief and Works Agency for Palestine Refugees in the Near East (UNRWA) to Palestinian refugees residing in Jordanian territories.

| Member State | External resources for health as % of total expenditure on health | | | | | Social security expenditure on health as % of general government expenditure on health | | | | | Out-of-pocket expenditure as % of private expenditure on health | | | | | Private prepaid plans as % of private expenditure on health | | | | |
|---|---|---|---|---|---|---|---|---|---|---|---|---|---|---|---|---|---|---|---|---|
| | 1999 | 2000 | 2001 | 2002 | 2003 | 1999 | 2000 | 2001 | 2002 | 2003 | 1999 | 2000 | 2001 | 2002 | 2003 | 1999 | 2000 | 2001 | 2002 | 2003 |
| Switzerland | 0 | 0 | 0 | 0 | 0 | 72.1 | 72.6 | 70.4 | 69.1 | 69.3 | 74.5 | 74.1 | 73.9 | 74.8 | 76 | 23.3 | 23.6 | 23.8 | 22.9 | 21.6 |
| Syrian Arab Republic | 0.1 | 0.1 | 0.2 | 0.3 | 0.2 | 0 | 0 | 0 | 0 | 0 | 100 | 100 | 100 | 100 | 100 | 0 | 0 | 0 | 0 | 0 |
| Tajikistan | 6.7 | 18.3 | 16.9 | 14.9 | 14.9 | 0 | 0 | 0 | 0 | 0 | 100 | 100 | 100 | 100 | 100 | 0 | 0 | 0 | 0 | 0 |
| Thailand | 0 | 0 | 0.1 | 0.2 | 0.3 | 29.5 | 30.2 | 34.4 | 30.8 | 32 | 76.4 | 76.8 | 75.7 | 76.3 | 74.8 | 12.6 | 12.8 | 13.6 | 13.4 | 14.6 |
| The former Yugoslav Republic of Macedonia | 3.7 | 2.7 | 2.5 | 1.8 | 1.7 | 97.4 | 97.4 | 97.1 | 97.4 | 97.8 | 100 | 100 | 100 | 100 | 100 | n/a | n/a | n/a | n/a | n/a |
| Timor-Leste^m | 47.9 | 56.4 | 55 | 45.8 | 48.7 | n/a | n/a | n/a | n/a | n/a | 30.9 | 30.9 | 25.6 | 25.6 | 25.6 | 0 | 0 | 0 | 0 | 0 |
| Togo^n | 4.9 | 7.1 | 4.8 | 11.4 | 2.3 | 8.1 | 13.4 | 11.6 | 14.4 | 14.6 | 87 | 86.6 | 87.8 | 87.7 | 88 | 5.1 | 5.4 | 4.3 | 4.3 | 4.1 |
| Tonga | 21.7 | 23.4 | 23.9 | 33.5 | 30.9 | 0 | 0 | 0 | 0 | 0 | 79 | 76.5 | 77.5 | 80 | 72.6 | 5.8 | 9.3 | 10.6 | 6 | 6 |
| Trinidad and Tobago | 8.5 | 7.3 | 7.3 | 6.6 | 1.4 | 0 | 0 | 0 | 0 | 0 | 85.8 | 86.3 | 86.4 | 85.8 | 88.6 | 7.5 | 7.2 | 7.2 | 7.5 | 6 |
| Tunisia | 0.7 | 0.7 | 0.7 | 0.2 | 0.4 | 23.3 | 26.7 | 22.3 | 24.5 | 23.5 | 83.8 | 81.7 | 82.6 | 83 | 83 | 14.4 | 16.6 | 15.7 | 15.3 | 15.3 |
| Turkey | 0 | 0 | 0 | 0 | 0 | 53 | 55.5 | 50.5 | 55 | 54.6 | 74.8 | 74.6 | 73.4 | 70.7 | 69.9 | 10.9 | 11.8 | 12.3 | 12.3 | 12.5 |
| Turkmenistan | 2 | 1 | 0.8 | 0.5 | 0.4 | 6.1 | 6.1 | 6.1 | 6.1 | 6.1 | 100 | 100 | 100 | 100 | 100 | 0 | 0 | 0 | 0 | 0 |
| Tuvalu^o | 3.5 | 39.9 | 95.7 | 68 | 70.5 | 0 | 0 | 0 | 0 | 0 | 13 | 13 | 13 | 13 | 13 | 0 | 0 | 0 | 0 | 0 |
| Uganda | 27.6 | 28.3 | 27.4 | 29.1 | 28.5 | 0 | 0 | 0 | 0 | 0 | 61.5 | 56.7 | 51.8 | 51 | 52.8 | 0.2 | 0.1 | 0.2 | 0.2 | 0.2 |
| Ukraine | 0.2 | 0.6 | 0.6 | 3.1 | 0.1 | 0 | 0 | 0 | 0 | 0 | 72.5 | 73 | 75.4 | 76.4 | 78.6 | 1 | 1.4 | 1.7 | 1.6 | 1.6 |
| United Arab Emirates | 0 | 0 | 0 | 0 | 0 | 0 | 0 | 0 | 0 | 0 | 70.5 | 68.7 | 69.4 | 70.6 | 70.4 | 19 | 21 | 20.2 | 18.8 | 19.1 |
| United Kingdom | 0 | 0 | 0 | 0 | 0 | 0 | 0 | 0 | 0 | 0 | 55.2 | 55 | 62.3 | 64.8 | 76.7 | 16.8 | 16.8 | 19 | 19.7 | 23.3 |
| United Republic of Tanzania | 29.3 | 32.1 | 34.1 | 29.6 | 21.9 | 0 | 0 | 5 | 3.2 | 2.6 | 83.5 | 83.6 | 83.8 | 83.5 | 81.1 | 4.5 | 4.5 | 4.5 | 4.7 | 5.4 |
| United States of America | 0 | 0 | 0 | 0 | 0 | 33.1 | 33.7 | 32.5 | 30.5 | 28.4 | 27 | 26.5 | 25.8 | 24.9 | 24.3 | 61.4 | 62.7 | 64.1 | 65.3 | 65.9 |
| Uruguay | 0.1 | 0.5 | 0.8 | 0.6 | 0.4 | 52.6 | 50 | 47.7 | 48.3 | 48.5 | 26.6 | 25.9 | 24.9 | 25 | 25 | 73.4 | 74.1 | 75.1 | 75 | 75 |
| Uzbekistan | 0.9 | 1.7 | 3.5 | 4.1 | 3 | 0 | 0 | 0 | 0 | 0 | 96.8 | 96.9 | 97.1 | 95.3 | 95.5 | 0 | 0 | 0 | 0 | 0 |
| Vanuatu | 23 | 25.8 | 18.6 | 18.3 | 25.4 | 0 | 0 | 0 | 0 | 0 | 47.8 | 49.9 | 46.3 | 45.8 | 45.8 | 0 | 0 | 0 | 0 | 0 |
| Venezuela, Bolivarian Republic of | 1 | 0.4 | 0.1 | 0.1 | 0.1 | 25 | 28.5 | 34.2 | 31.4 | 25.2 | 88.5 | 87 | 87.4 | 87.3 | 95.5 | 4 | 3.7 | 3.7 | 4.1 | 4.5 |
| Viet Nam | 3.4 | 2.7 | 2.8 | 3.5 | 2.6 | 9.5 | 10.5 | 13.7 | 15.8 | 16.6 | 86.5 | 87.1 | 83.6 | 80.8 | 74.2 | 3.7 | 4.1 | 2.2 | 2.3 | 3.1 |
| Yemen | 8.2 | 8.9 | 9.7 | 7.3 | 8.8 | n/a | n/a | n/a | n/a | n/a | 96.3 | 96.1 | 96.6 | 96.7 | 95.5 | n/a | n/a | n/a | n/a | n/a |
| Zambia | 8.9 | 18.2 | 13.7 | 18.3 | 44.7 | 0 | 0 | 0 | 0 | 0 | 82 | 81.1 | 74.9 | 72.7 | 68.2 | n/a | n/a | n/a | n/a | n/a |
| Zimbabwe | 15.7 | 11.7 | 5.6 | 1.4 | 6.8 | 0 | 0 | 0 | 0 | 0 | 44.9 | 46.7 | 50.7 | 51.7 | 56.7 | 39.6 | 31.1 | 29 | 25.9 | 21 |

[h]Expenditures, previously recorded as social security spending, were re-evaluated as extrabudgetary agency spending.

[i]THE:GDP ratio in 2001 is high because newly accessed information shows that WHO, NZAID and AusAID provided US$ 2 million for renovation of a hospital in 2001–2002.

[j]Series adjusted for the removal of a double count in previous years.

[k]The estimates for 1999 to 2003 do not include the expenditures of the provinces of Kosovo and Metohia, which are under the administration of the United Nations.

[l]Social security includes the expenditure by the Instituto Nacional de la Salud in the Comunidades autónomas up to 2002. The expenditure is now channelled through the Comunidades autónomas except for the Ceuta and Melilla Ciudades Autónomas, the civil servants, and those related to work injuries and sickness.

[m]The country came into existence in August 1999.

[n]Togo data on health research and development and training were adjusted to harmonize with the standard methodology used for World Health Reports.

[o]In 2002, an additional 9.3 million Tuvaluan $, mostly coming from external sources, were spent for construction of a new hospital.

n/a Used when the information accessed indicates that a cell should have an entry but no estimates could be made.

0 Used when no evidence of the schemes to which the cell relates exist. Some estimates yielding a ratio below 0.04% are shown as '0'.

## Annex Table 3 Selected national health accounts indicators: measured levels of per capita expenditure on health, 1999–2003
Figures computed by WHO to assure comparability;[a] they are not necessarily the official statistics of Member States, which may use alternative methods.

| Member State | Per capita total expenditure on health at average exchange rate (US$) | | | | | Per capita total expenditure on health at international dollar rate | | | | | Per capita government expenditure on health at average exchange rate (US$) | | | | | Per capita government expenditure on health at international dollar rate | | | | |
|---|---|---|---|---|---|---|---|---|---|---|---|---|---|---|---|---|---|---|---|---|
| | 1999 | 2000 | 2001 | 2002 | 2003 | 1999 | 2000 | 2001 | 2002 | 2003 | 1999 | 2000 | 2001 | 2002 | 2003 | 1999 | 2000 | 2001 | 2002 | 2003 |
| Afghanistan | 4 | 3 | 3 | 11 | 11 | 19 | 9 | 9 | 24 | 26 | <1 | <1 | <1 | 4 | 4 | <1 | <1 | <1 | 10 | 10 |
| Albania | 77 | 78 | 88 | 99 | 118 | 289 | 299 | 336 | 360 | 366 | 35 | 33 | 37 | 41 | 49 | 131 | 127 | 142 | 150 | 153 |
| Algeria | 61 | 63 | 68 | 75 | 89 | 137 | 132 | 149 | 174 | 186 | 43 | 46 | 53 | 60 | 71 | 99 | 97 | 115 | 137 | 150 |
| Andorra[b] | 1359 | 1287 | 1296 | 1549 | 2039 | 1749 | 1895 | 1936 | 2219 | 2453 | 913 | 841 | 891 | 1066 | 1399 | 1176 | 1239 | 1331 | 1527 | 1683 |
| Angola | 15 | 16 | 21 | 18 | 26 | 43 | 34 | 48 | 41 | 49 | 7 | 13 | 18 | 15 | 22 | 20 | 28 | 41 | 33 | 41 |
| Antigua and Barbuda | 389 | 397 | 425 | 495 | 426 | 423 | 437 | 472 | 555 | 477 | 281 | 286 | 301 | 359 | 300 | 305 | 314 | 334 | 402 | 336 |
| Argentina | 706 | 689 | 687 | 233 | 305 | 1135 | 1121 | 1157 | 934 | 1067 | 399 | 382 | 369 | 121 | 148 | 641 | 621 | 621 | 487 | 518 |
| Armenia | 36 | 39 | 45 | 46 | 55 | 181 | 205 | 241 | 253 | 302 | 8 | 6 | 9 | 9 | 11 | 41 | 31 | 49 | 51 | 61 |
| Australia | 1849 | 1832 | 1744 | 1961 | 2519 | 2204 | 2406 | 2531 | 2693 | 2874 | 1286 | 1262 | 1183 | 1336 | 1699 | 1533 | 1657 | 1716 | 1835 | 1939 |
| Austria | 2029 | 1812 | 1776 | 1923 | 2358 | 2051 | 2170 | 2162 | 2240 | 2306 | 1374 | 1235 | 1189 | 1305 | 1595 | 1388 | 1479 | 1448 | 1520 | 1560 |
| Azerbaijan | 27 | 26 | 27 | 28 | 32 | 115 | 112 | 121 | 128 | 140 | 6 | 6 | 6 | 6 | 8 | 24 | 24 | 27 | 27 | 33 |
| Bahamas | 1051 | 1075 | 1088 | 1128 | 1121 | 1164 | 1166 | 1187 | 1205 | 1220 | 491 | 507 | 517 | 548 | 533 | 545 | 550 | 564 | 586 | 579 |
| Bahrain | 473 | 463 | 484 | 514 | 555 | 750 | 656 | 739 | 787 | 813 | 328 | 310 | 327 | 349 | 384 | 519 | 440 | 499 | 534 | 562 |
| Bangladesh | 12 | 12 | 12 | 13 | 14 | 50 | 54 | 57 | 61 | 68 | 3 | 3 | 3 | 4 | 4 | 14 | 14 | 15 | 18 | 21 |
| Barbados | 574 | 604 | 638 | 674 | 691 | 870 | 918 | 976 | 1021 | 1050 | 375 | 398 | 431 | 461 | 479 | 570 | 604 | 659 | 699 | 729 |
| Belarus | 73 | 64 | 82 | 94 | 99 | 459 | 501 | 582 | 601 | 570 | 59 | 51 | 62 | 69 | 71 | 372 | 401 | 439 | 444 | 406 |
| Belgium | 2108 | 1926 | 1945 | 2172 | 2796 | 2108 | 2282 | 2420 | 2616 | 2828 | 1462 | 1335 | 1376 | 1528 | 1880 | 1462 | 1582 | 1713 | 1840 | 1902 |
| Belize | 148 | 155 | 165 | 174 | 174 | 258 | 262 | 295 | 290 | 309 | 72 | 74 | 75 | 82 | 86 | 125 | 126 | 133 | 138 | 152 |
| Benin | 16 | 15 | 16 | 16 | 20 | 34 | 34 | 38 | 37 | 36 | 7 | 7 | 7 | 7 | 9 | 15 | 15 | 18 | 16 | 16 |
| Bhutan | 11 | 11 | 14 | 10 | 10 | 67 | 66 | 88 | 64 | 59 | 9 | 9 | 12 | 9 | 9 | 60 | 58 | 79 | 54 | 49 |
| Bolivia | 63 | 61 | 61 | 60 | 61 | 149 | 150 | 161 | 170 | 176 | 37 | 37 | 36 | 37 | 39 | 87 | 90 | 95 | 107 | 113 |
| Bosnia and Herzegovina | 134 | 112 | 110 | 126 | 168 | 302 | 286 | 285 | 295 | 327 | 76 | 58 | 54 | 62 | 85 | 171 | 149 | 139 | 145 | 166 |
| Botswana | 138 | 152 | 132 | 144 | 232 | 259 | 294 | 284 | 312 | 375 | 75 | 87 | 67 | 78 | 135 | 141 | 168 | 143 | 169 | 218 |
| Brazil | 243 | 263 | 224 | 199 | 212 | 543 | 558 | 584 | 592 | 597 | 104 | 108 | 96 | 89 | 96 | 232 | 228 | 250 | 265 | 270 |
| Brunei Darussalam | 480 | 443 | 430 | 428 | 466 | 641 | 609 | 643 | 657 | 681 | 351 | 370 | 331 | 336 | 372 | 469 | 508 | 495 | 516 | 545 |
| Bulgaria | 97 | 97 | 123 | 155 | 191 | 342 | 381 | 476 | 561 | 573 | 63 | 58 | 69 | 88 | 104 | 223 | 226 | 267 | 317 | 312 |
| Burkina Faso | 15 | 12 | 12 | 15 | 19 | 55 | 54 | 55 | 62 | 68 | 6 | 5 | 5 | 6 | 9 | 24 | 23 | 22 | 27 | 32 |
| Burundi | 4 | 3 | 3 | 3 | 3 | 14 | 14 | 15 | 15 | 15 | 1 | 1 | 1 | 1 | 1 | 3 | 3 | 3 | 3 | 4 |
| Cambodia | 29 | 31 | 31 | 33 | 33 | 147 | 162 | 168 | 179 | 188 | 3 | 4 | 5 | 6 | 6 | 15 | 23 | 25 | 31 | 36 |
| Cameroon | 31 | 29 | 29 | 32 | 37 | 62 | 58 | 62 | 66 | 64 | 8 | 8 | 8 | 9 | 11 | 15 | 16 | 17 | 18 | 19 |
| Canada | 1916 | 2071 | 2129 | 2225 | 2669 | 2400 | 2509 | 2705 | 2841 | 2989 | 1347 | 1457 | 1493 | 1551 | 1866 | 1687 | 1765 | 1897 | 1980 | 2090 |
| Cape Verde | 61 | 55 | 61 | 66 | 78 | 148 | 163 | 186 | 193 | 185 | 45 | 41 | 46 | 50 | 57 | 110 | 119 | 141 | 145 | 135 |
| Central African Republic | 10 | 10 | 10 | 11 | 12 | 44 | 50 | 49 | 51 | 47 | 4 | 4 | 4 | 4 | 5 | 17 | 20 | 19 | 21 | 18 |
| Chad | 11 | 11 | 12 | 12 | 16 | 37 | 40 | 43 | 44 | 51 | 4 | 4 | 5 | 4 | 7 | 12 | 17 | 18 | 16 | 20 |
| Chile | 342 | 299 | 272 | 265 | 282 | 697 | 631 | 665 | 686 | 707 | 133 | 139 | 131 | 127 | 137 | 272 | 293 | 320 | 329 | 345 |
| China | 39 | 43 | 47 | 54 | 61 | 169 | 192 | 212 | 247 | 278 | 16 | 17 | 17 | 19 | 22 | 69 | 74 | 75 | 88 | 101 |
| Colombia | 195 | 152 | 147 | 141 | 138 | 572 | 485 | 498 | 497 | 522 | 148 | 123 | 118 | 116 | 116 | 436 | 392 | 399 | 408 | 439 |
| Comoros | 11 | 8 | 7 | 10 | 11 | 30 | 25 | 21 | 27 | 25 | 6 | 4 | 3 | 6 | 6 | 18 | 14 | 10 | 16 | 14 |
| Congo | 17 | 17 | 16 | 16 | 19 | 25 | 20 | 23 | 22 | 23 | 11 | 11 | 10 | 11 | 12 | 16 | 13 | 15 | 15 | 15 |
| Cook Islands | 154 | 171 | 176 | 203 | 294 | 275 | 354 | 373 | 378 | 425 | 134 | 150 | 154 | 177 | 258 | 240 | 312 | 327 | 329 | 373 |
| Costa Rica | 249 | 258 | 280 | 295 | 305 | 457 | 487 | 532 | 572 | 616 | 194 | 204 | 219 | 235 | 240 | 356 | 385 | 418 | 455 | 486 |
| Côte d'Ivoire | 39 | 30 | 24 | 25 | 28 | 87 | 79 | 65 | 62 | 57 | 7 | 6 | 4 | 8 | 8 | 15 | 16 | 12 | 20 | 16 |
| Croatia | 386 | 380 | 370 | 392 | 494 | 742 | 829 | 801 | 792 | 838 | 333 | 330 | 317 | 325 | 413 | 640 | 719 | 688 | 655 | 701 |
| Cuba | 164 | 176 | 187 | 199 | 211 | 196 | 212 | 226 | 239 | 251 | 140 | 151 | 161 | 172 | 183 | 167 | 182 | 194 | 206 | 218 |
| Cyprus | 700 | 675 | 697 | 794 | 1038 | 905 | 1000 | 934 | 1101 | 1143 | 299 | 280 | 295 | 356 | 510 | 386 | 415 | 395 | 495 | 561 |
| Czech Republic | 379 | 358 | 408 | 517 | 667 | 920 | 962 | 1065 | 1186 | 1302 | 347 | 327 | 373 | 471 | 600 | 842 | 879 | 973 | 1080 | 1172 |
| Democratic People's Republic of Korea[c] | 22 | 28 | 29 | <1 | <1 | 54 | 67 | 70 | 72 | 74 | 20 | 25 | 26 | <1 | <1 | 48 | 62 | 64 | 66 | 68 |
| Democratic Republic of Congo | 8 | 10 | 4 | 3 | 4 | 12 | 13 | 10 | 11 | 14 | 1 | 1 | <1 | <1 | 1 | 1 | 1 | 1 | 1 | 3 |
| Denmark | 2767 | 2478 | 2565 | 2835 | 3534 | 2297 | 2381 | 2556 | 2654 | 2762 | 2275 | 2043 | 2120 | 2352 | 2931 | 1888 | 1963 | 2113 | 2201 | 2292 |
| Djibouti | 40 | 41 | 42 | 43 | 47 | 61 | 63 | 64 | 67 | 72 | 26 | 27 | 27 | 28 | 31 | 40 | 42 | 41 | 44 | 48 |

| Member State | Per capita total expenditure on health at average exchange rate (US$) | | | | | Per capita total expenditure on health at international dollar rate | | | | | Per capita government expenditure on health at average exchange rate (US$) | | | | | Per capita government expenditure on health at international dollar rate | | | | |
|---|---|---|---|---|---|---|---|---|---|---|---|---|---|---|---|---|---|---|---|---|
| | 1999 | 2000 | 2001 | 2002 | 2003 | 1999 | 2000 | 2001 | 2002 | 2003 | 1999 | 2000 | 2001 | 2002 | 2003 | 1999 | 2000 | 2001 | 2002 | 2003 |
| Dominica | 214 | 216 | 203 | 206 | 212 | 313 | 323 | 302 | 313 | 320 | 159 | 159 | 145 | 147 | 151 | 232 | 237 | 216 | 223 | 228 |
| Dominican Republic | 129 | 162 | 179 | 186 | 132 | 248 | 301 | 323 | 356 | 335 | 39 | 52 | 57 | 60 | 44 | 75 | 97 | 103 | 115 | 111 |
| Ecuador[d] | 65 | 54 | 81 | 95 | 109 | 173 | 157 | 193 | 206 | 220 | 26 | 17 | 27 | 37 | 42 | 68 | 49 | 65 | 79 | 85 |
| Egypt | 68 | 71 | 63 | 71 | 55 | 173 | 190 | 208 | 231 | 235 | 23 | 26 | 25 | 30 | 24 | 59 | 69 | 83 | 99 | 100 |
| El Salvador | 162 | 168 | 167 | 175 | 183 | 343 | 352 | 347 | 366 | 378 | 70 | 76 | 71 | 78 | 84 | 149 | 159 | 147 | 164 | 174 |
| Equatorial Guinea | 46 | 54 | 67 | 85 | 96 | 125 | 106 | 152 | 193 | 179 | 28 | 37 | 47 | 61 | 65 | 76 | 72 | 107 | 139 | 121 |
| Eritrea | 8 | 8 | 8 | 7 | 8 | 47 | 48 | 53 | 51 | 50 | 6 | 5 | 5 | 4 | 4 | 33 | 32 | 31 | 26 | 23 |
| Estonia | 243 | 220 | 223 | 263 | 366 | 524 | 531 | 540 | 589 | 682 | 197 | 170 | 176 | 203 | 282 | 424 | 412 | 424 | 454 | 526 |
| Ethiopia | 5 | 5 | 5 | 5 | 5 | 17 | 19 | 21 | 21 | 20 | 3 | 3 | 3 | 3 | 3 | 9 | 10 | 11 | 12 | 12 |
| Fiji | 85 | 80 | 78 | 93 | 104 | 194 | 203 | 205 | 234 | 220 | 56 | 52 | 52 | 62 | 64 | 126 | 133 | 136 | 155 | 135 |
| Finland | 1713 | 1549 | 1622 | 1831 | 2307 | 1641 | 1716 | 1857 | 2012 | 2108 | 1290 | 1164 | 1231 | 1397 | 1766 | 1236 | 1289 | 1409 | 1535 | 1613 |
| France | 2285 | 2070 | 2107 | 2339 | 2981 | 2306 | 2469 | 2616 | 2762 | 2902 | 1738 | 1569 | 1600 | 1780 | 2273 | 1754 | 1872 | 1986 | 2101 | 2213 |
| Gabon | 165 | 164 | 148 | 158 | 196 | 250 | 229 | 235 | 244 | 255 | 113 | 120 | 108 | 111 | 130 | 171 | 167 | 171 | 171 | 170 |
| Gambia | 24 | 25 | 23 | 20 | 21 | 76 | 88 | 92 | 84 | 96 | 8 | 10 | 9 | 8 | 8 | 24 | 36 | 37 | 34 | 38 |
| Georgia | 17 | 28 | 31 | 33 | 35 | 90 | 143 | 158 | 173 | 174 | 6 | 8 | 9 | 10 | 8 | 32 | 41 | 47 | 50 | 42 |
| Germany | 2730 | 2404 | 2425 | 2637 | 3204 | 2566 | 2674 | 2772 | 2912 | 3001 | 2143 | 1889 | 1901 | 2072 | 2506 | 2014 | 2101 | 2173 | 2288 | 2348 |
| Ghana | 22 | 13 | 12 | 14 | 16 | 100 | 102 | 94 | 95 | 98 | 8 | 5 | 4 | 4 | 5 | 35 | 36 | 27 | 29 | 31 |
| Greece | 1114 | 1032 | 1091 | 1182 | 1556 | 1469 | 1628 | 1767 | 1847 | 1997 | 595 | 543 | 591 | 610 | 798 | 785 | 856 | 958 | 953 | 1025 |
| Grenada | 206 | 238 | 296 | 282 | 289 | 333 | 470 | 485 | 464 | 473 | 151 | 176 | 231 | 206 | 212 | 244 | 347 | 378 | 338 | 348 |
| Guatemala | 79 | 96 | 100 | 104 | 112 | 188 | 228 | 229 | 223 | 235 | 38 | 38 | 38 | 38 | 44 | 91 | 91 | 87 | 83 | 93 |
| Guinea | 20 | 18 | 17 | 19 | 22 | 74 | 76 | 81 | 90 | 95 | 3 | 2 | 3 | 3 | 4 | 10 | 10 | 15 | 13 | 16 |
| Guinea-Bissau | 8 | 6 | 6 | 9 | 9 | 45 | 38 | 38 | 49 | 45 | 2 | 2 | 1 | 4 | 4 | 13 | 9 | 8 | 20 | 21 |
| Guyana | 40 | 52 | 52 | 55 | 53 | 236 | 299 | 306 | 291 | 283 | 33 | 44 | 43 | 45 | 44 | 195 | 253 | 253 | 242 | 233 |
| Haiti | 34 | 31 | 31 | 29 | 26 | 75 | 76 | 79 | 84 | 84 | 12 | 11 | 12 | 12 | 10 | 27 | 27 | 30 | 33 | 32 |
| Honduras | 49 | 60 | 63 | 67 | 72 | 131 | 154 | 161 | 172 | 184 | 25 | 34 | 35 | 37 | 41 | 66 | 86 | 88 | 95 | 104 |
| Hungary | 345 | 326 | 375 | 496 | 684 | 819 | 857 | 975 | 1115 | 1269 | 250 | 231 | 258 | 348 | 495 | 593 | 606 | 673 | 783 | 919 |
| Iceland | 2858 | 2780 | 2500 | 2960 | 3821 | 2549 | 2627 | 2742 | 2943 | 3110 | 2389 | 2296 | 2068 | 2464 | 3191 | 2131 | 2169 | 2268 | 2450 | 2598 |
| India | 23 | 23 | 23 | 23 | 27 | 69 | 71 | 74 | 75 | 82 | 6 | 6 | 6 | 6 | 7 | 17 | 17 | 18 | 18 | 20 |
| Indonesia | 17 | 18 | 21 | 26 | 30 | 76 | 80 | 102 | 109 | 113 | 5 | 5 | 7 | 9 | 11 | 23 | 23 | 36 | 38 | 40 |
| Iran, Islamic Republic of[e] | 53 | 66 | 81 | 116 | 131 | 373 | 364 | 415 | 410 | 498 | 22 | 28 | 36 | 44 | 62 | 153 | 157 | 184 | 155 | 235 |
| Iraq | 14 | 17 | 12 | 11 | 23 | 50 | 49 | 54 | 48 | 64 | 6 | 5 | 3 | 2 | 12 | 20 | 14 | 15 | 8 | 33 |
| Ireland | 1590 | 1568 | 1835 | 2191 | 2860 | 1624 | 1800 | 2097 | 2322 | 2496 | 1171 | 1158 | 1382 | 1698 | 2256 | 1196 | 1329 | 1580 | 1800 | 1968 |
| Israel | 1492 | 1637 | 1682 | 1520 | 1514 | 1717 | 1869 | 2028 | 1968 | 1911 | 1037 | 1111 | 1139 | 1021 | 1032 | 1193 | 1268 | 1373 | 1322 | 1303 |
| Italy | 1602 | 1519 | 1574 | 1750 | 2139 | 1859 | 2044 | 2150 | 2262 | 2266 | 1153 | 1116 | 1193 | 1320 | 1607 | 1338 | 1502 | 1630 | 1706 | 1703 |
| Jamaica | 161 | 191 | 169 | 157 | 164 | 196 | 232 | 210 | 192 | 216 | 81 | 100 | 77 | 80 | 83 | 99 | 122 | 96 | 98 | 109 |
| Japan | 2601 | 2827 | 2558 | 2450 | 2662 | 1829 | 1971 | 2092 | 2139 | 2244 | 2109 | 2298 | 2089 | 1997 | 2158 | 1483 | 1602 | 1708 | 1743 | 1818 |
| Jordan | 149 | 156 | 165 | 169 | 177 | 361 | 389 | 415 | 425 | 440 | 71 | 71 | 75 | 78 | 80 | 173 | 176 | 189 | 196 | 199 |
| Kazakhstan | 48 | 50 | 50 | 59 | 73 | 231 | 251 | 243 | 284 | 315 | 25 | 25 | 28 | 31 | 42 | 120 | 128 | 137 | 151 | 180 |
| Kenya | 16 | 18 | 18 | 19 | 20 | 60 | 61 | 62 | 66 | 65 | 7 | 8 | 8 | 8 | 8 | 25 | 28 | 27 | 29 | 25 |
| Kiribati | 46 | 58 | 59 | 65 | 96 | 137 | 197 | 215 | 211 | 253 | 46 | 57 | 59 | 64 | 89 | 135 | 196 | 213 | 209 | 233 |
| Kuwait | 521 | 521 | 525 | 565 | 580 | 583 | 494 | 558 | 588 | 567 | 402 | 408 | 408 | 441 | 449 | 450 | 387 | 434 | 459 | 440 |
| Kyrgyzstan | 13 | 12 | 14 | 16 | 20 | 123 | 116 | 126 | 144 | 161 | 6 | 6 | 6 | 7 | 8 | 59 | 54 | 54 | 59 | 66 |
| Lao People's Democratic Republic | 7 | 8 | 9 | 10 | 11 | 35 | 38 | 42 | 49 | 56 | 3 | 3 | 3 | 4 | 4 | 14 | 15 | 17 | 22 | 22 |
| Latvia | 193 | 195 | 216 | 248 | 301 | 464 | 477 | 549 | 611 | 678 | 114 | 107 | 110 | 129 | 155 | 274 | 263 | 281 | 318 | 348 |
| Lebanon | 578 | 574 | 582 | 566 | 573 | 656 | 700 | 720 | 671 | 730 | 159 | 164 | 176 | 171 | 168 | 181 | 200 | 217 | 202 | 214 |
| Lesotho | 28 | 28 | 24 | 25 | 31 | 91 | 100 | 103 | 125 | 106 | 23 | 23 | 20 | 21 | 25 | 74 | 83 | 84 | 104 | 84 |
| Liberia | 10 | 8 | 7 | 7 | 6 | 26 | 23 | 21 | 20 | 17 | 6 | 5 | 3 | 3 | 4 | 18 | 13 | 10 | 10 | 10 |
| Libyan Arab Jamahiriya | 211 | 200 | 286 | 182 | 171 | 234 | 220 | 391 | 360 | 327 | 107 | 116 | 209 | 119 | 108 | 119 | 128 | 286 | 235 | 206 |
| Lithuania | 193 | 212 | 220 | 263 | 351 | 501 | 557 | 591 | 660 | 754 | 145 | 148 | 160 | 197 | 267 | 375 | 388 | 429 | 495 | 573 |
| Luxembourg | 2889 | 2702 | 2835 | 3423 | 4112 | 2767 | 2963 | 3169 | 3712 | 3680 | 2595 | 2439 | 2574 | 3120 | 3734 | 2485 | 2674 | 2877 | 3383 | 3341 |

## Annex Table 3 Selected national health accounts indicators: measured levels of per capita expenditure on health, 1999–2003

Figures computed by WHO to assure comparability;[a] they are not necessarily the official statistics of Member States, which may use alternative methods.

| Member State | Per capita total expenditure on health at average exchange rate (US$) | | | | | Per capita total expenditure on health at international dollar rate | | | | | Per capita government expenditure on health at average exchange rate (US$) | | | | | Per capita government expenditure on health at international dollar rate | | | | |
|---|---|---|---|---|---|---|---|---|---|---|---|---|---|---|---|---|---|---|---|---|
| | 1999 | 2000 | 2001 | 2002 | 2003 | 1999 | 2000 | 2001 | 2002 | 2003 | 1999 | 2000 | 2001 | 2002 | 2003 | 1999 | 2000 | 2001 | 2002 | 2003 |
| Madagascar[f] | 5 | 5 | 5 | 7 | 8 | 20 | 20 | 19 | 24 | 24 | 3 | 3 | 3 | 5 | 5 | 11 | 10 | 12 | 15 | 15 |
| Malawi | 16 | 13 | 15 | 15 | 13 | 47 | 41 | 48 | 44 | 46 | 6 | 4 | 7 | 5 | 5 | 17 | 12 | 22 | 15 | 16 |
| Malaysia | 112 | 130 | 138 | 146 | 163 | 261 | 294 | 329 | 342 | 374 | 58 | 68 | 77 | 81 | 95 | 134 | 154 | 184 | 190 | 218 |
| Maldives | 116 | 127 | 125 | 121 | 136 | 267 | 293 | 306 | 311 | 364 | 99 | 110 | 110 | 106 | 121 | 228 | 255 | 268 | 273 | 324 |
| Mali | 11 | 11 | 11 | 12 | 16 | 27 | 32 | 32 | 35 | 39 | 5 | 5 | 5 | 6 | 9 | 11 | 16 | 16 | 18 | 22 |
| Malta | 700 | 772 | 766 | 918 | 1104 | 1163 | 1209 | 1380 | 1421 | 1436 | 529 | 591 | 596 | 731 | 884 | 879 | 925 | 1073 | 1133 | 1150 |
| Marshall Islands | 301 | 275 | 232 | 229 | 255 | 554 | 507 | 437 | 431 | 477 | 292 | 266 | 223 | 221 | 247 | 538 | 492 | 421 | 415 | 461 |
| Mauritania | 10 | 9 | 10 | 14 | 17 | 32 | 32 | 38 | 53 | 59 | 7 | 6 | 7 | 10 | 13 | 21 | 20 | 26 | 39 | 46 |
| Mauritius | 113 | 127 | 132 | 143 | 172 | 281 | 331 | 373 | 398 | 430 | 70 | 74 | 80 | 87 | 105 | 174 | 194 | 226 | 242 | 261 |
| Mexico | 273 | 323 | 369 | 381 | 372 | 463 | 499 | 545 | 559 | 582 | 130 | 150 | 165 | 171 | 172 | 221 | 232 | 245 | 251 | 270 |
| Micronesia, Federated States of | 138 | 140 | 145 | 143 | 147 | 242 | 260 | 266 | 267 | 270 | 121 | 121 | 126 | 126 | 130 | 213 | 225 | 231 | 236 | 238 |
| Monaco[b] | 3471 | 3097 | 3103 | 3344 | 4587 | 3508 | 3709 | 3862 | 3938 | 4487 | 2407 | 2190 | 2230 | 2445 | 3480 | 2433 | 2623 | 2775 | 2880 | 3403 |
| Mongolia | 20 | 26 | 30 | 29 | 33 | 99 | 130 | 140 | 132 | 140 | 15 | 17 | 20 | 20 | 21 | 72 | 86 | 93 | 92 | 90 |
| Morocco | 56 | 54 | 57 | 60 | 72 | 167 | 175 | 196 | 205 | 218 | 17 | 17 | 18 | 19 | 24 | 50 | 54 | 64 | 67 | 72 |
| Mozambique | 11 | 12 | 10 | 11 | 12 | 34 | 40 | 39 | 45 | 45 | 7 | 8 | 6 | 7 | 7 | 21 | 27 | 26 | 30 | 28 |
| Myanmar[g] | 134 | 183 | 228 | 315 | 394 | 21 | 28 | 30 | 44 | 51 | 15 | 25 | 29 | 58 | 77 | 2 | 4 | 4 | 8 | 10 |
| Namibia | 127 | 126 | 107 | 95 | 145 | 328 | 340 | 323 | 318 | 359 | 93 | 87 | 75 | 65 | 101 | 240 | 235 | 224 | 218 | 252 |
| Nauru | 700 | 645 | 584 | 654 | 798 | 951 | 820 | 742 | 776 | 763 | 624 | 573 | 518 | 580 | 706 | 848 | 729 | 658 | 689 | 675 |
| Nepal | 11 | 11 | 12 | 12 | 12 | 55 | 56 | 64 | 67 | 64 | 3 | 3 | 4 | 4 | 3 | 14 | 14 | 20 | 21 | 18 |
| Netherlands | 2102 | 1916 | 2067 | 2411 | 3088 | 2124 | 2270 | 2517 | 2777 | 2987 | 1318 | 1209 | 1298 | 1506 | 1926 | 1332 | 1432 | 1581 | 1735 | 1863 |
| New Zealand | 1155 | 1054 | 1056 | 1255 | 1618 | 1527 | 1600 | 1698 | 1844 | 1893 | 895 | 823 | 807 | 978 | 1267 | 1183 | 1248 | 1298 | 1437 | 1483 |
| Nicaragua | 45 | 57 | 62 | 61 | 60 | 142 | 180 | 203 | 208 | 208 | 24 | 30 | 30 | 30 | 29 | 77 | 94 | 98 | 103 | 101 |
| Niger | 8 | 6 | 6 | 7 | 9 | 27 | 25 | 26 | 27 | 30 | 4 | 3 | 3 | 4 | 5 | 14 | 13 | 14 | 15 | 16 |
| Nigeria | 17 | 18 | 19 | 19 | 22 | 48 | 39 | 50 | 49 | 51 | 5 | 6 | 6 | 5 | 6 | 14 | 13 | 16 | 12 | 13 |
| Niue | 440 | 367 | 1710 | 506 | 655 | 103 | 102 | 529 | 154 | 153 | 427 | 355 | 1700 | 499 | 644 | 100 | 98 | 526 | 151 | 150 |
| Norway | 3325 | 3156 | 3333 | 4143 | 4976 | 2816 | 3083 | 3286 | 3617 | 3809 | 2745 | 2604 | 2785 | 3458 | 4167 | 2325 | 2543 | 2745 | 3019 | 3189 |
| Oman | 232 | 254 | 248 | 265 | 278 | 378 | 352 | 376 | 411 | 419 | 193 | 206 | 204 | 219 | 231 | 315 | 285 | 309 | 340 | 348 |
| Pakistan | 16 | 14 | 12 | 13 | 13 | 66 | 51 | 49 | 50 | 48 | 5 | 5 | 4 | 5 | 4 | 22 | 17 | 16 | 18 | 13 |
| Palau[h] | 567 | 593 | 598 | 586 | 607 | 696 | 740 | 770 | 761 | 798 | 502 | 528 | 533 | 511 | 526 | 616 | 659 | 685 | 664 | 691 |
| Panama | 271 | 306 | 303 | 322 | 315 | 450 | 524 | 527 | 559 | 555 | 180 | 208 | 203 | 222 | 209 | 298 | 357 | 354 | 386 | 368 |
| Papua New Guinea | 25 | 26 | 24 | 22 | 23 | 127 | 129 | 138 | 133 | 132 | 23 | 23 | 21 | 20 | 20 | 113 | 114 | 124 | 119 | 118 |
| Paraguay | 105 | 119 | 102 | 80 | 75 | 298 | 345 | 351 | 336 | 301 | 47 | 48 | 36 | 27 | 24 | 134 | 139 | 124 | 112 | 95 |
| Peru | 98 | 96 | 93 | 93 | 98 | 227 | 227 | 223 | 225 | 233 | 52 | 51 | 48 | 45 | 47 | 120 | 120 | 113 | 109 | 112 |
| Philippines | 36 | 34 | 30 | 29 | 31 | 166 | 171 | 162 | 157 | 174 | 16 | 16 | 13 | 12 | 14 | 73 | 82 | 72 | 63 | 76 |
| Poland | 249 | 246 | 292 | 328 | 354 | 564 | 587 | 646 | 732 | 745 | 177 | 172 | 210 | 234 | 248 | 401 | 411 | 464 | 521 | 521 |
| Portugal | 985 | 951 | 995 | 1092 | 1348 | 1424 | 1595 | 1688 | 1754 | 1791 | 665 | 661 | 702 | 770 | 940 | 962 | 1108 | 1192 | 1237 | 1249 |
| Qatar | 773 | 816 | 808 | 871 | 862 | 834 | 690 | 745 | 868 | 685 | 569 | 612 | 599 | 640 | 637 | 614 | 518 | 552 | 639 | 506 |
| Republic of Korea | 463 | 513 | 550 | 607 | 705 | 729 | 771 | 932 | 975 | 1074 | 206 | 237 | 286 | 305 | 348 | 324 | 356 | 484 | 490 | 531 |
| Republic of Moldova | 19 | 20 | 22 | 28 | 34 | 123 | 122 | 132 | 160 | 177 | 9 | 10 | 11 | 16 | 18 | 56 | 63 | 67 | 92 | 96 |
| Romania | 87 | 91 | 101 | 124 | 159 | 368 | 386 | 429 | 491 | 540 | 54 | 59 | 65 | 79 | 100 | 231 | 253 | 277 | 314 | 340 |
| Russian Federation | 74 | 102 | 119 | 141 | 167 | 385 | 449 | 476 | 534 | 551 | 43 | 57 | 70 | 84 | 98 | 223 | 252 | 280 | 317 | 325 |
| Rwanda | 11 | 10 | 8 | 9 | 7 | 33 | 32 | 31 | 35 | 32 | 5 | 3 | 3 | 4 | 3 | 16 | 11 | 12 | 17 | 14 |
| Saint Kitts and Nevis | 415 | 453 | 456 | 466 | 467 | 606 | 649 | 652 | 669 | 670 | 249 | 289 | 293 | 295 | 298 | 364 | 413 | 419 | 424 | 427 |
| Saint Lucia | 201 | 212 | 214 | 216 | 221 | 266 | 280 | 285 | 285 | 294 | 138 | 148 | 148 | 148 | 150 | 183 | 195 | 196 | 195 | 200 |
| Saint Vincent and the Grenadines | 164 | 164 | 169 | 191 | 194 | 311 | 318 | 329 | 371 | 384 | 100 | 105 | 109 | 127 | 131 | 189 | 203 | 212 | 248 | 259 |
| Samoa | 84 | 83 | 78 | 84 | 94 | 198 | 209 | 208 | 215 | 209 | 63 | 62 | 58 | 66 | 74 | 149 | 157 | 155 | 169 | 165 |
| San Marino[b] | 2322 | 2103 | 2304 | 2473 | 2957 | 2695 | 2830 | 3147 | 3197 | 3133 | 1807 | 1627 | 1829 | 1958 | 2328 | 2097 | 2190 | 2498 | 2531 | 2467 |
| Sao Tome and Principe | 34 | 29 | 35 | 31 | 34 | 94 | 84 | 107 | 95 | 93 | 30 | 25 | 30 | 26 | 29 | 82 | 72 | 92 | 81 | 78 |
| Saudi Arabia | 329 | 372 | 387 | 373 | 366 | 560 | 578 | 637 | 607 | 578 | 251 | 285 | 304 | 291 | 277 | 426 | 444 | 501 | 474 | 439 |
| Senegal[i] | 21 | 18 | 20 | 23 | 29 | 44 | 45 | 51 | 55 | 58 | 8 | 7 | 8 | 9 | 12 | 16 | 16 | 19 | 22 | 24 |

| Member State | Per capita total expenditure on health at average exchange rate (US$) | | | | | Per capita total expenditure on health at international dollar rate | | | | | Per capita government expenditure on health at average exchange rate (US$) | | | | | Per capita government expenditure on health at international dollar rate | | | | |
|---|---|---|---|---|---|---|---|---|---|---|---|---|---|---|---|---|---|---|---|---|
| | 1999 | 2000 | 2001 | 2002 | 2003 | 1999 | 2000 | 2001 | 2002 | 2003 | 1999 | 2000 | 2001 | 2002 | 2003 | 1999 | 2000 | 2001 | 2002 | 2003 |
| Serbia-Montenegro | 76 | 53 | 80 | 118 | 181 | 290 | 253 | 257 | 294 | 373 | 45 | 34 | 54 | 86 | 136 | 172 | 160 | 173 | 214 | 282 |
| Seychelles | 431 | 405 | 403 | 456 | 522 | 548 | 555 | 535 | 554 | 599 | 322 | 304 | 301 | 342 | 382 | 410 | 417 | 400 | 415 | 439 |
| Sierra Leone | 5 | 5 | 6 | 7 | 7 | 19 | 24 | 25 | 32 | 34 | 2 | 3 | 3 | 4 | 4 | 9 | 13 | 13 | 21 | 20 |
| Singapore | 847 | 820 | 888 | 894 | 964 | 961 | 925 | 1079 | 1101 | 1156 | 325 | 290 | 321 | 290 | 348 | 369 | 328 | 390 | 357 | 417 |
| Slovakia | 218 | 208 | 216 | 256 | 360 | 577 | 597 | 641 | 716 | 777 | 196 | 186 | 193 | 228 | 318 | 517 | 533 | 573 | 638 | 687 |
| Slovenia | 831 | 823 | 889 | 982 | 1218 | 1211 | 1421 | 1571 | 1616 | 1669 | 628 | 640 | 683 | 751 | 930 | 915 | 1105 | 1208 | 1237 | 1274 |
| Solomon Islands | 44 | 41 | 40 | 31 | 28 | 110 | 103 | 98 | 89 | 87 | 41 | 38 | 37 | 28 | 26 | 103 | 96 | 92 | 83 | 81 |
| Somalia | 9 | 8 | 8 | n/a | n/a | 18 | 18 | 18 | n/a | n/a | 4 | 4 | 4 | n/a | n/a | 8 | 8 | 8 | n/a | n/a |
| South Africa | 257 | 236 | 216 | 198 | 295 | 595 | 579 | 626 | 649 | 669 | 105 | 100 | 89 | 80 | 114 | 244 | 245 | 258 | 263 | 258 |
| Spain | 1133 | 1038 | 1083 | 1211 | 1541 | 1459 | 1529 | 1618 | 1735 | 1853 | 816 | 743 | 771 | 864 | 1098 | 1051 | 1095 | 1152 | 1237 | 1321 |
| Sri Lanka | 28 | 29 | 28 | 30 | 31 | 104 | 113 | 114 | 120 | 121 | 14 | 14 | 13 | 13 | 14 | 50 | 55 | 53 | 54 | 55 |
| Sudan | 13 | 13 | 15 | 17 | 21 | 42 | 40 | 44 | 47 | 54 | 3 | 5 | 6 | 7 | 9 | 11 | 14 | 16 | 18 | 23 |
| Suriname | 157 | 163 | 138 | 175 | 182 | 246 | 261 | 287 | 304 | 309 | 80 | 80 | 66 | 81 | 83 | 126 | 127 | 137 | 141 | 142 |
| Swaziland | 87 | 83 | 73 | 68 | 107 | 305 | 302 | 308 | 315 | 324 | 51 | 48 | 42 | 40 | 61 | 180 | 177 | 178 | 187 | 185 |
| Sweden | 2396 | 2280 | 2173 | 2495 | 3149 | 2119 | 2273 | 2404 | 2596 | 2704 | 2054 | 1936 | 1845 | 2123 | 2684 | 1816 | 1929 | 2040 | 2210 | 2305 |
| Switzerland | 3881 | 3572 | 3774 | 4220 | 5035 | 3016 | 3177 | 3357 | 3658 | 3776 | 2148 | 1986 | 2156 | 2444 | 2945 | 1669 | 1767 | 1917 | 2118 | 2209 |
| Syrian Arab Republic[i] | 59 | 59 | 57 | 58 | 59 | 113 | 106 | 107 | 108 | 116 | 24 | 26 | 26 | 26 | 28 | 46 | 46 | 48 | 50 | 56 |
| Tajikistan | 7 | 5 | 6 | 6 | 11 | 41 | 39 | 44 | 48 | 71 | 2 | 1 | 2 | 2 | 2 | 11 | 11 | 13 | 13 | 15 |
| Thailand | 71 | 68 | 62 | 68 | 76 | 217 | 223 | 226 | 242 | 260 | 39 | 38 | 35 | 41 | 47 | 119 | 125 | 127 | 146 | 160 |
| The former Yugoslav Republic of Macedonia | 115 | 108 | 103 | 127 | 161 | 312 | 320 | 313 | 356 | 389 | 98 | 91 | 86 | 107 | 136 | 266 | 270 | 260 | 302 | 329 |
| Timor-Leste | 37 | 37 | 41 | 38 | 39 | 101 | 101 | 111 | 108 | 125 | 25 | 28 | 30 | 27 | 30 | 69 | 76 | 80 | 78 | 95 |
| Togo | 16 | 11 | 13 | 13 | 16 | 59 | 49 | 58 | 54 | 62 | 7 | 3 | 3 | 2 | 4 | 24 | 14 | 15 | 10 | 15 |
| Tonga | 101 | 97 | 94 | 87 | 102 | 256 | 277 | 309 | 286 | 300 | 76 | 73 | 71 | 65 | 87 | 193 | 207 | 234 | 212 | 255 |
| Trinidad and Tobago | 204 | 235 | 245 | 265 | 316 | 354 | 389 | 393 | 459 | 532 | 88 | 95 | 98 | 99 | 120 | 153 | 157 | 157 | 171 | 201 |
| Tunisia | 122 | 114 | 118 | 120 | 137 | 343 | 367 | 396 | 396 | 409 | 60 | 55 | 59 | 57 | 63 | 169 | 178 | 196 | 187 | 187 |
| Turkey | 179 | 194 | 158 | 190 | 257 | 395 | 453 | 463 | 470 | 528 | 109 | 122 | 108 | 132 | 184 | 242 | 285 | 316 | 327 | 378 |
| Turkmenistan | 31 | 49 | 59 | 67 | 89 | 171 | 233 | 217 | 195 | 221 | 21 | 36 | 41 | 43 | 60 | 120 | 169 | 150 | 125 | 149 |
| Tuvalu | 137 | 165 | 107 | 600 | 142 | 113 | 149 | 99 | 377 | 74 | 121 | 149 | 93 | 581 | 119 | 100 | 135 | 86 | 365 | 62 |
| Uganda | 16 | 16 | 17 | 18 | 18 | 55 | 60 | 70 | 75 | 75 | 5 | 4 | 5 | 5 | 5 | 17 | 16 | 19 | 23 | 23 |
| Ukraine | 35 | 32 | 39 | 47 | 60 | 197 | 194 | 222 | 255 | 305 | 19 | 18 | 24 | 29 | 40 | 105 | 113 | 135 | 159 | 201 |
| United Arab Emirates | 681 | 704 | 737 | 650 | 661 | 727 | 634 | 713 | 631 | 623 | 528 | 539 | 577 | 487 | 493 | 564 | 485 | 558 | 473 | 465 |
| United Kingdom | 1755 | 1756 | 1837 | 2031 | 2428 | 1700 | 1840 | 2044 | 2231 | 2389 | 1415 | 1420 | 1524 | 1693 | 2081 | 1370 | 1488 | 1696 | 1860 | 2047 |
| United Republic of Tanzania | 11 | 12 | 12 | 12 | 12 | 23 | 25 | 27 | 28 | 29 | 5 | 6 | 6 | 6 | 7 | 10 | 12 | 13 | 15 | 16 |
| United States of America | 4335 | 4588 | 4934 | 5324 | 5711 | 4335 | 4588 | 4934 | 5324 | 5711 | 1897 | 2017 | 2212 | 2387 | 2548 | 1897 | 2017 | 2212 | 2387 | 2548 |
| Uruguay | 668 | 631 | 597 | 373 | 323 | 972 | 962 | 976 | 832 | 824 | 233 | 211 | 202 | 117 | 88 | 338 | 322 | 330 | 260 | 224 |
| Uzbekistan | 42 | 32 | 26 | 21 | 21 | 143 | 142 | 149 | 155 | 159 | 20 | 14 | 12 | 10 | 9 | 69 | 65 | 68 | 69 | 68 |
| Vanuatu | 57 | 49 | 46 | 48 | 54 | 121 | 114 | 111 | 112 | 110 | 43 | 36 | 34 | 36 | 40 | 92 | 83 | 83 | 84 | 81 |
| Venezuela, Bolivarian Republic of | 253 | 299 | 258 | 183 | 146 | 354 | 369 | 320 | 278 | 231 | 131 | 162 | 112 | 84 | 65 | 184 | 201 | 139 | 128 | 102 |
| Viet Nam | 18 | 21 | 23 | 22 | 26 | 111 | 129 | 145 | 143 | 164 | 6 | 6 | 7 | 6 | 7 | 36 | 36 | 42 | 40 | 46 |
| Yemen | 18 | 24 | 26 | 27 | 32 | 61 | 68 | 78 | 78 | 89 | 7 | 10 | 11 | 10 | 13 | 22 | 29 | 33 | 30 | 37 |
| Zambia | 17 | 17 | 19 | 20 | 21 | 45 | 46 | 51 | 53 | 51 | 8 | 9 | 11 | 11 | 11 | 23 | 23 | 29 | 30 | 26 |
| Zimbabwe | 36 | 44 | 65 | 132 | 40 | 185 | 168 | 184 | 161 | 132 | 17 | 21 | 25 | 50 | 14 | 91 | 81 | 71 | 61 | 47 |

[a]See explanatory notes for sources and methods.
[b]Andorra, Monaco, and San Marino: international dollar exchange rates for Spain, France and Italy, respectively, were used.
[c]Exchange rate changed from 2.15 Won in 2001 to 152 Won in 2002.
[d]Ecuador dollarized its economy in 2000. The time series has been recalculated from 1998 in dollar terms.
[e]Exchange rate changed in 2002 from multiple to a managed floating exchange rate. Inter-bank market rate used prior to 2002.
[f]The currency now called Ariary is worth one fifth of the Francs previously used.
[g]The official exchange was used although marked difference exists between this and the rates on the open market.
[h]Currency was changed from Australian dollar to US dollar in 1996. The series was revised for this report.
[i]The exchange rate used for Syrian Arab Republic is the rate for non-commercial transactions from the Central Bank of Syria.
n/a Used when the information accessed indicates that a cell should have an entry but no estimates could be made.

**Annex Table 4 Global distribution of health workers in WHO Member States**
Figures computed by WHO to ensure comparability;[a] they are not necessarily the official statistics of Member States, which may use alternative rigorous methods.

| Country | Physicians Number | Density per 1000 | Year | Nurses Number | Density per 1000 | Year | Midwives Number | Density per 1000 | Year | Dentists Number | Density per 1000 | Year | Pharmacists Number | Density per 1000 | Year |
|---|---|---|---|---|---|---|---|---|---|---|---|---|---|---|---|
| Afghanistan | 4104 | 0.19 | 2001 | 4752 | 0.22 | 2001 | | | | 630 | 0.03 | 2001 | 525 | 0.02 | 2001 |
| Albania | 4100 | 1.31 | 2002 | 11473 | 3.62 | 2003 | 1891 | 0.59 | 1994 | 1390 | 0.45 | 1998 | 1300 | 0.40 | 1994 |
| Algeria | 35368 | 1.13 | 2002 | 68950 | 2.21 | 2002 | 799 | 0.03 | 2002 | 9553 | 0.31 | 2002 | 6333 | 0.20 | 2002 |
| Andorra | 244 | 3.70 | 2003 | 205 | 3.11 | 2003 | 10 | 0.15 | 2003 | 44 | 0.67 | 2003 | 68 | 1.03 | 2003 |
| Angola | 881 | 0.08 | 1997 | 13135 | 1.15 | 1997 | 492 | 0.04 | 1997 | 2 | 0.00 | 1997 | 24 | 0.00 | 1997 |
| Antigua and Barbuda | 12 | 0.17 | 1999 | 233 | 3.28 | 1999 | | | | 13 | 0.19 | 1997 | | | |
| Argentina | 108800 | 3.01 | 1998 | 29000 | 0.80 | 1998 | | | | 28900 | 0.80 | 1998 | 15300 | 0.42 | 1998 |
| Armenia | 10983 | 3.59 | 2003 | 13320 | 4.35 | 2003 | 1433 | 0.47 | 2003 | 802 | 0.26 | 2003 | 126 | 0.04 | 2003 |
| Australia | 47875 | 2.47 | 2001 | 187837 | 9.71 | 2001 | | | | 21296 | 1.10 | 2001 | 13956 | 0.72 | 2001 |
| Austria | 27413 | 3.38 | 2003 | 76161 | 9.38 | 2003 | 1671 | 0.21 | 2003 | 4037 | 0.50 | 2003 | 4869 | 0.60 | 2003 |
| Azerbaijan | 29687 | 3.55 | 2003 | 59531 | 7.11 | 2003 | 9803 | 1.17 | 2003 | 2272 | 0.27 | 2003 | 1842 | 0.22 | 2003 |
| Bahamas | 312 | 1.05 | 1998 | 1323 | 4.47 | 1998 | | | | 21 | 0.07 | 1998 | | | |
| Bahrain | 803 | 1.09 | 2004 | 3153 | 4.27 | 2004 | 396 | 0.54 | 2004 | 342 | 0.46 | 2004 | 460 | 0.62 | 2004 |
| Bangladesh | 38485 | 0.26 | 2004 | 20334 | 0.14 | 2004 | 26460 | 0.18 | 2004 | 2537 | 0.02 | 2004 | 9411 | 0.06 | 2004 |
| Barbados | 322 | 1.21 | 1999 | 988 | 3.70 | 1999 | | | | 63 | 0.24 | 1999 | | | |
| Belarus | 45027 | 4.55 | 2003 | 115116 | 11.63 | 2003 | 5182 | 0.52 | 2003 | 4315 | 0.44 | 2003 | 2901 | 0.29 | 2003 |
| Belgium | 46268 | 4.49 | 2002 | 60142 | 5.83 | 2003 | 6603 | 0.64 | 2001 | 8322 | 0.81 | 2002 | 11775 | 1.14 | 2002 |
| Belize | 251 | 1.05 | 2000 | 303 | 1.26 | 2000 | | | | 32 | 0.13 | 2000 | | | |
| Benin | 311 | 0.04 | 2004 | 5789 | 0.84 | 2004 | | | | 12 | 0.00 | 2004 | 11 | 0.00 | 2004 |
| Bhutan | 118 | 0.05 | 2004 | 330 | 0.14 | 2004 | 185 | 0.08 | 2004 | 58 | 0.02 | 2004 | 79 | 0.03 | 2004 |
| Bolivia | 10329 | 1.22 | 2001 | 27063 | 3.19 | 2001 | 96 | 0.01 | 2001 | 5997 | 0.71 | 2001 | 4670 | 0.55 | 2001 |
| Bosnia and Herzegovina | 5576 | 1.34 | 2003 | 17170 | 4.13 | 2003 | 1229 | 0.30 | 2003 | 690 | 0.17 | 2003 | 363 | 0.09 | 2003 |
| Botswana | 715 | 0.40 | 2004 | 4753 | 2.65 | 2004 | | | | 38 | 0.02 | 2004 | 333 | 0.19 | 2004 |
| Brazil | 198153 | 1.15 | 2000 | 659111 | 3.84 | 2000 | | | | 190448 | 1.11 | 2000 | 51317 | 0.30 | 2000 |
| Brunei Darussalam | 336 | 1.01 | 2000 | 892 | 2.67 | 2000 | 404 | 1.21 | 2000 | 48 | 0.14 | 2000 | 90 | 0.27 | 2000 |
| Bulgaria | 28128 | 3.56 | 2003 | 29650 | 3.75 | 2003 | 3456 | 0.44 | 2003 | 6475 | 0.82 | 2003 | 1020 | 0.13 | 2001 |
| Burkina Faso | 789 | 0.06 | 2004 | 5518 | 0.41 | 2004 | 1732 | 0.13 | 2004 | 58 | 0.00 | 2004 | 343 | 0.03 | 2004 |
| Burundi | 200 | 0.03 | 2004 | 1348 | 0.19 | 2004 | | | | 14 | 0.00 | 2004 | 76 | 0.01 | 2004 |
| Cambodia | 2047 | 0.16 | 2000 | 8085 | 0.61 | 2000 | 3040 | 0.23 | 2000 | 209 | 0.02 | 2000 | 564 | 0.04 | 2000 |
| Cameroon | 3124 | 0.19 | 2004 | 26042 | 1.60 | 2004 | | | | 147 | 0.01 | 2004 | 700 | 0.04 | 2004 |
| Canada | 66583 | 2.14 | 2003 | 309576 | 9.95 | 2003 | | | | 18265 | 0.59 | 2003 | 20765 | 0.67 | 2003 |
| Cape Verde | 231 | 0.49 | 2004 | 410 | 0.87 | 2004 | | | | 11 | 0.02 | 2004 | 43 | 0.09 | 2004 |
| Central African Republic | 331 | 0.08 | 2004 | 1188 | 0.30 | 2004 | 519 | 0.13 | 2004 | 13 | 0.00 | 2004 | 17 | 0.00 | 2004 |
| Chad | 345 | 0.04 | 2004 | 2387 | 0.27 | 2004 | 112 | 0.01 | 2004 | 15 | 0.00 | 2004 | 37 | 0.00 | 2004 |
| Chile | 17250 | 1.09 | 2003 | 10000 | 0.63 | 2003 | | | | 6750 | 0.43 | 2003 | | | |
| China | 1364000 | 1.06 | 2001 | 1358000 | 1.05 | 2001 | 42000 | 0.03 | 2001 | 136520 | 0.11 | 2001 | 359000 | 0.28 | 2001 |
| Colombia | 58761 | 1.35 | 2002 | 23940 | 0.55 | 2002 | | | | 33951 | 0.78 | 2002 | | | |
| Comoros | 115 | 0.15 | 2004 | 588 | 0.74 | 2004 | | | | 29 | 0.04 | 2004 | 41 | 0.05 | 2004 |
| Congo | 756 | 0.20 | 2004 | 3672 | 0.96 | 2004 | | | | 12 | 0.00 | 2004 | 99 | 0.03 | 2004 |
| Cook Islands | 14 | 0.78 | 2001 | 49 | 2.72 | 2001 | 3 | 0.17 | 2001 | 10 | 0.56 | 2001 | 2 | 0.11 | 2001 |
| Costa Rica | 5204 | 1.32 | 2000 | 3631 | 0.92 | 2000 | 22 | 0.01 | 2000 | 1905 | 0.48 | 2000 | 2101 | 0.53 | 2000 |
| Côte d'Ivoire | 2081 | 0.12 | 2004 | 10180 | 0.60 | 2004 | | | | 339 | 0.02 | 2004 | 1015 | 0.06 | 2004 |
| Croatia | 10820 | 2.44 | 2003 | 22372 | 5.05 | 2003 | 1476 | 0.33 | 2003 | 3085 | 0.70 | 2003 | 2348 | 0.53 | 2003 |
| Cuba | 66567 | 5.91 | 2002 | 83880 | 7.44 | 2002 | | | | 9841 | 0.87 | 2002 | | | |
| Cyprus | 1864 | 2.34 | 2002 | 2994 | 3.76 | 2002 | | | | 650 | 0.82 | 2002 | 144 | 0.18 | 2002 |

| Public and environmental health workers | | | Community health workers | | | Lab technicians | | | Other health workers | | | Health management and support workers | | |
|---|---|---|---|---|---|---|---|---|---|---|---|---|---|---|
| Number | Density per 1000 | Year | Number | Density per 1000 | Year | Number | Density per 1000 | Year | Number | Density per 1000 | Year | Number | Density per 1000 | Year |
| 2534 | 0.08 | 2002 | 1062 | 0.03 | 2002 | 8838 | 0.28 | 2002 | 5088 | 0.16 | 2002 | 60882 | 1.95 | 2002 |
| | | | | | | | | | | | | | | |
| | | | 3812 | 0.20 | 2001 | 8326 | 0.43 | 2001 | 35710 | 1.85 | 2001 | 490942 | 25.37 | 2001 |
| 294 | 0.40 | 2004 | 0 | 0.00 | 2004 | 479 | 0.65 | 2004 | 1278 | 1.73 | 2004 | 1433 | 1.94 | 2004 |
| 5743 | 0.04 | 2004 | 46202 | 0.31 | 2004 | 3794 | 0.03 | 2004 | 5847 | 0.04 | 2004 | | | |
| 178 | 0.03 | 2004 | 88 | 0.01 | 2004 | 477 | 0.07 | 2004 | 128 | 0.02 | 2004 | 3281 | 0.47 | 2004 |
| 71 | 0.03 | 2004 | 464 | 0.20 | 2004 | 136 | 0.06 | 2004 | 121 | 0.05 | 2004 | 1219 | 0.52 | 2004 |
| | | | | | | | | | 3939 | 0.46 | 2001 | 9648 | 1.14 | 2001 |
| 172 | 0.10 | 2004 | | | | 277 | 0.15 | 2004 | | | | 829 | 0.46 | 2004 |
| 167080 | 0.97 | 2000 | | | | 44095 | 0.26 | 2000 | 237100 | 1.38 | 2000 | 839376 | 4.89 | 2000 |
| 46 | 0.00 | 2004 | 1291 | 0.10 | 2004 | 424 | 0.03 | 2004 | 975 | 0.07 | 2004 | 325 | 0.02 | 2004 |
| | | | 657 | 0.09 | 2004 | 147 | 0.02 | 2004 | 1186 | 0.17 | 2004 | 2087 | 0.30 | 2004 |
| 28 | 0.00 | 2004 | | | | 1793 | 0.11 | 2004 | 16 | 0.00 | 2004 | 5902 | 0.36 | 2004 |
| 9 | 0.02 | 2004 | 65 | 0.14 | 2004 | 78 | 0.16 | 2004 | 42 | 0.09 | 2004 | 74 | 0.16 | 2004 |
| 55 | 0.01 | 2004 | 211 | 0.05 | 2004 | 48 | 0.01 | 2004 | 367 | 0.09 | 2004 | 167 | 0.04 | 2004 |
| 230 | 0.03 | 2004 | 268 | 0.03 | 2004 | 317 | 0.04 | 2004 | 153 | 0.02 | 2004 | 1502 | 0.17 | 2004 |
| | | | 109000 | 0.08 | 2001 | 203000 | 0.16 | 2001 | 1061000 | 0.82 | 2001 | 1077000 | 0.83 | 2001 |
| 17 | 0.02 | 2004 | 41 | 0.05 | 2004 | 63 | 0.08 | 2004 | 9 | 0.01 | 2004 | 272 | 0.34 | 2004 |
| 9 | 0.00 | 2004 | 124 | 0.03 | 2004 | 554 | 0.15 | 2004 | 957 | 0.25 | 2004 | 987 | 0.26 | 2004 |
| 1266 | 0.32 | 2000 | | | | | | | 7379 | 1.88 | 2000 | 23477 | 5.98 | 2000 |
| 155 | 0.01 | 2004 | | | | 1165 | 0.07 | 2004 | 172 | 0.01 | 2004 | 2107 | 0.12 | 2004 |

## Annex Table 4 Global distribution of health workers in WHO Member States

Figures computed by WHO to ensure comparability;[a] they are not necessarily the official statistics of Member States, which may use alternative rigorous methods.

| Country | Physicians | | | Nurses | | | Midwives | | | Dentists | | | Pharmacists | | |
|---|---|---|---|---|---|---|---|---|---|---|---|---|---|---|---|
| | Number | Density per 1000 | Year | Number | Density per 1000 | Year | Number | Density per 1000 | Year | Number | Density per 1000 | Year | Number | Density per 1000 | Year |
| Czech Republic | 35960 | 3.51 | 2003 | 99351 | 9.71 | 2003 | 4772 | 0.47 | 2003 | 6737 | 0.66 | 2003 | 5610 | 0.55 | 2003 |
| Democratic People's Republic of Korea | 74597 | 3.29 | 2003 | 87330 | 3.85 | 2003 | 6084 | 0.27 | 2003 | 8315 | 0.37 | 2003 | 13497 | 0.60 | 2003 |
| Democratic Republic of the Congo | 5827 | 0.11 | 2004 | 28789 | 0.53 | 2004 | | | | 159 | 0.00 | 2004 | 1200 | 0.02 | 2004 |
| Denmark | 15653 | 2.93 | 2002 | 55425 | 10.36 | 2002 | 1200 | 0.22 | 2002 | 4437 | 0.83 | 2002 | 2638 | 0.49 | 2002 |
| Djibouti | 129 | 0.18 | 2004 | 257 | 0.36 | 2004 | 39 | 0.05 | 2004 | 10 | 0.01 | 2004 | 18 | 0.03 | 2004 |
| Dominica | 38 | 0.50 | 1997 | 317 | 4.17 | 1997 | | | | 4 | 0.05 | 1997 | | | |
| Dominican Republic | 15670 | 1.88 | 2000 | 15352 | 1.84 | 2000 | | | | 7000 | 0.84 | 2000 | 3330 | 0.40 | 2000 |
| Ecuador | 18335 | 1.48 | 2000 | 19549 | 1.57 | 2000 | 1037 | 0.08 | 2000 | 2062 | 0.17 | 2000 | | | |
| Egypt | 38485 | 0.54 | 2003 | 146761 | 2.00 | 2004 | | | | 9917 | 0.14 | 2004 | 7119 | 0.10 | 2004 |
| El Salvador | 7938 | 1.24 | 2002 | 5103 | 0.80 | 2002 | | | | 3465 | 0.54 | 2002 | | | |
| Equatorial Guinea | 153 | 0.30 | 2004 | 228 | 0.45 | 2004 | 43 | 0.08 | 2004 | 15 | 0.03 | 2004 | 130 | 0.26 | 2004 |
| Eritrea | 215 | 0.05 | 2004 | 2505 | 0.58 | 2004 | | | | 16 | 0.00 | 2004 | 107 | 0.02 | 2004 |
| Estonia | 6118 | 4.48 | 2000 | 11618 | 8.50 | 2000 | 469 | 0.34 | 2000 | 1747 | 1.28 | 2000 | 580 | 0.42 | 2000 |
| Ethiopia | 1936 | 0.03 | 2003 | 14893 | 0.21 | 2003 | 651 | 0.01 | 2003 | 93 | 0.00 | 2003 | 1343 | 0.02 | 2003 |
| Fiji | 271 | 0.34 | 1999 | 1576 | 1.96 | 1999 | | | | 32 | 0.04 | 1999 | 59 | 0.07 | 1999 |
| Finland | 16446 | 3.16 | 2002 | 74450 | 14.33 | 2002 | 3952 | 0.76 | 2002 | 6674 | 1.28 | 2002 | 5829 | 1.12 | 2002 |
| France | 203487 | 3.37 | 2004 | 437525 | 7.24 | 2004 | 15684 | 0.26 | 2003 | 40904 | 0.68 | 2004 | 63909 | 1.06 | 2003 |
| Gabon | 395 | 0.29 | 2004 | 6974 | 5.16 | 2004 | | | | 66 | 0.05 | 2004 | 63 | 0.05 | 2004 |
| Gambia | 156 | 0.11 | 2003 | 1719 | 1.21 | 2003 | 162 | 0.11 | 2003 | 43 | 0.03 | 2003 | 48 | 0.03 | 2003 |
| Georgia | 20962 | 4.09 | 2003 | 17807 | 3.47 | 2003 | 1495 | 0.29 | 2003 | 1438 | 0.28 | 2003 | 352 | 0.07 | 2003 |
| Germany | 277885 | 3.37 | 2003 | 801677 | 9.72 | 2003 | 8559 | 0.10 | 2002 | 64609 | 0.78 | 2003 | 47956 | 0.58 | 2003 |
| Ghana | 3240 | 0.15 | 2004 | 19707 | 0.92 | 2004 | | | | 393 | 0.02 | 2004 | 1388 | 0.06 | 2004 |
| Greece | 47944 | 4.38 | 2001 | 42129 | 3.86 | 2000 | 1916 | 0.18 | 2001 | 12394 | 1.13 | 2001 | 8977 | 0.82 | 2000 |
| Grenada | 41 | 0.50 | 1997 | 303 | 3.70 | 1997 | | | | 7 | 0.09 | 1997 | | | |
| Guatemala | 9965 | 0.90 | 1999 | 44986 | 4.05 | 1999 | | | | 2046 | 0.18 | 1999 | | | |
| Guinea | 987 | 0.11 | 2004 | 4757 | 0.55 | 2004 | 64 | 0.01 | 2004 | 60 | 0.01 | 2004 | 530 | 0.06 | 2004 |
| Guinea-Bissau | 188 | 0.12 | 2004 | 1037 | 0.67 | 2004 | 35 | 0.02 | 2004 | 22 | 0.01 | 2004 | 40 | 0.03 | 2004 |
| Guyana | 366 | 0.48 | 2000 | 1738 | 2.29 | 2000 | | | | 30 | 0.04 | 2000 | | | |
| Haiti | 1949 | 0.25 | 1998 | 834 | 0.11 | 1998 | | | | 94 | 0.01 | 1998 | | | |
| Honduras | 3676 | 0.57 | 2000 | 8333 | 1.29 | 2000 | 195 | 0.03 | 2000 | 1371 | 0.21 | 2000 | 926 | 0.14 | 2000 |
| Hungary | 32877 | 3.33 | 2003 | 87381 | 8.85 | 2003 | 2032 | 0.21 | 2003 | 5364 | 0.54 | 2003 | 5125 | 0.52 | 2003 |
| Iceland | 1056 | 3.62 | 2004 | 3954 | 13.63 | 2003 | 200 | 0.69 | 2003 | 283 | 1.00 | 2000 | 374 | 1.30 | 2002 |
| India | 645825 | 0.60 | 2005 | 865135 | 0.80 | 2004 | 506924 | 0.47 | 2004 | 61424 | 0.06 | 2004 | 592577 | 0.56 | 2003 |
| Indonesia | 29499 | 0.13 | 2003 | 135705 | 0.62 | 2003 | 44254 | 0.20 | 2003 | 6896 | 0.03 | 2003 | 7580 | 0.03 | 2003 |
| Iran, Islamic Republic of | 31394 | 0.45 | 2004 | 91365 | 1.31 | 2004 | 4897 | 0.07 | 2004 | 6587 | 0.09 | 2004 | 6229 | 0.09 | 2004 |
| Iraq | 17022 | 0.66 | 2004 | 32304 | 1.25 | 2004 | 1701 | 0.07 | 2004 | 11489 | 0.44 | 2004 | 13775 | 0.53 | 2004 |
| Ireland | 11141 | 2.79 | 2004 | 60774 | 15.20 | 2004 | 16486 | 4.27 | 2001 | 2237 | 0.56 | 2004 | 3898 | 0.97 | 2004 |
| Israel | 24577 | 3.82 | 2003 | 40280 | 6.26 | 2003 | 1202 | 0.19 | 2003 | 7510 | 1.17 | 2003 | 4480 | 0.70 | 2003 |
| Italy | 241000 | 4.20 | 2004 | 312377 | 5.44 | 2003 | 16523 | 0.29 | 1982 | 33000 | 0.58 | 2004 | 66119 | 1.15 | 2003 |
| Jamaica | 2253 | 0.85 | 2003 | 4374 | 1.65 | 2003 | | | | 212 | 0.08 | 2003 | | | |
| Japan | 251889 | 1.98 | 2002 | 993628 | 7.79 | 2002 | 24511 | 0.19 | 2000 | 90510 | 0.71 | 2002 | 154428 | 1.21 | 2002 |
| Jordan | 11398 | 2.03 | 2004 | 18196 | 3.24 | 2004 | | | | 7270 | 1.29 | 2004 | 17654 | 3.14 | 2004 |
| Kazakhstan | 54613 | 3.54 | 2003 | 92773 | 6.01 | 2003 | 8018 | 0.52 | 2003 | 5215 | 0.34 | 2003 | 10390 | 0.67 | 2003 |
| Kenya | 4506 | 0.14 | 2004 | 37113 | 1.14 | 2004 | | | | 1340 | 0.04 | 2004 | 3094 | 0.01 | 2004 |
| Kiribati | 24 | 0.30 | 1998 | 191 | 2.36 | 1998 | | | | 4 | 0.05 | 1998 | 4 | 0.05 | 1998 |

| Public and environmental health workers | | | Community health workers | | | Lab technicians | | | Other health workers | | | Health management and support workers | | |
|---|---|---|---|---|---|---|---|---|---|---|---|---|---|---|
| Number | Density per 1000 | Year | Number | Density per 1000 | Year | Number | Density per 1000 | Year | Number | Density per 1000 | Year | Number | Density per 1000 | Year |
| 2685 | 0.12 | 2003 | | | | 950 | 0.04 | 2003 | 67957 | 3.00 | 2003 | | | |
| | | | | | | 512 | 0.01 | 2004 | 1042 | 0.02 | 2004 | 15013 | 0.28 | 2004 |
| | | | 23 | 0.03 | 2004 | 84 | 0.12 | 2004 | 159 | 0.22 | 2004 | 232 | 0.33 | 2004 |
| | | | | | | | | | | | | | | |
| 9531 | 0.13 | 2004 | | | | 20011 | 0.27 | 2004 | 3694 | 0.05 | 2004 | 5167 | 0.07 | 2004 |
| 18 | 0.04 | 2004 | 1275 | 2.51 | 2004 | 75 | 0.15 | 2004 | | | | 74 | 0.15 | 2004 |
| 88 | 0.02 | 2004 | | | | 248 | 0.06 | 2004 | 56 | 0.01 | 2004 | 765 | 0.18 | 2004 |
| 115 | 0.08 | 2000 | 44 | 0.03 | 2000 | | | | 597 | 0.44 | 2000 | 16057 | 11.75 | 2000 |
| 1347 | 0.02 | 2003 | 18652 | 0.26 | 2003 | 2703 | 0.04 | 2003 | 7354 | 0.10 | 2003 | | | |
| | | | | | | 10119 | 1.95 | 2002 | 19202 | 3.69 | 2002 | | | |
| 150 | 0.11 | 2004 | | | | 276 | 0.20 | 2004 | 1 | 0.00 | 2004 | 144 | 0.11 | 2004 |
| 33 | 0.02 | 2003 | 968 | 0.68 | 2003 | 99 | 0.07 | 2003 | 3 | 0.00 | 2003 | 391 | 0.27 | 2003 |
| | | | | | | 899 | 0.04 | 2004 | 7132 | 0.33 | 2004 | 19151 | 0.90 | 2004 |
| 135 | 0.02 | 2004 | 93 | 0.01 | 2004 | 268 | 0.03 | 2004 | 17 | 0.00 | 2004 | 511 | 0.06 | 2004 |
| 13 | 0.01 | 2004 | 4486 | 2.92 | 2004 | 230 | 0.15 | 2004 | 61 | 0.04 | 2004 | 38 | 0.02 | 2004 |
| 215 | 0.03 | 2000 | | | | | | | 2936 | 0.45 | 2000 | | | |
| 325263 | 0.38 | 1991 | 50393 | 0.05 | 2004 | 15886 | 0.02 | 1991 | 818301 | 0.76 | 2005 | | | |
| 6493 | 0.03 | 2003 | 0 | 0.00 | 2003 | 8882 | 0.04 | 2003 | 21178 | 0.10 | 2003 | 228095 | 1.04 | 2003 |
| 10004 | 0.14 | 2004 | 25242 | 0.36 | 2004 | 17618 | 0.25 | 2004 | 84207 | 1.21 | 2004 | 72905 | 1.04 | 2004 |
| 2601 | 0.10 | 2004 | 1968 | 0.08 | 2004 | 12103 | 0.47 | 2004 | 20421 | 0.79 | 2004 | 34273 | 1.33 | 2004 |
| 1412 | 0.25 | 2004 | 1000 | 0.18 | 2004 | 5630 | 1.00 | 2004 | 6529 | 1.16 | 2004 | 17708 | 3.15 | 2004 |
| 6496 | 0.20 | 2004 | | | | 7000 | 0.22 | 2004 | 5610 | 0.17 | 2004 | 1797 | 0.06 | 2004 |

## Annex Table 4 Global distribution of health workers in WHO Member States

Figures computed by WHO to ensure comparability;[a] they are not necessarily the official statistics of Member States, which may use alternative rigorous methods.

| Country | Physicians Number | Density per 1000 | Year | Nurses Number | Density per 1000 | Year | Midwives Number | Density per 1000 | Year | Dentists Number | Density per 1000 | Year | Pharmacists Number | Density per 1000 | Year |
|---|---|---|---|---|---|---|---|---|---|---|---|---|---|---|---|
| Kuwait | 3589 | 1.53 | 2001 | 9197 | 3.91 | 2001 | | | | 673 | 0.29 | 2001 | 722 | 0.31 | 2001 |
| Kyrgyzstan | 12902 | 2.51 | 2003 | 31557 | 6.14 | 2003 | 2663 | 0.52 | 2003 | 992 | 0.19 | 2003 | 158 | 0.03 | 2003 |
| Lao People's Democratic Republic | 2812 | 0.59 | 1996 | 4931 | 1.03 | 1996 | | | | 196 | 0.04 | 1996 | | | |
| Latvia | 6940 | 3.01 | 2003 | 12150 | 5.27 | 2003 | 482 | 0.21 | 2003 | 1287 | 0.56 | 2003 | | | |
| Lebanon | 11505 | 3.25 | 2001 | 4157 | 1.18 | 2001 | | | | 4283 | 1.21 | 2001 | 3359 | 0.95 | 2001 |
| Lesotho | 89 | 0.05 | 2003 | 1123 | 0.62 | 2003 | | | | 16 | 0.01 | 2003 | 62 | 0.03 | 2003 |
| Liberia | 103 | 0.03 | 2004 | 613 | 0.18 | 2004 | 422 | 0.12 | 2004 | 13 | 0.00 | 2004 | 35 | 0.01 | 2004 |
| Libyan Arab Jamahiriya | 6371 | 1.29 | 1997 | 17779 | 3.60 | 1997 | | | | 693 | 0.14 | 1997 | 1225 | 0.25 | 1997 |
| Lithuania | 13682 | 3.97 | 2003 | 26229 | 7.62 | 2003 | 1132 | 0.33 | 2003 | 2372 | 0.69 | 2003 | 2390 | 0.69 | 2003 |
| Luxembourg | 1206 | 2.66 | 2003 | 4151 | 9.16 | 2003 | 114 | 0.25 | 2003 | 323 | 0.71 | 2003 | 371 | 0.82 | 2003 |
| Madagascar | 5201 | 0.29 | 2004 | 5661 | 0.32 | 2004 | | | | 410 | 0.02 | 2004 | 175 | 0.01 | 2004 |
| Malawi | 266 | 0.02 | 2004 | 7264 | 0.59 | 2004 | | | | | | | | | |
| Malaysia | 16146 | 0.70 | 2000 | 31129 | 1.35 | 2000 | 7711 | 0.34 | 2000 | 2144 | 0.09 | 2000 | 2333 | 0.10 | 2000 |
| Maldives | 302 | 0.92 | 2004 | 886 | 2.70 | 2004 | | | | 14 | 0.04 | 2004 | 241 | 0.73 | 2004 |
| Mali | 1053 | 0.08 | 2004 | 6538 | 0.49 | 2004 | 573 | 0.04 | 2004 | 84 | 0.01 | 2004 | 351 | 0.03 | 2004 |
| Malta | 1254 | 3.18 | 2003 | 2298 | 5.83 | 2003 | 125 | 0.32 | 2003 | 167 | 0.42 | 2003 | 800 | 2.03 | 2003 |
| Marshall Islands | 24 | 0.47 | 2000 | 152 | 2.98 | 2000 | | | | 4 | 0.08 | 2000 | 2 | 0.04 | 2000 |
| Mauritania | 313 | 0.11 | 2004 | 1893 | 0.64 | 2004 | | | | 64 | 0.02 | 2004 | 81 | 0.03 | 2004 |
| Mauritius | 1303 | 1.06 | 2004 | 4550 | 3.69 | 2004 | 54 | 0.04 | 2004 | 233 | 0.19 | 2004 | 1428 | 1.16 | 2004 |
| Mexico | 195897 | 1.98 | 2000 | 88678 | 0.90 | 2000 | | | | 78281 | 0.79 | 2000 | 3189 | 0.03 | 2000 |
| Micronesia, Federated States of | 64 | 0.60 | 2000 | 410 | 3.83 | 2000 | 7 | 0.07 | 2000 | 14 | 0.13 | 2000 | | | |
| Monaco | 186 | 5.81 | 1995 | 454 | 14.19 | 1995 | 10 | 0.31 | 1995 | 34 | 1.06 | 1995 | 61 | 1.91 | 1995 |
| Mongolia | 6732 | 2.63 | 2002 | 8012 | 3.13 | 2002 | 612 | 0.24 | 2002 | 337 | 0.13 | 2002 | 1093 | 0.43 | 2002 |
| Morocco | 15991 | 0.51 | 2004 | 24328 | 0.78 | 2004 | | | | 3091 | 0.10 | 2004 | 7366 | 0.24 | 2004 |
| Mozambique | 514 | 0.03 | 2004 | 3954 | 0.21 | 2004 | 2229 | 0.12 | 2004 | 159 | 0.01 | 2004 | 618 | 0.03 | 2004 |
| Myanmar | 17791 | 0.36 | 2004 | 19254 | 0.38 | 2004 | 30087 | 0.60 | 2004 | 1396 | 0.03 | 2004 | 127 | 0.00 | 2004 |
| Namibia | 598 | 0.30 | 2004 | 6145 | 3.06 | 2004 | | | | 113 | 0.06 | 2004 | 288 | 0.14 | 2004 |
| Nauru | 16 | 1.45 | 1995 | 60 | 5.45 | 1995 | | | | | | | | | |
| Nepal | 5384 | 0.21 | 2004 | 5664 | 0.22 | 2004 | 6161 | 0.24 | 2004 | 359 | 0.01 | 2004 | 358 | 0.01 | 2004 |
| Netherlands | 50854 | 3.15 | 2003 | 221783 | 13.73 | 2003 | 1940 | 0.12 | 2003 | 7759 | 0.48 | 2003 | 3134 | 0.19 | 2003 |
| New Zealand | 9027 | 2.37 | 2001 | 31128 | 8.16 | 2001 | 2121 | 0.56 | 2001 | 2586 | 0.68 | 2001 | 3495 | 0.92 | 2001 |
| Nicaragua | 2045 | 0.37 | 2003 | 5862 | 1.07 | 2003 | | | | 243 | 0.04 | 2003 | | | |
| Niger | 377 | 0.03 | 2004 | 2716 | 0.22 | 2004 | 21 | 0.00 | 2004 | 15 | 0.00 | 2004 | 20 | 0.00 | 2004 |
| Nigeria | 34923 | 0.28 | 2003 | 210306 | 1.70 | 2003 | | | | 2482 | 0.02 | 2003 | 6344 | 0.05 | 2004 |
| Niue | 3 | 1.50 | 1996 | 11 | 5.50 | 1996 | 2 | 1.00 | 1996 | 2 | 1.00 | 1996 | 1 | 0.50 | 1996 |
| Norway | 14200 | 3.13 | 2003 | 67274 | 14.84 | 2003 | 2243 | 0.49 | 2003 | 3733 | 0.82 | 2003 | 1675 | 0.37 | 2003 |
| Oman | 3871 | 1.32 | 2004 | 10273 | 3.50 | 2004 | 16 | 0.01 | 2004 | 544 | 0.19 | 2004 | 1551 | 0.53 | 2004 |
| Pakistan | 116298 | 0.74 | 2004 | 71764 | 0.46 | 2004 | | | | 7862 | 0.05 | 2004 | 8102 | 0.05 | 2004 |
| Palau | 20 | 1.11 | 1998 | 26 | 1.44 | 1998 | 1 | 0.06 | 1998 | 2 | 0.11 | 1998 | 1 | 0.06 | 1998 |
| Panama | 4431 | 1.50 | 2000 | 4545 | 1.54 | 2000 | | | | 2231 | 0.76 | 2000 | 2526 | 0.86 | 2000 |
| Papua New Guinea | 275 | 0.05 | 2000 | 2841 | 0.53 | 2000 | | | | 90 | 0.02 | 2000 | | | |
| Paraguay | 6355 | 1.11 | 2002 | 9727 | 1.69 | 2002 | 534 | 0.09 | 2002 | 3182 | 0.55 | 2002 | 1868 | 0.33 | 2002 |
| Peru | 29799 | 1.17 | 1999 | 17108 | 0.67 | 1999 | | | | 2809 | 0.11 | 1999 | | | |
| Philippines | 44287 | 0.58 | 2000 | 127595 | 1.69 | 2000 | 33963 | 0.45 | 2000 | 8564 | 0.11 | 2000 | 2482 | 0.03 | 2000 |
| Poland | 95272 | 2.47 | 2003 | 188898 | 4.90 | 2003 | 21997 | 0.57 | 2002 | 11451 | 0.30 | 2003 | 25397 | 0.66 | 2003 |

| | Public and environmental health workers | | | Community health workers | | | Lab technicians | | | Other health workers | | | Health management and support workers | | |
|---|---|---|---|---|---|---|---|---|---|---|---|---|---|---|---|
| | Number | Density per 1000 | Year | Number | Density per 1000 | Year | Number | Density per 1000 | Year | Number | Density per 1000 | Year | Number | Density per 1000 | Year |
| | 55 | 0.03 | 2003 | | | | 146 | 0.08 | 2003 | 23 | 0.01 | 2003 | 18 | 0.01 | 2003 |
| | 150 | 0.04 | 2004 | 142 | 0.04 | 2004 | 218 | 0.06 | 2004 | 540 | 0.15 | 2004 | 518 | 0.15 | 2004 |
| | 130 | 0.01 | 2004 | 385 | 0.02 | 2004 | 172 | 0.01 | 2004 | 530 | 0.03 | 2004 | 6036 | 0.34 | 2004 |
| | 26 | 0.00 | 2004 | | | | 46 | 0.00 | 2004 | 707 | 0.06 | 2004 | | | |
| | | | | 919 | 2.80 | 2004 | 168 | 0.51 | 2004 | 14 | 0.04 | 2004 | | | |
| | 231 | 0.02 | 2004 | 1295 | 0.01 | 2004 | 264 | 0.02 | 2004 | 377 | 0.03 | 2004 | 652 | 0.05 | 2004 |
| | | | | 429 | 0.14 | 2004 | 106 | 0.04 | 2004 | 48 | 0.02 | 2004 | 1056 | 0.35 | 2004 |
| | 238 | 0.19 | 2004 | 236 | 0.19 | 2004 | 324 | 0.26 | 2004 | 134 | 0.11 | 2004 | 2038 | 1.65 | 2004 |
| | | | | | | | | | | 282343 | 2.85 | 2000 | 412319 | 4.17 | 2000 |
| | 85 | 0.03 | 2002 | | | | | | | 3389 | 1.32 | 2002 | 3758 | 1.47 | 2002 |
| | 737 | 0.02 | 2004 | | | | 1470 | 0.05 | 2004 | 975 | 0.03 | 2004 | 6448 | 0.21 | 2004 |
| | 564 | 0.03 | 2004 | | | | 941 | 0.05 | 2004 | 1633 | 0.09 | 2004 | 9517 | 0.50 | 2004 |
| | 1757 | 0.04 | 2004 | 49531 | 0.99 | 2004 | 2241 | 0.04 | 2004 | 2077 | 0.04 | 2004 | 49661 | 0.99 | 2004 |
| | 240 | 0.12 | 2004 | | | | 481 | 0.24 | 2004 | 597 | 0.30 | 2004 | 7782 | 3.87 | 2004 |
| | 172 | 0.01 | 2004 | 16206 | 0.63 | 2004 | 3209 | 0.12 | 2004 | 1892 | 0.07 | 2004 | | | |
| | | | | | | | 3696 | 0.97 | 2001 | 16863 | 4.42 | 2001 | 30987 | 8.12 | 2001 |
| | 268 | 0.02 | 2004 | | | | 294 | 0.02 | 2004 | 213 | 0.02 | 2004 | 513 | 0.04 | 2004 |
| | | | | 115761 | 0.91 | 2004 | 690 | 0.01 | 2004 | 1220 | 0.01 | 2004 | | | |
| | 173 | 0.06 | 2004 | | | | 1049 | 0.36 | 2004 | 1256 | 0.43 | 2004 | 3898 | 1.33 | 2004 |
| | 106 | 0.00 | 2004 | 65999 | 0.42 | 2004 | 9744 | 0.06 | 2004 | 19082 | 0.12 | 2004 | 203337 | 1.29 | 2004 |
| | 948 | 0.32 | 2000 | | | | | | | 870 | 0.29 | 2000 | 8221 | 2.79 | 2000 |
| | 133 | 0.02 | 2002 | | | | | | | 2235 | 0.39 | 2002 | 6598 | 1.15 | 2002 |
| | | | | | | | | | | 90788 | 1.20 | 2000 | | | |

## Annex Table 4 Global distribution of health workers in WHO Member States

Figures computed by WHO to ensure comparability;[a] they are not necessarily the official statistics of Member States, which may use alternative rigorous methods.

| Country | Physicians | | | Nurses | | | Midwives | | | Dentists | | | Pharmacists | | |
|---|---|---|---|---|---|---|---|---|---|---|---|---|---|---|---|
| | Number | Density per 1000 | Year | Number | Density per 1000 | Year | Number | Density per 1000 | Year | Number | Density per 1000 | Year | Number | Density per 1000 | Year |
| Portugal | 34440 | 3.42 | 2003 | 43860 | 4.36 | 2003 | 824 | 0.08 | 2000 | 5510 | 0.55 | 2003 | 9543 | 0.95 | 2003 |
| Qatar | 1310 | 2.22 | 2001 | 2917 | 4.94 | 2001 | | | | 220 | 0.37 | 2001 | 530 | 0.90 | 2001 |
| Republic of Korea | 75045 | 1.57 | 2003 | 83333 | 1.75 | 2003 | 8728 | 0.19 | 2000 | 16033 | 0.34 | 2003 | 50623 | 1.08 | 2000 |
| Republic of Moldova | 11246 | 2.64 | 2003 | 25848 | 6.06 | 2003 | 991 | 0.23 | 2003 | 1403 | 0.33 | 2003 | 2061 | 0.48 | 2003 |
| Romania | 42538 | 1.90 | 2003 | 86802 | 3.89 | 2003 | 5571 | 0.25 | 2003 | 4919 | 0.22 | 2003 | 1275 | 0.06 | 2003 |
| Russian Federation | 609043 | 4.25 | 2003 | 1153683 | 8.05 | 2003 | 67403 | 0.47 | 2003 | 45972 | 0.32 | 2003 | 11404 | 0.08 | 2003 |
| Rwanda | 401 | 0.05 | 2004 | 3593 | 0.42 | 2004 | 54 | 0.01 | 2004 | 21 | 0.00 | 2004 | 278 | 0.03 | 2004 |
| Saint Kitts and Nevis | 51 | 1.19 | 1997 | 216 | 5.02 | 1997 | | | | 8 | 0.19 | 1997 | | | |
| Saint Lucia | 749 | 5.17 | 1999 | 331 | 2.28 | 1999 | | | | 9 | 0.06 | 1999 | | | |
| Saint Vincent and the Grenadines | 101 | 0.87 | 1997 | 276 | 2.38 | 1997 | | | | 6 | 0.05 | 1997 | | | |
| Samoa | 120 | 0.70 | 1999 | 346 | 2.02 | 1999 | 3 | 0.02 | 1999 | 30 | 0.18 | 1999 | 5 | 0.03 | 1999 |
| San Marino | 1089 | 47.35 | 1990 | 2196 | 95.48 | 1990 | | | | 8 | 0.35 | 1990 | 23 | 1.00 | 1990 |
| Sao Tome and Principe | 81 | 0.49 | 2004 | 256 | 1.55 | 2004 | 52 | 0.32 | 2004 | 11 | 0.07 | 2004 | 24 | 0.15 | 2004 |
| Saudi Arabia | 34261 | 1.37 | 2004 | 74114 | 2.97 | 2004 | | | | 4235 | 0.17 | 2004 | 5485 | 0.22 | 2004 |
| Senegal | 594 | 0.06 | 2004 | 3287 | 0.32 | 2004 | | | | 97 | 0.01 | 2004 | 85 | 0.01 | 2004 |
| Serbia and Montenegro | 21738 | 2.06 | 2002 | 48875 | 4.64 | 2002 | 2864 | 0.27 | 2002 | 3792 | 0.36 | 2002 | 1980 | 0.19 | 2002 |
| Seychelles | 121 | 1.51 | 2004 | 634 | 7.93 | 2004 | | | | 94 | 1.17 | 2004 | 61 | 0.76 | 2004 |
| Sierra Leone | 168 | 0.03 | 2004 | 1841 | 0.36 | 2004 | | | | 5 | 0.00 | 2004 | 340 | 0.07 | 2004 |
| Singapore | 5747 | 1.40 | 2001 | 17398 | 4.24 | 2001 | | | | 1087 | 0.26 | 2001 | 1141 | 0.28 | 2001 |
| Slovakia | 17172 | 3.18 | 2003 | 36569 | 6.77 | 2003 | 1456 | 0.27 | 2003 | 2364 | 0.44 | 2003 | 2783 | 0.52 | 2003 |
| Slovenia | 4475 | 2.25 | 2002 | 14327 | 7.21 | 2002 | 654 | 0.33 | 2001 | 1199 | 0.60 | 2002 | 790 | 0.40 | 2002 |
| Solomon Islands | 54 | 0.13 | 1999 | 338 | 0.80 | 1999 | 23 | 0.05 | 1999 | 26 | 0.06 | 1999 | 28 | 0.07 | 1999 |
| Somalia | 310 | 0.04 | 1997 | 1486 | 0.19 | 1997 | | | | 15 | 0.00 | 1997 | 8 | 0.00 | 1997 |
| South Africa | 34829 | 0.77 | 2004 | 184459 | 4.08 | 2004 | | | | 5995 | 0.13 | 2004 | 12521 | 0.28 | 2004 |
| Spain | 135300 | 3.30 | 2003 | 315200 | 7.68 | 2003 | 6291 | 0.15 | 2001 | 20005 | 0.49 | 2003 | 35800 | 0.87 | 2003 |
| Sri Lanka | 10479 | 0.55 | 2004 | 30318 | 1.58 | 2004 | 3113 | 0.16 | 2004 | 1245 | 0.06 | 2004 | 1066 | 0.06 | 2004 |
| Sudan | 7552 | 0.22 | 2004 | 28704 | 0.84 | 2004 | 2792 | 0.08 | 2004 | 1082 | 0.03 | 2004 | 3558 | 0.10 | 2004 |
| Suriname | 191 | 0.45 | 2000 | 688 | 1.62 | 2000 | | | | 4 | 0.01 | 2000 | | | |
| Swaziland | 171 | 0.16 | 2004 | 6828 | 6.30 | 2004 | | | | 32 | 0.03 | 2004 | 70 | 0.06 | 2004 |
| Sweden | 29122 | 3.28 | 2002 | 90758 | 10.24 | 2002 | 6247 | 0.70 | 2002 | 7270 | 0.82 | 2002 | 5885 | 0.66 | 2002 |
| Switzerland | 25921 | 3.61 | 2002 | 77120 | 10.75 | 2000 | 2033 | 0.28 | 2000 | 3598 | 0.50 | 2003 | 4322 | 0.60 | 2003 |
| Syrian Arab Republic | 23742 | 1.40 | 2001 | 32938 | 1.94 | 2001 | | | | 12206 | 0.72 | 2001 | 8862 | 0.52 | 2001 |
| Tajikistan | 12697 | 2.03 | 2003 | 28586 | 4.58 | 2003 | 3780 | 0.61 | 2003 | 945 | 0.15 | 2003 | 680 | 0.11 | 2003 |
| Thailand | 22435 | 0.37 | 2000 | 171605 | 2.82 | 2000 | 872 | 0.01 | 2000 | 10459 | 0.17 | 2000 | 15480 | 0.25 | 2000 |
| The former Yugoslav Republic of Macedonia | 4459 | 2.19 | 2001 | 10553 | 5.19 | 2001 | 1456 | 0.72 | 2001 | 1125 | 0.55 | 2001 | 309 | 0.15 | 2001 |
| Timor-Leste | 79 | 0.10 | 2004 | 1468 | 1.79 | 2004 | 327 | 0.40 | 2004 | 45 | 0.05 | 2004 | 14 | 0.02 | 2004 |
| Togo | 225 | 0.04 | 2004 | 2141 | 0.43 | 2004 | 5 | 0.00 | 2004 | 19 | 0.00 | 2004 | 134 | 0.03 | 2004 |
| Tonga | 35 | 0.34 | 2001 | 322 | 3.16 | 2001 | 19 | 0.19 | 2001 | 33 | 0.32 | 2001 | 17 | 0.17 | 2001 |
| Trinidad and Tobago | 1004 | 0.79 | 1997 | 3653 | 2.87 | 1997 | | | | 107 | 0.08 | 1997 | | | |
| Tunisia | 13330 | 1.34 | 2004 | 28537 | 2.87 | 2004 | | | | 2452 | 0.25 | 2004 | 2909 | 0.29 | 2004 |
| Turkey | 96000 | 1.35 | 2003 | 121000 | 1.70 | 2003 | | | | 17200 | 0.24 | 2003 | 22500 | 0.32 | 2003 |
| Turkmenistan | 20032 | 4.18 | 2002 | 43359 | 9.04 | 2002 | | | | 876 | 0.18 | 2002 | 1626 | 0.34 | 2002 |
| Tuvalu | 6 | 0.55 | 2002 | 29 | 2.64 | 2002 | 10 | 0.91 | 2002 | 2 | 0.18 | 2002 | 1 | 0.09 | 2002 |
| Uganda | 2209 | 0.08 | 2004 | 16221 | 0.61 | 2004 | 3104 | 0.12 | 2004 | 363 | 0.01 | 2004 | 688 | 0.03 | 2004 |
| Ukraine | 143202 | 2.95 | 2003 | 369755 | 7.62 | 2003 | 24496 | 0.50 | 2003 | 19354 | 0.40 | 2003 | 23576 | 0.48 | 2001 |

| Public and environmental health workers | | | Community health workers | | | Lab technicians | | | Other health workers | | | Health management and support workers | | |
|---|---|---|---|---|---|---|---|---|---|---|---|---|---|---|
| Number | Density per 1000 | Year | Number | Density per 1000 | Year | Number | Density per 1000 | Year | Number | Density per 1000 | Year | Number | Density per 1000 | Year |
| 72515 | 0.50 | 2000 | | | | | | | 670768 | 4.61 | 2000 | 435093 | 2.99 | 2000 |
| 101 | 0.01 | 2004 | 12000 | 1.41 | 2004 | 39 | 0.00 | 2004 | 521 | 0.06 | 2004 | 1419 | 0.17 | 2004 |
| 19 | 0.12 | 2004 | 374 | 2.27 | 2004 | 51 | 0.31 | 2004 | 291 | 1.76 | 2004 | 288 | 1.75 | 2004 |
| | | | | | | | | | 39073 | 1.57 | 2004 | | | |
| 705 | 0.07 | 2004 | | | | 66 | 0.01 | 2004 | 704 | 0.07 | 2004 | 564 | 0.05 | 2004 |
| 77 | 0.96 | 2004 | | | | 59 | 0.74 | 2004 | 35 | 0.44 | 2004 | | | |
| 136 | 0.03 | 2004 | 1227 | 0.24 | 2004 | | | | | | | 4 | 0.00 | 2004 |
| 2529 | 0.06 | 2004 | 9160 | 0.20 | 2004 | 1968 | 0.04 | 2004 | 40526 | 0.90 | 2004 | 28005 | 0.62 | 2004 |
| 1541 | 0.08 | 2004 | | | | 1252 | 0.07 | 2004 | 1546 | 0.08 | 2004 | 112 | 0.01 | 2004 |
| 2897 | 0.08 | 2004 | 5797 | 0.17 | 2004 | 3115 | 0.09 | 2004 | 8667 | 0.25 | 2004 | 35374 | 1.03 | 2004 |
| 110 | 0.10 | 2004 | 4700 | 4.34 | 2004 | 78 | 0.07 | 2004 | 551 | 0.51 | 2004 | 374 | 0.35 | 2004 |
| 2151 | 0.04 | 2000 | 3601 | 0.06 | 2000 | | | | 14117 | 0.23 | 2000 | 153563 | 2.52 | 2000 |
| 22 | 0.03 | 2004 | 1657 | 2.02 | 2004 | 36 | 0.04 | 2004 | 18 | 0.02 | 2004 | 184 | 0.22 | 2004 |
| 289 | 0.06 | 2004 | 475 | 0.09 | 2004 | 528 | 0.11 | 2004 | 397 | 0.08 | 2004 | 1335 | 0.27 | 2004 |
| 890 | 0.09 | 2004 | | | | 3936 | 0.40 | 2004 | 10478 | 1.05 | 2004 | 16276 | 1.64 | 2004 |
| | | | | | | | | | 7846 | 1.64 | 2002 | | | |
| 1042 | 0.04 | 2004 | | | | 1702 | 0.06 | 2004 | 3617 | 0.14 | 2004 | 6499 | 0.24 | 2004 |

**Annex Table 4 Global distribution of health workers in WHO Member States**

Figures computed by WHO to ensure comparability;[a] they are not necessarily the official statistics of Member States, which may use alternative rigorous methods.

| Country | Physicians | | | Nurses | | | Midwives | | | Dentists | | | Pharmacists | | |
|---|---|---|---|---|---|---|---|---|---|---|---|---|---|---|---|
| | Number | Density per 1000 | Year | Number | Density per 1000 | Year | Number | Density per 1000 | Year | Number | Density per 1000 | Year | Number | Density per 1000 | Year |
| United Arab Emirates | 5825 | 2.02 | 2001 | 12045 | 4.18 | 2001 | | | | 954 | 0.33 | 2001 | 1086 | 0.38 | 2001 |
| United Kingdom | 133641 | 2.30 | 1997 | 704332 | 12.12 | 1997 | 36399 | 0.63 | 1997 | 58729 | 1.01 | 1997 | 29726 | 0.51 | 1997 |
| United Republic of Tanzania | 822 | 0.02 | 2002 | 13292 | 0.37 | 2002 | | | | 267 | 0.01 | 2002 | 365 | 0.01 | 2002 |
| United States of America | 730801 | 2.56 | 2000 | 2669603 | 9.37 | 2000 | | | | 463663 | 1.63 | 2000 | 249642 | 0.88 | 2000 |
| Uruguay | 12384 | 3.65 | 2002 | 2880 | 0.85 | 2002 | | | | 3936 | 1.16 | 2002 | | | |
| Uzbekistan | 71623 | 2.74 | 2003 | 256183 | 9.82 | 2003 | 21270 | 0.82 | 2003 | 3606 | 0.14 | 2003 | 899 | 0.03 | 2003 |
| Vanuatu | 20 | 0.11 | 1997 | 428 | 2.35 | 1997 | | | | | | | | | |
| Venezuela, Bolivarian Republic of | 48000 | 1.94 | 2001 | | | | | | | 13680 | 0.55 | 2001 | | | |
| Viet Nam | 42327 | 0.53 | 2001 | 44539 | 0.56 | 2001 | 14662 | 0.19 | 2001 | | | | 5977 | 0.08 | 2001 |
| Yemen | 6739 | 0.33 | 2004 | 13506 | 0.65 | 2004 | 240 | 0.01 | 2004 | 850 | 0.04 | 2004 | 2638 | 0.13 | 2004 |
| Zambia | 1264 | 0.12 | 2004 | 19014 | 1.74 | 2004 | 2996 | 0.27 | 2004 | 491 | 0.04 | 2004 | 1039 | 0.01 | 2004 |
| Zimbabwe | 2086 | 0.16 | 2004 | 9357 | 0.72 | 2004 | | | | 310 | 0.02 | 2004 | 883 | 0.07 | 2004 |

[a] See explanatory notes for sources and methods.

| | Public and environmental health workers | | | Community health workers | | | Lab technicians | | | Other health workers | | | Health management and support workers | | |
|---|---|---|---|---|---|---|---|---|---|---|---|---|---|---|---|
| | Number | Density per 1000 | Year | Number | Density per 1000 | Year | Number | Density per 1000 | Year | Number | Density per 1000 | Year | Number | Density per 1000 | Year |
| | 14439 | 0.25 | 1997 | | | | 20035 | 0.34 | 1997 | 161490 | 2.78 | 1997 | 1231666 | 21.20 | 1997 |
| | 1831 | 0.05 | 2002 | | | | 1520 | 0.04 | 2002 | 29722 | 0.82 | 2002 | 689 | 0.02 | 2002 |
| | | | | | | | 611993 | 2.15 | 2000 | 4177609 | 14.66 | 2000 | 7056080 | 24.76 | 2000 |
| | | | | | | | | | | | | | | | |
| | | | | | | | | | | | | | | | |
| | 792 | 0.04 | 2004 | 6025 | 0.29 | 2004 | 4709 | 0.23 | 2004 | 4580 | 0.22 | 2004 | 10902 | 0.53 | 2004 |
| | 1027 | 0.09 | 2004 | | | | 1415 | 0.13 | 2004 | 3330 | 0.30 | 2004 | 10853 | 0.99 | 2004 |
| | 1803 | 0.14 | 2004 | | | | 917 | 0.07 | 2004 | 743 | 0.06 | 2004 | 581 | 0.04 | 2004 |

# *index*

Note: this index does not include the Statistical Annexes and their explanatory notes.